Third Edition

Appleton & Lange's Review for the
DENTAL ASSISTANT

Emily Andujo, RDH, BS, MS
Department Chairperson
Dental Hygiene Education
Pima Community College
Tucson, Arizona

APPLETON & LANGE
Norwalk, Connecticut

0-8385-0135-4

Copyright © 1992 by Appleton & Lange
Simon & Schuster Business and Professional Group

Copyright © 1978, 1983 by Arco Publishing, Inc.
Published by Appleton & Lange, a division of Prentice Hall.

95 96 / 10 9 8 7 6 5

Prentice Hall International (UK) Limited, *London*
Prentice Hall of Australia Pty. Limited, *Sydney*
Prentice Hall Canada, Inc., *Toronto*
Prentice Hall Hispanoamericana, S.A., *Mexico*
Prentice Hall of India Private Limited, *New Delhi*
Prentice Hall of Japan, Inc., *Tokyo*
Simon & Schuster Asia Pte. Ltd., *Singapore*
Editora Prentice Hall do Brasil Ltda., *Rio de Janeiro*
Prentice Hall, *Englewood Cliffs, New Jersey*

Library of Congress Cataloging-in-Publication Data

Appleton & Lange's review for the dental assistant / [edited by] Emily
  Andujo.—3rd ed.
        p.   cm.
    Rev. ed of: Dental assistant review / Stuart M. Hirsch, Michael
Ostrofsky; edited by Marie E. Gallagher. 2nd ed. c1983.
    ISBN 0-8385-0135-4
    1. Dental assistants—Examinations, questions, etc. 2. Dentistry—
Examinations, questions, etc. I. Anjudo, Emily. II. Hirsch,
Stuart M. Dental assistant review. III. Title: Review for the
dental assistant.
    [DNLM: 1. Dental Assistants—examination questions. WU 18.5
A6491]
RK60.5.H57 1992
617.6'0233076—dc20
DNLM/DLC
for Library of Congress   92-6994
                                                              CIP

Acquisitions Editor: Jamie L. Mount
Production Editor: Sasha Kintzler
Designer: Penny Kindzierski

PRINTED IN THE UNITED STATES OF AMERICA

This book is dedicated
to all dental assistants and
dental assisting students who aspire to
excel in their chosen profession

In Memoriam
Doni Corbin, CDA, RDH
and Thomas Schott, DDS
They enjoyed life and teaching to the fullest

Contributors

Doni Corbin, CDA, RDA, RDH, BS[†]
Instructor, Dental Radiology
Department of Dental Assisting—Dental Hygiene
Cypress Community College
Cypress, California
DENTAL RADIOLOGY

Stephanie Dante, CDA, RDA, AS
Instructor, Dental Practice Management
Department of Dental Assisting
Cerritos Community College
Norwalk, California
DENTAL PRACTICE MANAGEMENT

Joleen Failor, CDA, RDA, BVE
Director, Department of Dental Assisting
Division of Health Occupations
Cerritos Community College
Norwalk, California
CHAIRSIDE ASSISTING

Edward D. Maggiore, DDS, MS, DrPH
Director, UCLA Venice Dental Center
Adjunct Associate Professor
University of California, Los Angeles, School of
  Dentistry
Los Angeles, California
BEHAVIORAL SCIENCES

Richard J. Nagy, DDS, BA
Director, Department of Periodontics
Veterans Administration Medical Center West Los
  Angeles
Lecturer
University of California, Los Angeles, School of
  Dentistry
Los Angeles, California
Staff Dentist
Rancho Los Amigos Hospital

Downey, California
BIOMEDICAL SCIENCES—Oral Pathology
MEDICAL EMERGENCIES

Joan Otomo-Corgel, DDS, MPH
Adjunct Assistant Professor, Department of
  Periodontics
University of California, Los Angeles, School
  of Dentistry
Los Angeles, California
Faculty, Staff Dentist
Veterans Administration Medical Center West
  Los Angeles
Staff Dentist
Rancho Los Amigos Hospital
Downey, California
PREVENTIVE DENTISTRY
BIOMEDICAL SCIENCES—Pharmacology, Oral
  Pathology
CHAIRSIDE ASSISTING—Periodontics

Virginia F. Santos, CDA, RDA, BVE
Director, Department of Dental Assisting
Division of Health Science
East Los Angeles Occupational Center
Los Angeles, California
CHAIRSIDE ASSISTING—Orthodontics
DENTAL PRACTICE MANAGEMENT—Ethics and
  Jurisprudence

Jane M. Watanabe, CDA, RDA, OSMA, MSEd
Program Coordinator, Oral and Maxillofacial Surgery
Surgical Assistant for Implant Program
Former Coordinator Department of Auxiliary
  Utilization
University of Southern California School of Dentistry
Los Angeles, California
CHAIRSIDE ASSISTING—Oral and Maxillofacial
  Surgery

[†]Deceased.

Donna J. Wedell, CDA, RDA, AS
Instructor, Radiology and Dental Science
Department of Dental Assisting
Cerritos Community College
Norwalk, California
DENTAL RADIOLOGY

Sheila D. Whetstone, RDH, BHS
Education Program Coordinator
Western Dental Education Center
Veterans Administration Medical Center West Los
   Angeles
Los Angeles, California

Instructor for Dental Assistants
Cerritos Community College
Norwalk, California
BIOMEDICAL SCIENCES
DENTAL RADIOLOGY

Rizkalla Zakhary, PhD
Associate Professor of Anatomy
Department of Basic Sciences
University of Southern California School of Dentistry
Los Angeles, California
GENERAL ANATOMY
DENTAL ANATOMY

Contents

Contents

Preface

The principal purpose in preparing a text of this nature is to furnish dental assistant students with a source of information to facilitate studying for examinations, particularly the National Dental Assistant Certification Examination. Based on the original work of Stuart M. Hirsch, DDS, and Michael Ostrofsky, DDS, and the invaluable contributions of their colleagues of the New York University College of Dentistry, this revised third edition of *Appleton & Lange's Review for the Dental Assistant* strives to continue to reflect this original premise.

New and revised sample practice test questions and the development of review questions for the Certification Specialty Examinations in Oral and Maxillofacial Surgery and Orthodontics are compiled in the style representative of the National Dental Assistant Certification Examination; thus offering a current viable study tool for all dental assistants and students. A team of authors and contributors from various specialty disciplines (academic and clinical) were organized to present to the reader the most complete and accurate review text possible.

Each of the chapters follows a basic format, consisting of an introductory dental subject synopsis review, sample practice test questions, answers and explanations, and a bibliography for additional current reference sources related to the testing subject matter. This text is not a course in dental assisting but should be used as a supplement and reference source in conjunction with other dental assisting course texts.

New areas have been added to the third edition to meet the changes in the content subject matter of the current Certification Examination. Emphasis on infection control in the dental environment, radiation health and safety, extraoral radiography techniques, specialty chairside assisting, dental materials, occupational safety, office medical emergencies, legal issues, and preventive dentistry are addressed. This information is presented to give the dental assistant a concise and comprehensive review in preparation for the National Dental Assistant Certification Examinations.

We wish you success on your examination and your future professional career endeavors.

Introduction

If you are preparing for the Dental Assisting National Board Certification Examination, for General Chairside and Radiation Health and Safety, the Specialty Certification Examinations in Oral and Maxillofacial Surgery Assisting, Orthodontic Assisting, or Dental Practice Management, *Appleton & Lange's Review for the Dental Assistant* is designed for you. Here, in one package, is a comprehensive review resource with over 1200 Board-type clinical science multiple-choice questions with keyed answers and detailed explanations. In addition, each chapter provides the reader with a brief synopsis of a specific designated dental subject area covered on the Dental Assistant National Certification Examination. A bibliography for further reference is included at the end of each chapter.

ORGANIZATION OF THIS BOOK

Appleton & Lange's Review of the Dental Assistant is divided into 10 chapters. The content areas are

1. **General Anatomy:** focusing on the basic health sciences of human anatomy, cytology, histology, and the human body systems
2. **Dental Anatomy:** including head and neck anatomy, tooth morphology, occlusion, and the structures of the periodontium
3. **Preventive Dentistry:** including plaque etiology, plaque control, nutrition, oral physiotherapy, and fluorides
4. **Biomedical Sciences:** focusing on infection control in the dental environment and the related sciences of microbiology, oral pathology, and pharmacology
5. **Chairside Assisting:** including dental charting, and specialty chairside assisting in oral maxillofacial surgery and orthodontics
6. **Dental Radiology:** focusing on radiation health and safety and related radiographic techniques, including film mounting, interpretation, processing techniques, and principles of radiology exposure

7. **Dental Materials:** focusing on the science of dental materials and the manipulation of laboratory and chairside dental materials
8. **Medical Emergencies:** including medical emergency office protocol, vital signs, artificial resuscitation techniques, and an overview of related dental emergencies
9. **Behavioral Sciences:** including patient motivation and patient management strategies, interoffice communication skills, special patient needs, and psychologic aspects of dental fear and anxiety
10. **Dental Practice Management:** including business office procedures, appointment control, records management, office inventory control, dental ethics, and legal jurisprudence

Each of the chapters is organized in the following order.

1. Course Synopsis
2. Question Section
3. Answers and Explanations
4. Bibliography

These sections and how to use them are described below.

Course Synopsis

The synopsis provides a detailed overview of the key designated dental subject areas represented on the certification examination. It is supplemented with illustrations and quick reference tables to facilitate the review process. The synopsis at the beginning of each chapter section is not a course in dental assisting but is designed to serve as a supplement that can be used in conjunction with other dental assisting course texts and study guides. Students should read each chapter, answer the questions to the best of their ability, and check their answers with the keyed answers and explanations provided. Additional reference materials and resources for each of the chapters can be located at the end of each section by referring to the bibliography.

Questions

Each of the 10 chapters contains a varying number of questions weighted in accordance with the percentage of examination questions for each of the subject areas on the Certification Examination. The questions have been prepared carefully and represent the question style format used on the Certification Examination. In view of the fact that the current Certified Dental Assistant Examination emphasizes test questions of a task-oriented or functional format rather than the rote memory or recall only format, a greater number of practice test questions are task-oriented to help prepare the candidate for the test. The four question styles include *one best answer—single item,* *complex multiple choice* or *K-type, negative format,* and *matching.* In some cases, a group of questions may be related to a dental charting exercise or dental condition for interpretation. Some of the items are stated in the negative. In such instances, the negative word is in capital letters (eg, "All of the following are correct EXCEPT," "Which of the following choices is NOT correct?" *and* "Which of the following is LEAST correct?"). Additionally, some questions have illustrative material (instruments, x-rays, tables) that will require further understanding and interpretation on your part.

One best answer—single item question. This type of question presents a problem or asks a question and is followed by four choices, only one of which is entirely correct. The directions preceding this type of question generally will appear as follows.

DIRECTIONS (Question 1): Each of the questions or incomplete statements in this section is followed by four suggested answers or completions. Select the ONE lettered answer or completion that is BEST in each case. Check your answers with the correct answers at the end of the chapter.

An example of this item type follows.

1. The most important reason for using alginate for preliminary impressions is the

   A. pleasant color and taste of the material
   B. speed and simplicity of mixing
   C. ability of alginate to withstand the pouring of multiple models from a single impression
   D. greater precision of alginate as compared to hydrocolloid

In this type of question, choices other than the correct answer may be partially correct, but there can only be one best answer. In Question 1, the key word is "most." Although alginate impression material is pleasant tasting, has a pleasing color, and is easy to mix, these factors do not account for using alginate impressions material for preliminary impression procedures. Hydrocolloid impression material is used for final impression procedures only and is not used to take preliminary working impressions. Thus, the most important reason can only be (C) ability of

---

BOX 1. STRATEGIES FOR ANSWERING ONE BEST ANSWER—SINGLE ITEM QUESTIONS

- Remember that only one choice can be the correct answer.
- Read the question carefully to be sure that you understand what is being asked.
- Quickly read each choice for familiarity. (This important step is often not done by test takers.)
- Go back and consider each choice individually.
- If a choice is partially correct, tentatively consider it to be incorrect. (This step will help you lessen your choices and increase your odds of choosing the correct answer.)
- Consider the remaining choices and select the one you think is the answer. At this point, you may want to quickly scan the stem to be sure you understand the question and your answer.
- Fill in the appropriate circle on the answer sheet. (Even if you do not know the answer, you should use your best judgment and make a selection. You are scored on the number of correct answers, so **do not leave any blanks**.)

---

alginate to withstand the pouring of multiple models from a single impression.

Complex multiple choice—K-Type. These questions are considered the most difficult and you should be certain that you understand and follow the code that always accompanies these questions:

DIRECTIONS (Question 2): For each of the items in this section, ONE or MORE of the numbered options is correct. Choose answer

   A if only 1, 2, and 3 are correct
   B if only 1 and 3 are correct
   C if only 2 and 4 are correct
   D if only 4 is correct
   E if all are correct

This code is always the same (ie, D would never say "if 3 is correct"), and it is repeated throughout this book whenever there are multiple complex—K-type item questions.

A sample question follows:

2. Some benefits of tray setups are

   1. they save time setting up
   2. the dentist sets them up for the assistant
   3. they eliminate delay in searching for instruments
   4. they are used only in restorative procedures

You first need to determine which choices are right and wrong and then which code corresponds to the correct numbers. In Question 2, statements 1 and 3 are true, and therefore (B) is the correct answer.

Negative format questions. This type of question is used to test the exception to a general rule or principle. These questions can be tricky, since they require a reverse logic of reasoning for the examinee.

BOX 2. STRATEGIES FOR ANSWERING COMPLEX MULTIPLE CHOICE—K-TYPE QUESTIONS
- Carefully read and become familiar with the accompanying directions to this tricky question type.
- Read the stem to be certain that you know what is being asked.
- Read through each of the numbered choices. If you can determine whether any of the choices is true or false, you may find it helpful to place a "+" (true) or a "−" (false) next to the number.
- Focus on the numbered choices and your true/false notations, and use the following sequence to logically determine the correct answer.
  1. Note that in the answer code choices 1 *and* 3 are *always* both either true or false together. If you are sure that either one is incorrect, your answer must be (C) or (D).
  2. If you are sure that choice 2 and either choice 2 *or* 3 are incorrect, your answer must be (D).
  3. If you are sure that choices 2 and 4 are incorrect, your answer must be (B).
- Only one circle on the answer sheet must be filled in.

DIRECTIONS (Question 3): Each of the items or incomplete statements in this section is followed by suggested answers or completions. Select the ONE lettered answer or completion that is the EXCEPTION or false statement.

An example of this item type follows.

3. All of the following statements apply to interdental brushes EXCEPT

   A. they are useful in removing interproximal plaque
   B. they are used where there is a space between the teeth
   C. they are useful even when it is possible to remove plaque with a toothbrush around healthy tissues
   D. they are useful in exposed furcation areas

Note that unlike the one best answer—single item question style, the negative format question is asking you to select the one answer that is false or the exception. Carefully read each of the choices to determine the positive options first. Remember that positive choices can be safely eliminated, since you are being asked to select the choice that is false. This process of elimination is sometimes easier to think through and allows the correct choice—the exception—to stand out quickly. In this particular case, option choices (A), (B), and (D) are positive or true in reference to interdental brushes and are, therefore, incorrect answer choices. By eliminating these three positive options, only choice (C) remains. Choice (C) is the correct answer because it is the exception, or false statement. If plaque can be removed easily with a toothbrush and the tissue is healthy, an interdental brush is not necessary.

BOX 3. STRATEGIES FOR ANSWERING NEGATIVE FORMAT QUESTIONS
- Remember that you are using reverse logic reasoning.
- Focus on words that are capitalized in the stem of the question.
- Consider each choice option individually. Note that the incorrect options of a negative format question are written in a positive form.
- Your circled answer is the option choice that is the exception or least correct.

Matching. These questions are essentially matching questions that are always accompanied by the following general directions.

DIRECTIONS (Questions 4 through 8): Match the items in Column A with their primary function in Column B.

A sample matching series follows.

COLUMN A	COLUMN B
4. spoon excavator	A. used to pack filling material
5. condenser	B. finishes or smooths restorations
6. scaler	C. effective in excavating soft caries
7. discoid–cleoid	D. used for removal of cement
8. ball burnisher	E. refines occlusal anatomy

A series of five questions usually is listed under Column A, with five answer choices under Column B. In this particular matching set, dental instruments are listed under Column A. Select the first item, question 4. spoon excavator, and systematically proceed to Column B, carefully reading all of the options and considering each choice individually. Continue this process with each item question 5, 6, 7, and 8. After reading each possible option in Column B, determine your correct choice on the answer sheet. As with single item questions, only one choice can be correct for a given question. For this reason, it is best to run through each question with all five option choices before entering your final answers. The correct answers for the matching set are as follows: 4 (C), 5 (A), 6 (D), 7 (E), 8 (B).

BOX 4. STRATEGIES FOR ANSWERING MATCHING QUESTIONS
- As with single item questions, these questions have only one best answer.
- Carefully read through each option in Column B with every item question in the matching set before selecting your final answer.
- Refer to strategies under One Best Answer—Single Item Questions for additional information.

Answers and Explanations, and Bibliography
In each of the chapters of this book, the question sections are followed by a section containing the answers, explanations, and references to the questions. This section (1) tells you the answer to each question; (2) gives you an explanation and review of why the answer is correct, background information on the subject matter, and why the other answers are incorrect; and (3) tells you where to find more in-depth information on the subject matter in other books or journals or both. We encourage you to use this section as a basis for further study and understanding.

If you choose the correct answer to a question, you can then read the explanation (1) for reinforcement and (2) to add to your knowledge about the subject matter (remember that the explanations usually tell not only why the answer is correct but also why the other choices are incorrect).

If you choose the wrong answer to a question, you can read the explanation for a learning/reviewing discussion of the material in the question. Furthermore, you can consult the reference sources cited in the Bibliography for further clarification and background information on that particular subject area.

HOW TO USE THIS BOOK

There are two logical ways to get the most value from this book. We call them Plan A and Plan B.

In **Plan A**, you go straight to the practice test in Chapter 5, Chairside Assisting, and follow the directions given at the beginning of the examination. After taking the practice test, you check your answers against the answer key provided and note the number of incorrect answers. The number of questions marked incorrectly will be a good indicator of your initial knowledge state. This will help you to identify your areas of relative weakness and point you in the right direction for further preparation and review.

Chapter 5 draws varied test questions from all 10 subject areas and requires a general knowledge of the other subject areas addressed in the remaining chapters of this book. At this point, you can begin reviewing each of the chapters, sample test questions, and answers and explanations sections to help you improve your areas of relative weakness.

In **Plan B**, you begin by systematically reading each chapter for a quick refresher and answering the sample test questions immediately following that section. Check off your answers and compare your choices with the answers and explanations section included in each chapter. *Under Plan B, you should cover Chapter 5* last, since this chapter draws practice test questions from subject content matter obtained from the other nine chapters of the book and will give you a good indicator of your initial review process. If you still have a major weakness, it should be apparent in time for you to take remedial action.

In Plan A, by taking the practice test first, you get quick feedback regarding your initial areas of strength and weakness. You may find that you know all of the material very well, indicating that perhaps only a cursory review of the other subject areas is necessary. This, of course, would be good to know early in your examination preparation. On the other hand, you may find that you have many areas of weakness (say, for example, in dental radiography or dental materials). In this case, you could then focus on these areas in your review—not just with this book but also with other dental textbooks on radiography and the dental sciences.

Plan B may be the preferred method of study because it will give you a more realistic test-type situation, since very few of us just sit down to a test without studying. In this case, you will have done some reviewing (from superficial to in-depth), and your practice test will reflect this studying time. If, after reviewing the 10 chapters and taking the practice test, your scores still indicate some weaknesses, you can go back into each of the subject areas covered on the examination and supplement your review with your texts.

If preparing for a Specialty Certification Examination only, you should begin by following the specific directions at the beginning of each of the specialty question sections. For example, to prepare for the Specialty Examination in Orthodontics you are advised to review Chapters 3, 4, 5, 6, 7, 8, and 10 before attempting the practice questions designed for that Specialty Certification Examination. You will also find specific directions to assist you in preparing for the Specialty Certification Examination in Oral Maxillofacial Surgery and Dental Practice Management and for the examination section covering Radiation Health and Safety.

SPECIFIC INFORMATION ABOUT THE CERTIFICATION EXAMINATION

The official source of all information with respect to the Dental Assistant Certification Examination is the Dental Assisting National Board (DANB), 216 E. Ontario Street, Chicago, IL 60611.

Qualification for certification must be met before sitting for the examination. Several eligibility pathways are defined by the certifying board, and the candidate must submit written proof of eligibility directly to the DANB. A formal application must be completed before the appropriate deadline and accompanied by the required fee in order to sit for the certification examination.

Approximate examination testing time is 4 hours and 15 minutes. Test results will require approximately 6 to 8 weeks from the date of testing to be processed and mailed. Examination results are not released by phone.

SCORING

Because there is no deduction for wrong answers, you should **answer every question**. The certification examination is not graded on a curve. Your test is scored in the following way.

1. The Certified Dental Assisting Examination consists of a total of 300 test questions; 200 questions are derived from general chairside assisting subject matter, and the remaining 100 questions are derived from dental radiography and radiation health and safety. The test candidate must answer a minimum number of questions correctly in *each of these two subject areas* in order to successfully pass the certification examination. These minimum passing standards are calculated according to the number of correctly answered questions, which are individually scored according to item subject matter content and value of importance.

2. The Specialty Certification Examination in Dental Practice Management and Orthodontics consists of a total of 275 test questions; 225 questions are specifically derived from that particular dental specialty. The remaining 50 questions are derived from dental radiography. The Specialty Certification Examination in Oral and Maxillofacial Surgery consists of a total of 300 test questions; 260 questions are derived specifically from that particular dental specialty. The remaining 40 questions are derived from dental radiography. The test candidate must answer a minimum number of questions based on the entire examination (total number of questions) correctly in order to successfully pass the specialty certification examinations. On these specialty examinations dental radiography is not scored separately. The specialty certification examinations are not scored on a curve.

The examination may be repeated if failed following guidelines established by the DANB. Examination results are released in writing and issued directly to the test candidate only. All test candidates who pass the certification examinations successfully will receive a certificate designating them as a Certified Dental Assistant or a credential certifying them in a particular dental assisting specialty.

PHYSICAL CONDITIONS

The DANB is very concerned that all their examinations be administered under uniform conditions in the numerous centers that are used. All test candidates are advised to protect the integrity of their answer choices. If the test candidate feels that the testing site facilities are too crowded or arranged in such a manner that would make it difficult to protect the answers, the candidate should inform the testing site test administrator immediately.

Except for a No. 2 pencil and eraser, you are not permitted to bring anything (books, notes, reference materials) into the test room. A calculator is permitted for the Dental Practice Management Specialty Examination only. All candidates are required to bring their assigned admission card on the day of the examination and appropriate identification. No questions concerning the content matter of the examination may be asked during the testing session. Furthermore, no visitors will be permitted during the examination session. Late comers may be admitted but will not be allowed to write beyond the allotted examination testing time period.

Acknowledgments

My sincere appreciation and thanks is expressed to Mr. Craig Percy for his patience and encouragement.

Additional thanks is extended to my friends, colleagues, and contributors for their suggestions, encouragement, support, and time spent away form their busy work schedules and families—in particular to Terry G. Hudson CDT, VA Dental Service, for his technical expertise and invaluable contributions to the chapter on Dental Radiology and to Isabel Jurado, Dental Assisting Supervisor of the UCLA Venice Dental Clinic, for her assistance and contributions. I also would like to thank Dr. W. H. Fragalla and staff for their support and contributions and Marie Downey for her very helpful input and assistance.

The demands of typing and formatting a text of this nature are especially challenging, and a special note of thanks is given to Deborah L. Martinez for undertaking this project and for her many long weekends and evenings spent at the keyboard. For typing assistance, thanks are given to Stephanie Ortiz and David Santos. Major credit for art work and coordination of illustrations goes to Arthur V. Dorame, Medical Illustrator, VA Medical Center.

Last but not least, a special note of thanks to my computer mentor for the extra patience displayed and the countless hours spent formatting, inputting, and editing this project to final perfecton for copy. Thanks, "D."

CHAPTER 1

General Anatomy

INTRODUCTION

In order to provide appropriate patient treatment and care, a fundamental knowledge of the interrelationship between general health and oral health is necessary. The dental auxiliary must have a firm foundation in the basic health sciences, including anatomy and physiology, to understand this relationship. This chapter provides an overview of the major systems of the human body, their physiologic functions, and their significance to dental health. A synopsis of the closely related health sciences of cytology and histology is presented.

CYTOLOGY AND HISTOLOGY

Cytology is the study of cells, and histology is the study of the structure and arrangement of the tissues of an organism. Cytology and histology are the basic sciences that deal with the fundamental building blocks of the oral tissues. The ability to recognize different types of tissues and to differentiate between normal and abnormal tissues enables the dentist and the assistant to treat and heal diseases of the oral cavity.

Cytology

The cell is the basic unit of life, and its morphology (structure) is composed of the following basic structures.

1. The *nucleus* is considered the brain of the cell, which controls all cellular functions.
2. *Mitochondria* are known as the powerhouses of the cell. They are responsible for energy production and respiration.
3. *Lysosomes* are vesicles that store many powerful digestive enzymes. They are called on to process bulk material that enters the cell and are enclosed within a membrane to prevent the release of these enzymes and to protect the cell from self-destruction.
4. The *endoplasmic reticulum* is a system of membranes within the cell that functions to transport various cellular material.
5. The *Golgi apparatus* consists of groups of small membranes that function in the storage and modification of secretory products.

6. *Centrioles* are paired cylindrical structures lying adjacent to the nucleus that have a role in cell division.
7. *Vacuoles* are fluid-filled sacs that contain food products and waste material. They play a part in the fluid balance of the cell.
8. The *cell membrane* defines the shape of the cell and permits certain materials to enter and leave the cell.
9. *Cytoplasm* is a gel-like substance in which the cell components are suspended.
10. *Cilia* or *flagella* enable cell movement by shifting the cytoplasm within the cell.

Cells have three major functions: respiration, reproduction, and locomotion. The respiratory process is carried out by a series of complex chemical reactions that produce the energy necessary to support cellular function. Mitosis is the process of cell division, specifically, a division of the nucleus and a division of the cytoplasm. The result of mitosis is the production of a second cell that contains identical genetic materials (chromosomes) to the original cell.

Histology

Individual cells that form an organ or specialized tissue are related and perform specialized functions. The four basic types of tissues are epithelial, connective, muscle, and nervous tissue. Epithelial tissues act as a covering or lining of a body system, and connective tissue supports or binds together body organs. Muscle tissue and nervous tissue are composed of highly specialized cells and serve to coordinate the motor and sensory functions of the human body.

SYSTEMS OF THE BODY

Skeletal System

Bone is a rigid form of connective tissue that contains cells in an intercellular matrix or ground substance. Three types of cells are associated with bone: osteoblasts, osteocytes, and osteoclasts. Osteoblasts are involved with bone formation and are found near those surfaces of bones where the intercellular matrix is deposited. Osteocytes, or matrix bone cells, are osteoblasts that have become

TABLE 1–1. SYSTEMS OF THE BODY

1. Skeletal system	6.	Respiratory system
2. Muscular system	7.	Digestive system
3. Nervous system	8.	Excretory system
4. Circulatory system	9.	Endocrine system
5. Lymphatic system	10.	Reproductive system

TABLE 1–2. CRANIAL NERVES

Cranial Nerves	Function
I Olfactory	Smell
II Optic	Sight
III Oculomotor	Movement of eyes
IV Trochlear	Movement of eyes
V Trigeminal	Chewing, conduction of sensation, and movement by the ophthalmic, maxillary, and mandibular nerves to the face
VI Abducens	Movement of eyes
VII Facial	Secretion of saliva, taste, facial expression
VIII Auditory (acoustic)	Hearing and balance
IX Glossopharyngeal	Taste, swallowing, secretion of saliva
X Vagus	Slowing of heart beat, increase in peristaltic movement
XI (Spinal) Accessory	Movement of shoulder and head
XII Hypoglossal	Movement of tongue, speech

trapped within the intercellular matrix. Osteoclasts are giant cells that possess many nuclei and are responsible for the breakdown of bone. Within bone is a substance known as bone marrow. Its function is the production of red blood cells, white blood cells, and platelets, which are the main components of blood.

The main functions of bone are support and protection. The skeleton, which consists of 206 bones, provides support for the body and enables a human to stand in an erect position. The bones protect many vital organs, provide locations for muscle attachments, and store minerals.

The skeleton is divided into two parts: axial and appendicular. The axial skeleton is comprised of the skull, vertebral column, and ribcage. The appendicular skeleton is comprised of bones associated with the body's appendages.

Bones are connected at joints or articulations. There are three types of joints: synarthrotic, amphiarthrotic, and diarthrotic. Synarthrotic joints do not move and join bones in close contact. Examples include the sutures, which are the joints between the bones in the skull. Amphiarthrotic joints have limited movement. Diarthrotic joints are freely movable and are the most common joints found in the body. Examples include the elbow, knee, and wrist. The temporomandibular joint, joining the maxilla and mandible, is a diarthrotic joint.

Muscular System

Muscle cells or fibers are grouped into bundles that are responsible for producing movement. Muscle fibers require a rich blood supply to work effectively. These blood vessels, as well as nerves, are carried in connective tissue, which also serves to bind the muscle fibers together. There are three types of muscle: striated, smooth, and cardiac.

Smooth muscles, also known as involuntary muscles, are not consciously controlled and are located within the wall structures of the organ systems, such as the digestive and respiratory systems.

Cardiac muscle is specialized muscle found in the heart. It is an involuntary muscle that is responsible for contraction of the heart and circulation of blood.

Muscle reflexes are actions causing an uncontrollable reaction, such as gagging, swallowing, and coughing.

Nervous System

Nervous tissue is distributed widely throughout the body. The nervous system consists of those tissues that collect stimuli from the environment, transform the stimuli into

impulses, and transmit these impulses to highly organized receptor areas, where they are interpreted, and the appropriate response is made.

There are two major segments of the nervous system: the central nervous system, composed of the brain and the spinal cord, and the peripheral nervous system, composed of all other nerves of the body.

The cranial nerves are 12 paired nerves that control many major functions of the body, including sight, smell, and taste (Table 1–2).

Also included in the peripheral nervous system is the autonomic nervous system, composed of neurons that innervate internal organs and that perform such basic life functions as digestion, respiration, and regulation of the heart. The autonomic nervous system is responsible for maintaining bodily homeostasis (equilibrium and physiologic stability) and is subdivided into the sympathetic and parasympathetic nervous systems.

When stimulated, the sympathetic nervous system accelerates the heart beat, produces thick, viscous saliva, and decreases motility and tone of the gastrointestinal tract. Conversely, when the parasympathetic nervous system is stimulated, the heart beat is slowed, watery saliva is produced, and motility and tone of the gastrointestinal system are increased. Although these two parts of the autonomic nervous system appear to be antagonistic in nature, it is their dual action that maintains homeostasis.

The nervous system is perhaps one of the most important systems related to dentistry, since stimuli, such as pain and anxiety, often occur. Nerve fibers are ubiquitous in the oral cavity. Therefore, any deviation from the norm usually results in an unpleasant situation. Of primary importance is the use of anesthesia to block the sensation of pain. A local anesthetic prevents a nerve fiber from firing when a stimulus is applied.

Paresthesia, a sensation of anesthesia caused by nerve damage, can result from trauma to a nerve during the administration of anesthesia or from the surgical removal of a tooth. It can be temporary or permanent.

Trigeminal neuralgia is a nerve disturbance involving the oral cavity and face. The etiologic factors are varied, but the clinical effect is searing or stabbing facial pain. This condition can be temporary or permanent.

Common diseases associated with the nervous system include Parkinson's disease, epilepsy, and Bell's palsy (paralysis of the facial nerve).

Circulatory System

The circulatory system is comprised of the heart, blood vessels, and the blood. The heart is the specialized organ of the body responsible for initiating the flow of the blood through the body. It is a pump composed of four chambers: left and right atria and left and right ventricles.

After blood leaves the heart, it travels through the arteries, capillaries, and veins. Arteries carry blood away from the heart to all other parts of the body. They are relatively thick elastic vessels that expand and contract as the heart pumps blood. The pulse rate is the number of heart contractions during a given period of time. When the heart contracts, systole occurs. When it is in a relaxed phase, diastole occurs. The measurement of arterial pressure generated during systole and diastole corresponds to the body's blood pressure. For example, the average normal pressure is 120/80, measured in millimeters of mercury (mm Hg), which means 120 systole and 80 diastole.

Veins carry blood back to the heart, are thinner than arteries, and possess small valves that prevent blood from flowing backward. Unlike the blood flow in arteries, the blood in veins flows smoothly.

Capillaries are the blood vessels that appear in the greatest number, and they are the smallest blood vessels. It is at the capillary level that the blood and cells exchange nutrients, oxygen, and waste products.

Blood. Each adult has 10 to 12 pints (4.7 to 5.6 liters) of blood. Blood is composed of a liquid component called plasma and of solid components that include red blood cells, white blood cells, and platelets.

Plasma is 90% water. The remaining 10% is divided among plasma proteins (globulin and fibrinogen), inorganic salts, and other products (hormones, antibodies, urea, oxygen, carbon dioxide, and products of digestion). Globulin functions in the body's defense system, and fibrinogen is an integral component in the clotting of blood.

The solid constituents of blood include the red blood cells, white blood cells, and platelets. Red blood cells, or erythrocytes, are donut-shaped discs that have no nuclei. They are produced in bone marrow and contain hemoglobin, an iron-containing protein responsible for transporting oxygen to the cells.

White blood cells, or leukocytes, are larger than red blood cells and include neutrophils, basophils, and lymphocytes. Some are formed in bone marrow and some in the lymphatic system. Neutrophils are the most common type of white blood cells. They are phagocytes (cell eaters), which function in areas of inflammation by ingesting foreign debris. Basophils are the second most common white blood cells, which function in the production of the anticoagulant heparin. Lymphocytes are an integral part of the body's defense mechanisms.

Platelets, which play a critical role in the clotting process, are actually fragments of larger cells called megakaryocytes, which are formed in bone marrow.

Blood type is inherited and remains unchanged throughout life. There are four basic blood types: A, B, AB, and O. These categories are based on the presence of certain antibodies and the degree to which the red blood cells agglutinate (clump together). In addition, blood types are subdivided by the presence or absence of certain groups of proteins or antigens.

Lymphatic System

The lymphatic system works in close association with the circulatory system. Its purpose is to return intercellular fluid and materials to the circulatory system. The fluid and returning materials are called *lymph*. The lymphatic system also serves to transport absorbed fats from the intestines to the blood and plays an integral part in the body's defense systems.

The organs of the lymphatic system include lymph nodes, tonsils, the thymus, and the spleen. Lymph nodes are encapsulated masses of lymph tissue that filter the lymph fluid and produce lymphocytes and monocytes, which destroy micoorganisms in the body. The tonsils and the thymus serve in similar capacities, although their function is still not completely understood. The spleen acts as a storage area for red blood cells and has other important functions.

If larger amounts of tissue fluid collect in an area because of a blockage in the lymphatic system or a change in the protein concentration of the surrounding intercellular fluid, a pathologic state termed *edema* results. Edema often is symptomatic of other bodily pathologies or of a reaction to a localized inflammatory process or both.

Lymphadenopathy, or swelling of the lymph nodes, should alert the dentist and dental assistant to an infectious process in the patient's body (Fig. 1–1).

Respiratory System

Respiration is the process whereby the oxygen required by each cell for the production of energy is introduced into the bloodstream and carbon dioxide, a waste product of cellular activity, is removed. This transfer of gases occurs in the lungs where thin-walled capillaries are in close proximity to the alveoli, the air sacs of the lungs. Air is inhaled through the nose and enters the nasal sinuses, where it is filtered, warmed, and moistened. The air then travels through the nasopharynx to the pharynx, past the glottis, which is the opening into the larynx and trachea. The epiglottis is a protective flap of tissue that prevents food from entering the lungs. After passing through the

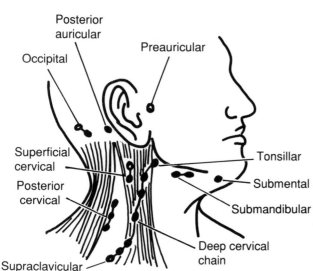

Figure 1-1. Lymph nodes of the head and neck.

glottis, air enters the larynx and subsequently enters the trachea, the major duct leading to the lungs. The trachea branches out into smaller ducts called bronchi, which in turn divide into bronchioles and subsequently alveoli, the smallest components of the respiratory system.

Air is inspired by expansion of the ribcage and diaphragm, causing a negative air pressure against the lungs. The lungs expand as air is drawn into them.

After the exchange of gases, air pressure around the lungs increases while the diaphragm and ribcage relax. As the air pressure increases, the air is forced out of the lungs.

Digestive System

The digestive system functions to reduce ingested food mechanically and chemically to a state in which it can be used by the body. This process occurs in the alimentary canal, which is composed of five organs: the oral cavity, esophagus, stomach, and small and large intestines. In addition to the alimentary canal, there are adjunct organs, including the salivary glands, liver, gallbladder, and pancreas, which assist in the digestive process.

Food enters the oral cavity, where it is acted on by teeth and saliva. The teeth function to break up food. Incisors are used for biting, canines for tearing, and molars for crushing food. The food bolus is lubricated by saliva, primarily produced in the parotid, submandibular, and sublingual glands.

Saliva is transported to the oral cavity through a system of ducts. In addition to lubricating the food bolus, saliva contains the digestive enzyme ptyalin, which begins the breakdown of starches in the mouth. The tongue pushes the food bolus downward into the esophagus, which is a long tube that connects the oral cavity to the stomach. Food moves quickly through the esophagus, assisted by waves of muscular contractions in a process called *peristalsis*. In the stomach, food is churned and acted on by a variety of gastric enzymes and hydrochloric

acid. Some absorption into the bloodstream takes place in the stomach, although this process is conducted mainly in the small intestine. Residual waste products not absorbed into the bloodstream enter the large intestine, or colon, where water is absorbed, and the solid waste products are conducted outward from the body. The liver is an adjunct organ of the digestive system involved in the formation of bile, which is important in the intestinal phases of fat digestion. The liver also metabolizes carbohydrates, fats, and proteins for storage or energy use. The importance of the liver as a detoxification organ cannot be overemphasized. It detoxifies harmful chemicals that enter the body. Many drugs used in dentistry (eg, local anesthetics) are broken down in the liver.

Excretory System

The excretory system functions to remove waste products from the body, thereby supporting the maintenance of homeostasis. Included in the excretory system are the skin, lungs, intestines, and urinary tract.

The chemical reactions taking place within cells produce certain waste products, such as water, carbon dioxide, and urea, as well as heat, which must be eliminated from the body. This elimination process must occur regularly. Otherwise, cell functioning will deteriorate, causing eventual death of the cell. The skin, which is the largest organ of the body, functions to eliminate water and various salts through perspiration. As water is eliminated, it evaporates, cooling the skin and lowering body temperature.

The lungs function to remove the carbon dioxide and water excreted during respiration. The intestines, both small and large, rid the body of solid and liquid waste products. Solid waste products include cellulose, roughage, and nondigestible material. Liquids excreted by the intestines are bile, calcium salts, and water.

The organs of the urinary system include the kidneys, ureters, bladder, and urethra. The two kidneys, located behind the abdominal cavity on each side of the spinal column, function in the balance of osmotic pressure of extracellular fluids. In addition, the kidneys control electrolyte balance and excretion of metabolic wastes, as well as regulating the pH level of body fluids.

Endocrine System

The endocrine system is responsible for secreting hormones, which regulate metabolic functions of the body. Hormones are chemicals that are specific in action, continuously secreted, and generally slow acting. Organs of the endocrine system include the pituitary, thyroid, parathyroid, pineal, and adrenal glands, the pancreas, and gonads. The pituitary, located in the cranial cavity, secretes several hormones.

The adrenal hormones are released through the influence of the pituitary hormone ACTH. The mineralocorticoids stimulate resorption of sodium in the kidneys, which in turn controls fluid balance in the body. The glucocorticoids predominantly act in the regulation of metabolism of carbohydrates, fats, and proteins. The adrenal gland also secretes epinephrine, which affects all structures of the body innervated by the sympathetic nervous system and thereby reinforces its action (cardiac acceleration, vasoconstriction, and rise in blood pressure).

The pancreas, located in the abdominal group of cells, the isles of Langerhans, secretes insulin. Insulin promotes the use of glucose in cells and thereby decreases blood glucose concentration. Insulin is essential for the maintenance of normal levels of blood glucose. A marked increase in the level of blood glucose is known as diabetes mellitus and is caused by an inadequate supply of insulin in the body. The pancreatic hormone glucagon increases the blood glucose level. Insulin and glucagon work together to maintain a normal blood glucose level.

A variety of hormones have numerous effects on the oral cavity. For instance, the development and eruption rate of teeth can be severely affected if there is an imbalance in the release of thyroid hormones. The abnormal release of epinephrine from the adrenals can have deleterious effects on the oral mucosa and pulp due to vasoconstriction. In addition, the female sex hormones estrogen and progesterone can exert harmful gingival effects, especially during pregnancy.

Reproductive System

Humans reproduce sexually. Fertilization is the fusion of the nuclei of the female egg and male sperm. Once a month, an ovum (egg) is emitted from a woman's ovary and enters one of the fallopian tubes. The egg then travels down toward the uterus. If the egg is not fertilized, it degenerates and is discharged from the body. If it is united with the sperm, it becomes what is known as a zygote.

An embryo in its later development is known as a fetus. Various physiologic developments occur at different time intervals. The face begins to develop between the third and twelfth weeks, teeth begin to develop around the sixth week, and the heart begins to form about the fourth week.

The embryo is nourished through the placenta, a membrane through which oxygen, food, and waste prod-

ucts are exchanged. During the final trimester, the fetus increases greatly in size and weight, and brain cells form rapidly. The fetus also acquires antibodies from the mother, and immunity is transferred. Birth takes place approximately 266 days after conception.

During pregnancy, certain changes occur in the oral cavity of the mother as a result of hormonal fluctuation. The gingiva can become smooth, reddened, and swollen. Increased pocket depth can occur, causing teeth to become loose. Drugs taken by a pregnant woman can have an effect on the developing fetus. For example, tetracycline taken during the last trimester can cause discoloration of the teeth of the newborn.

It is particularly important to ascertain whether a woman is pregnant before radiographs are taken. The fetus is most vulnerable during the first trimester. If radiographs are necessary, the pregnant woman should be draped with a lead-lined apron and exposed to the least amount of radiation possible.

GENETICS

Genetics is the study of heredity and patterns of transmission of a given trait (eg, blue eyes or brown hair) from parent to offspring.

Chromosomes are filamentous structures in the cell nucleus along which genes are located. Genes are the basic units of heredity and are capable of self-replication.

Deoxyribonucleic acid (DNA) is the basic carrier of genetic information in the cells. It is included in every cell of the human body.

Examples of genetic manifestations are sex determination, blood type, hemophilia, cleft palate, tooth hardness, saliva flow, and missing teeth. Significant developmental and growth disturbances in the oral cavity have definite genetic implications. Disturbances in the development and growth of teeth, bones, and soft tissues are an important aspect in the study of dentistry.

Questions

DIRECTIONS (Questions 1 through 44): Each of the questions or incomplete statements in this section is followed by four suggested answers or completions. Select the ONE lettered answer or completion that is BEST in each case. Check your answers with the correct answers at the end of the chapter.

1. The cells that produce bone are

   (A) ameloblasts
   (B) osteoblasts
   (C) fibroblasts
   (D) fibrocytes

2. The function of bone marrow is to

   (A) produce blood cells
   (B) add resiliency to bones
   (C) decrease the weight of bones
   (D) aid in muscular attachments

3. A joint is the

   (A) center of ossification
   (B) overlapping of muscles
   (C) junction of bones
   (D) point of intersection of muscle and bone

4. Joints that do not move are called

   (A) hinge joints
   (B) ball-and-socket joints
   (C) gliding joints
   (D) sutures

5. Histology is the study of

   (A) the history of the human species
   (B) artifacts
   (C) tissue anatomy
   (D) internal body pressure

6. Muscle tissue is present in all of the body systems EXCEPT

   (A) circulatory
   (B) digestive

   (C) respiratory
   (D) cytology

7. Which tissue has the poorest regenerative capability?

   (A) muscle
   (B) nerve
   (C) connective
   (D) epithelial

8. Tendons attach

   (A) muscle to bone
   (B) bone to bone
   (C) muscle to nerve
   (D) nerve to bone

9. A reflex is

   (A) an action that can always be controlled
   (B) always hormonal in nature
   (C) an involuntary response to a stimulus
   (D) a response that bypasses the central nervous system

10. The condition that exists when a muscle loses its ability to contract is

    (A) exhaustion
    (B) reflex
    (C) fatigue
    (D) hyperextension

11. The central nervous system is covered by a membrane called the

    (A) hyaline membrane
    (B) meninges
    (C) Nasmyth membrane
    (D) primary cuticle

12. A nerve impulse is transmitted from nerve to nerve via

    (A) foramina
    (B) the myoneural junction

(C) ligament to muscle
(D) the synaptic junction

13. Neurons conducting impulses away from the central nervous system are called

(A) afferent nerves
(B) sensory nerves
(C) motor nerves
(D) accessory nerves

14. The cranial nerve controlling tongue movements is the

(A) olfactory
(B) trigeminal
(C) vagus
(D) hypoglossal

15. Involuntary nervous control of the body is determined by the

(A) cerebellum
(B) fifth cranial nerve
(C) autonomic nervous system
(D) accessory nerves

16. The passage of the respiratory tract is trachea to

(A) alveoli
(B) bronchi
(C) sinus
(D) larynx

17. The function of the epiglottis is to

(A) control the tidal volume of air
(B) support the thyroid gland
(C) regulate the CO_2 and O_2 ratio of inspired air
(D) prevent liquids and solids from entering the respiratory system

18. Where does gaseous exchange take place in the lungs?

(A) alveoli
(B) bronchi
(C) bronchioles
(D) larynx

19. Inspiration is caused by

(A) a decrease in size of alveoli
(B) expansion of the pleural cavity
(C) relaxation of the diaphragm
(D) contraction of the chest

20. The function of hemoglobin is to

(A) carry nutrients
(B) fight infection
(C) transport oxygen
(D) stimulate endocrine glands

21. The fluid portion of blood is known as

(A) erythrocytes
(B) plasma
(C) lymph
(D) platelets

22. Blood platelets are necessary in

(A) allergic reactions
(B) antigen-antibody reactions
(C) CO_2 elimination
(D) blood clotting

23. The blood vessels that contain valves are

(A) veins
(B) arteries
(C) capillaries
(D) platelets

24. Leukocytes are

(A) called red blood cells
(B) a defense mechanism of the body
(C) part of the oxygen transport system
(D) part of the excretory system

25. The number of chambers in the human heart is

(A) one
(B) two
(C) three
(D) four

26. The blood vessel that conducts blood from the heart to the body is

(A) the right atrium
(B) the right pulmonary vein
(C) the aorta
(D) the superior vena cava

27. Valves between the chambers of the heart

(A) supply blood to the heart muscles
(B) prevent the backflow of blood
(C) are vestigial organs
(D) regulate the electrical potential of the pressure

28. The arterial pulse indicates the

(A) blood pressure
(B) number of times the heart is contracting
(C) temperature of the blood
(D) cardiac output

29. The diastolic blood pressure is the pressure exerted by blood on the walls of

   (A) arteries when the heart is at rest
   (B) veins when the heart pumps
   (C) arteries when the heart pumps
   (D) veins when the heart is at rest

30. Lymph nodes function to

   (A) transport nutrients
   (B) produce plasma
   (C) produce lymphocytes
   (D) store leukocytes

31. What is the fate of lymph?

   (A) secreted as saliva
   (B) absorbed by the body
   (C) swallowed and digested
   (D) enters the bloodstream

32. Water comprises what percentage of body weight?

   (A) 10 to 20%
   (B) 20 to 40%
   (C) 50 to 70%
   (D) 70 to 90%

33. Digestion begins in the

   (A) large intestine
   (B) oral cavity
   (C) small intestine
   (D) stomach

34. The rhythmic movement of the esophagus that moves the food bolus onward is known as

   (A) churning
   (B) digestion
   (C) swallowing
   (D) peristalsis

35. The major function of the large intestine is to

   (A) lubricate the food bolus
   (B) store nutrients
   (C) aid in water absorption
   (D) aid in protein metabolism

36. Absorption of most nutrients occurs in the

   (A) small intestine
   (B) stomach
   (C) large intestine
   (D) esophagus

37. Embryology is the study of

   (A) humans and their environment
   (B) the human organism in the uterus
   (C) the endocrine system
   (D) genetics

38. Congenital refers to

   (A) a condition at birth
   (B) a condition that worsens during aging
   (C) diseases of the genitalia
   (D) missing teeth

39. A hereditary blood disease that can lead to uncontrolled bleeding is

   (A) epidermal dysplasia
   (B) sickle cell anemia
   (C) A and B blood types
   (D) hemophilia

40. Genetics is the study of

   (A) the reproductive system
   (B) heredity
   (C) tissue composition
   (D) intercellular fluids

41. Chromosomes are made up of

   (A) fats
   (B) carbohydrates
   (C) nucleic acids
   (D) glycogen

42. Endocrine glands affect the body by chemical mediators called

   (A) catalysts
   (B) hormones
   (C) impulses
   (D) genes

43. The hormone released during times of dental stress is

   (A) epinephrine
   (B) estrogen
   (C) testosterone
   (D) thyroxine

44. The presence of bacteria in the urine indicates

   (A) a possible infection in the urinary tract
   (B) hormone dysfunction
   (C) normal functioning
   (D) hypotension

DIRECTIONS (Questions 45 through 57): For each of the items in this section, ONE or MORE of the numbered options is correct. Choose answer

   A   if only 1, 2, and 3 are correct
   B   if only 1 and 3 are correct
   C   if only 2 and 4 are correct
   D   if only 4 is correct
   E   if all are correct

45. Metabolism is the combined process of

   (1) osmosis
   (2) catabolism
   (3) passive diffusion
   (4) anabolism

46. The axial skeleton refers to bones of the

   (1) head
   (2) neck
   (3) ribs
   (4) arms

47. The union of egg and sperm is known as

   (1) an embryo
   (2) a yolk sac
   (3) a fetus
   (4) fertilization

48. Blood normally transports

   (1) nutrients
   (2) hormones
   (3) oxygen
   (4) infection-fighting components

49. Which of the following are endocrine glands?

   (1) pituitary
   (2) thyroid
   (3) gonads
   (4) kidneys

50. The primary female hormones are

   (1) estrogen
   (2) thyroxine
   (3) progesterone
   (4) testosterone

51. What type of tissues make up the heart?

   (1) muscle
   (2) epithelial
   (3) nervous
   (4) connective

52. The types of muscle tissues are

   (1) cardiac
   (2) smooth
   (3) striated
   (4) elastic

53. The lungs are considered a part of which two systems?

   (1) circulatory
   (2) respiratory
   (3) urinary
   (4) excretory

54. The liver functions to

   (1) metabolize fat
   (2) detoxify harmful substances
   (3) manufacture bile
   (4) manufacture genes

55. Components of the urinary system are the

   (1) bladder
   (2) ureters
   (3) urethra
   (4) uterus

56. Organs found in the excretory system are the

   (1) skin
   (2) kidneys
   (3) lungs
   (4) intestines

57. The portions of the brain are

   (1) cerebrum
   (2) cerebellum
   (3) medulla oblongata
   (4) spinal nerves

Answers and Explanations

1. **(B)** Cells involved in the production, maintenance, and resorption of bone are osteoblasts, osteocytes, and osteoclasts, respectively. Osteoblasts produce a prebony matrix that is then calcified. They then become osteocytes, which are responsible for maintaining bone. Osteoclasts cause the resorption of bone by secreting enzymes that dissolve the bony matrix.

2. **(A)** Bone marrow functions to form red blood cells, some white blood cells, and platelets and to destroy old red blood cells.

3. **(C)** A joint is the junction of bones. The types of joints are synarthroses, which do not move, such as those found in the skull, amphiarthroses, those with limited movements, such as those between vertebrae, and diarthroses, the most mobile, such as the temporomandibular joint.

4. **(D)** A suture is a type of joint that does not move.

5. **(C)** Histology is the microscopic study of tissue anatomy.

6. **(D)** Muscle tissue is present in all body systems including the circulatory in vessel walls and the heart, the digestive in the oral cavity and in the wall along the entire length of the tract, and the respiratory in the diaphragm and intercostal muscles. Cytology is the study of cells.

7. **(B)** Nerve tissue has the poorest regenerative capability of any tissue. A severed nerve may regenerate only if its nerve body is not injured.

8. **(A)** Tendons are made up of fibrous tissue that attaches skeletal muscle to bone. Ligaments are fibrous tissues that attach bone to bone, limiting movement.

9. **(C)** The simplest type of reflex is the stimulation of an afferent neuron, which transmits an impulse to an efferent neuron, which stimulates an effector to respond involuntarily to the initial stimulation. An example of this is the jerking of a hand from a hot object.

10. **(C)** Fatigue is the condition in which the ability of a muscle to contract is impaired. It is caused by the accumulation of lactic acid, which is removed by respiration.

11. **(B)** The central nervous system is protected by tough coverings called the meninges. The meninges are made up of three membranes: the dura mater, the arachnoid, and the pia mater.

12. **(D)** A nerve impulse is transmitted from the axon of one nerve to the dendrite of the next nerve over a synaptic junction. The transmission is caused by a chemical released from the axon that can excite or inhibit the next neuron. A neuron is a nerve cell.

13. **(C)** Neurons can be classified as motor or efferent, which conduct impulses away from the central nervous system; sensory or afferent, which conduct impulses toward the central nervous system; and internuncial, which connect sensory and motor neurons.

14. **(D)** The hypoglossal nerve controls tongue movement.

15. **(C)** Involuntary nervous control of the body is mediated through the autonomic nervous system. The system attempts to maintain homeostasis in the body. It is further broken down into the sympathetic and parasympathetic division. The sympathetic is most active during times of stress, and the parasympathetic is most active during quieter times.

16. **(B)** The passage of the respiratory tract is nose→ pharynx→ larynx→ trachea→ bronchi→ bronchioles→ alveolar duct→ alveolar sac.

17. **(D)** The epiglottis prevents solids and liquids from entering the respiratory system by closing the entrance of the larynx.

18. **(A)** In the lungs, gaseous exchange takes place between the alveoli and the pulmonary capillaries. Gas diffuses from areas of higher concentration to areas of lower concentration. Therefore, oxygen, which has a higher concentration in the lungs, diffuses into the blood, and carbon dioxide, which has a higher concentration in the blood, diffuses into the alveoli. Blood reaching the cells has a higher concentration of oxygen. Therefore, the oxygen will diffuse into the cell. The cell has a higher concentration of carbon dioxide, and the carbon dioxide will, therefore, diffuse into the blood.

19. **(B)** Inspiration is caused by expansion of the pleural cavity. This is accomplished by the contraction of the diaphragm and the intercostal muscles, causing the alveoli to expand and create a vacuum. Expiration is the reverse of inspiration.

20. **(C)** Hemoglobin is a red pigment in red blood cells that transports oxygen to cells and helps remove carbon dioxide from cells.

21. **(B)** Plasma is made up of 90% water. The other 10% includes proteins, glucose, fats, wastes, dissolved gases, hormones, enzymes, and many other components.

22. **(D)** The sequence in blood clotting is
    a. broken blood vessels → breakdown of platelets→ platelet factors→
    b. platelet factors + antihemophilic factor→ thromboplastin
    c. prothrombin + thromboplastin→ thrombin
    d. fibrinogen + thrombin→ fibrin

23. **(A)** Large veins contain valves to stop the backflow of blood. Valves are found most commonly in veins of the extremities. If the valves are not able to stop the backflow of blood, the veins become dilated and are known as varicose veins.

24. **(B)** Leukocytes, also known as white blood cells, function as a protection against infection. There are two groups of leukocytes: granular and nongranular. Leukocytes are transported to the area in which they are needed by blood vessels. They then leave the circulatory system and move to the area of infection to begin the reparative process.

25. **(D)** The heart is composed of four chambers: two atria and two ventricles. The atria have thinner walls and are collecting chambers, receiving blood from the body and the lungs. The ventricles contain more muscle tissue and pump the blood to the lungs and the body.

26. **(C)** The aorta conducts the blood from the left ventricle of the heart to the body. The aorta may be

divided into the following parts: ascending aorta, aortic arch, thoracic aorta, and abdominal aorta.

27. **(B)** Heart valves are used to regulate the flow of blood through the heart and prevent blood from flowing backward.

28. **(B)** The arterial pulse normally indicates the number of times the heart is contracting. Other characteristics of the pulse, such as rhythm and strength, are indications of the cardiac condition.

29. **(A)** Diastolic blood pressure is the pressure exerted by blood on the walls of arteries when the heart is at rest. Systolic blood pressure is the pressure exerted on the walls of arteries when the heart contracts. In healthy young adults, the average blood pressure is 120/80.

30. **(C)** Lymph nodes function to filter lymph and to produce lymphocytes and antibodies.

31. **(D)** Lymph moves from smaller to larger vessels and eventually enters the venous system. The function of the lymphatic system is to return to the bloodstream water, proteins, and products of cellular metabolism not previously picked up by the bloodstream.

32. **(C)** Water comprises 50 to 70% of human body weight. Some functions of water in the body are to serve as a solvent, allow chemical reactions to occur, ionize chemicals, and regulate body temperature.

33. **(B)** Digestion begins in the oral cavity. The enzyme ptyalin, contained in the saliva, begins the digestion of starch and lubricates the food bolus. The tongue pushes the food bolus downward into the esophagus, which connects the oral cavity to the stomach.

34. **(D)** The movement of food in the digestive tract is caused by peristalsis. The amount of peristalsis is controlled by the autonomic nervous system. Parasympathetic control increases the amount of peristalsis, and sympathetic control decreases the amount of peristalsis.

35. **(C)** The function of the large intestine is to absorb water.

36. **(A)** Absorption of most nutrients occurs in the small intestine. The surface area of the small intestine is greatly enlarged by the number of surface projections, called villi.

37. **(B)** Embryology is the study of the human organism developing in the uterus.

38. **(A)** Congenital refers to a condition that exists at or before birth. Some common congenital defects of the

oral cavity are missing teeth, alterations in the enamel and dentin, cleft palate, and many facial defects.

39. **(D)** A hereditary blood disease that can lead to uncontrolled bleeding is hemophilia. The dental team must take special precautions when treating the hemophiliac. Medical histories must be thoroughly reviewed before treatment for appropriate premedication and factor replacement therapy. Consult with patient's physician or hematologist or both before scheduled dental appointments. Appropriate infection control measures are necessary due to the high risk of hepatitis and AIDS found in hemophiliac patients, who must receive numerous blood transfusions.

40. **(B)** Genetics is the study of heredity.

41. **(C)** Chromosomes are made up of genes, which carry the hereditary message. Genes are made of deoxyribonucleic acid (DNA).

42. **(B)** Endocrine glands produce chemical mediators called hormones. Hormones are proteins distributed via the circulatory system.

43. **(A)** Epinephrine is produced by the medullary portion of the adrenal glands during times of stress. It increases the heart rate, constricts most arterioles, and increases the blood pressure. The effects of epinephrine are similar to the effects of the sympathetic division of the autonomic nervous system.

44. **(A)** Bacteria in freshly drawn urine could indicate an infection in the urinary tract and should be further investigated. Other abnormal constituents of the urine that are indications of problems are blood, pus, albumin, and large amounts of glucose.

45. **(C)** Metabolism is the combined process catabolism (breakdown of body materials) and anabolism (build-up of body materials). Growth is dependent on the anabolic reactions exceeding the catabolic reactions.

46. **(A)** The axial skeleton consists of the head, neck, vertebrae, ribs, and sternum.

47. **(D)** The union of an egg and a sperm is known as fertilization, which occurs in the fallopian tubes. The fertilized egg is known as a zygote.

48. **(E)** Blood transports gases, hormones, nutrients, waste products, and infection-fighting components.

49. **(A)** The endocrine glands are the pituitary, thyroid, gonads, parathyroid, adrenals, pancreas, and pineal.

50. **(B)** The primary female hormones include estrogen, and progesterone, which play an important role in the female reproductive system.

51. **(E)** Heart tissue is made up of muscle (cardiac), epithelial (pericardium), nervous, and connective tissues.

52. **(A)** The three types of muscle tissue are striated or voluntary, smooth or involuntary, and cardiac.

53. **(C)** The lungs are considered a part of the respiratory system by the exchange of gases and the excretory system by expelling waste products (primarily carbon dioxide and water vapor).

54. **(A)** The liver functions to metabolize fats, carbohydrates, and proteins, to produce bile and blood proteins, to detoxify harmful substances, to produce body heat, and to store vitamins.

55. **(A)** The urinary system consists of two kidneys, which produce urine, two ureters, which transport it from the kidneys to the bladder, the urinary bladder, which stores urine, and the urethra, through which urination occurs.

56. **(E)** The organs of the excretory system are the skin, which removes water, minerals, and nitrogenous wastes, the lungs, which remove water and carbon dioxide, the digestive tract, which removes solid nondigestible materials and some water, and the urinary system, which removes water, toxins, nitrogenous wastes, and minerals.

57. **(A)** The brain can be divided into three parts: the hindbrain, including the medulla oblongata, pons, and cerebellum, the midbrain, and the forebrain, including the cerebrum, thalamus, and hypothalamus.

BIBLIOGRAPHY

Alexander G, Alexander DG. *Biology,* 9th ed. New York: Harper & Row Publishers Inc, 1970.

Anthony CP, Thibodeau GA. *Basic Concepts in Anatomy and Physiology: A Programmed Presentation,* 4th ed. St. Louis: CV Mosby Co, 1979.

Anthony CP, Thibodeau GA. *Structure and Function of the Body,* 6th ed. St. Louis: CV Mosby Co, 1980.

Chen PS. *Chemistry: Inorganic, Organic and Biological,* 2nd ed. New York: Harper & Row Publisher Inc, 1980.

Goss CM. *Gray's Anatomy,* 30th ed. Philadelphia: Lea & Febiger Publishers, 1985.

Ham AW. *Histology,* 8th ed. Philadelphia: JB Lippincott Co, 1979.

Keeton WT. *Biological Science,* 3rd ed. New York: WW Norton and Co, 1980.

Miller F. *College Physics,* 6th ed. New York: Harcourt Brace Jovanovich, Inc, 1987.

Ross G. *Essentials of Human Physiology,* Chicago: Year Book Medical Publishers Inc, 1978.

Torres H, Ehrlich A. *Modern Dental Assisting,* 4th ed. Philadelphia: WB Saunders Co, 1990.

CHAPTER 2

Dental Anatomy

INTRODUCTION

A dental assistant must be aware of the fundamentals of head and neck anatomy, oral embryology, and tooth morphology in order to perform delegated dental procedures with a better understanding. This chapter presents the basic hard and soft tissue anatomic landmarks of the skull and oral cavity. A synopsis of the development of teeth and individual tooth morphology descriptions of the permanent dentition are given.

ANATOMIC LANDMARKS OF THE SKULL

The skull is a bony structure composed of 22 bones. It is divided into the cranium (Table 2–1), which protects the brain, and the skeleton of the face. All the bones of the skull except the mandible, are joined by immovable joints, called sutures (Fig. 2–1).

The upper jaw, or maxilla, contains the upper teeth. This irregularly shaped bone helps form the boundaries of the roof of the mouth, the floor and lateral walls of the nose, the floor of the orbit, and the maxillary sinus (Fig. 2–2) (Table 2–2).

The lower jaw, or mandible, contains the lower teeth. This horseshoe-shaped bone, the largest and strongest bone of the face, consists of the horizontal structure (body) and a pair of vertical structures (rami). Each ramus has

two processes (extensions): the condylar process and the coronoid process. Soft tissue attachments (muscles and ligaments) to these processes enable the jaw to be opened and closed (Figs. 2–3, 2–4).

The range of motion of the mandible is defined by the temporomandibular joint, which is both a hinge joint and a gliding joint. This joint is a complex articulator composed of several ligaments that contribute to its functioning.

SOFT TISSUE LANDMARKS OF THE ORAL CAVITY

The oral cavity is the beginning of the digestive system. It is composed of the vestibule, bounded by the lips and cheeks externally and by the gums internally. The oral cavity proper is bounded by the alveolar arches, teeth, isthmus of fauces, hard and soft palate, and the tongue. It receives secretions from the salivary glands (Fig. 2–5).

The roof of the mouth is formed by the palate, which is divided into two areas: the hard palate and the soft palate. The hard palate separates the oral and nasal cavities and is bound by the alveolar arches and gingiva anteriorly and by the soft palate posteriorly. The soft palate is mostly muscular in origin and functions in speech and deglutition. Its posterior border hangs free and acts as a separation between the mouth and pharynx.

THE SALIVARY GLANDS

The oral cavity contains three major paired glands that produce saliva. Saliva is a liquid medium that distributes basic digestive enzymes, lubricates the oral tissues and ingested food, and functions to maintain the balance of oral bacteria.

The parotid glands are located in front of and just below each ear. Their secretions enter the oral cavity through the parotid ducts (Stensen's), opening into the cheeks opposite the second maxillary molars.

The submandibular glands are located on the inner surface at the angle of the mandible. Their secretions enter the oral cavity through the submandibular (Wharton's)

TABLE 2–1. BONES OF THE CRANIUM

Bones	Anatomic Landmarks
Frontal (1)	Superior anterior and roof of the skull; contains the frontal sinuses
Parietal (2)	Superior medial sides and roof of the skull
Temporal (2)	Medial sides of the skull; contains the middle ear, inner ear
Occipital (1)	Posterior base of the skull; posterior wall and posterior floor of cranial cavity
Sphenoid (1)	Anterior base of skull behind orbits
Ethmoid (1)	Part of nose, orbits, and floor of cranial cavity

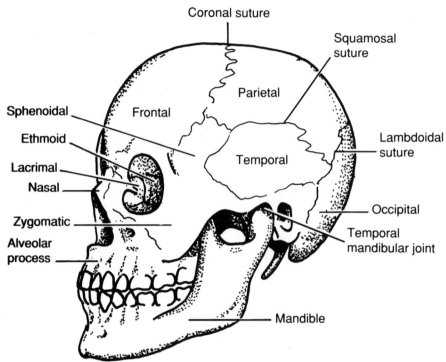

Figure 2–1. Bones of the cranium (lateral view).

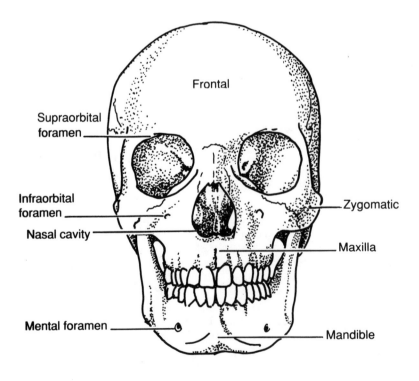

Figure 2–2. Bones of the face (frontal view).

TABLE 2–2. BONES OF THE FACE

Bones	Anatomic Landmarks
Zygomatic (2)	Forms the prominence of the cheeks, lateral wall, and floor of the orbit
Maxilla (2)	Helps form the boundaries of the roof of the mouth, provides support for teeth of the upper arch; contains the maxillary sinus
Nasal (2)	Bridge of the nose
Lacrimal (2)	Anterior part of medial wall of the orbit
Palatine (2)	Floor of nasal cavity, floor of the orbit
Vomer (1)	Posterior and inferior portion of nasal septum
Inferior concha (2)	Lateral wall of nasal cavity
Mandible (1)	Consists of body, ramus, and angle; forms lower jaw and provides support for teeth; range of motion is defined by temporomandibular joint

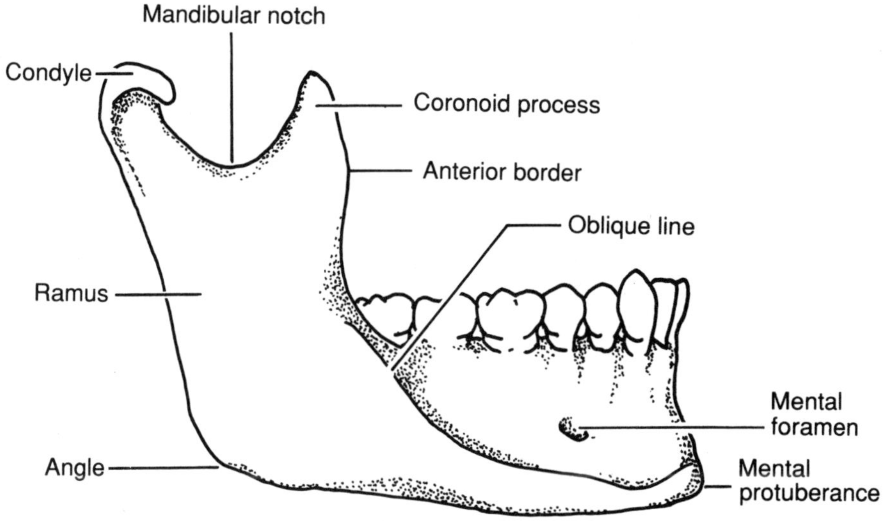

Condyle · Mandibular notch · Coronoid process · Anterior border · Oblique line · Ramus · Mental foramen · Angle · Mental protuberance

Figure 2–3. External aspect of mandible.

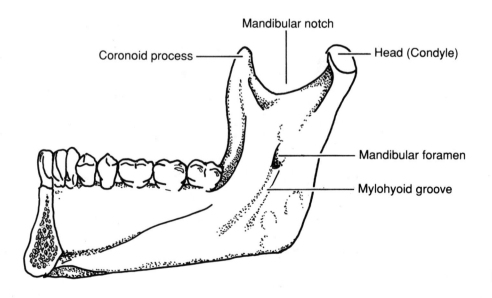

Mandibular notch · Coronoid process · Head (Condyle) · Mandibular foramen · Mylohyoid groove

Figure 2–4. Internal aspect of mandible.

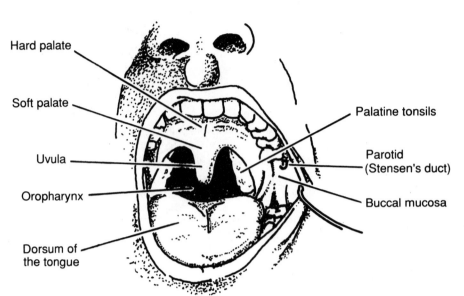

Figure 2–5. Soft tissue landmarks of the oral cavity.

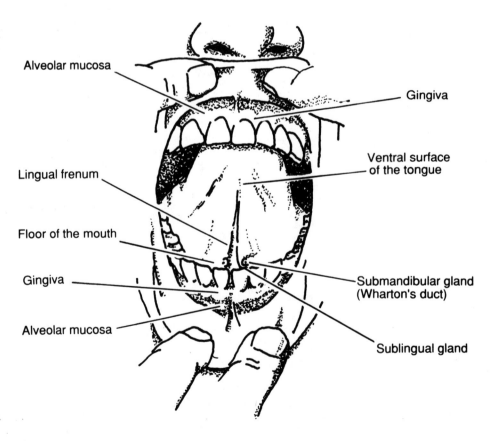

Figure 2–6. Oral cavity: salivary glands.

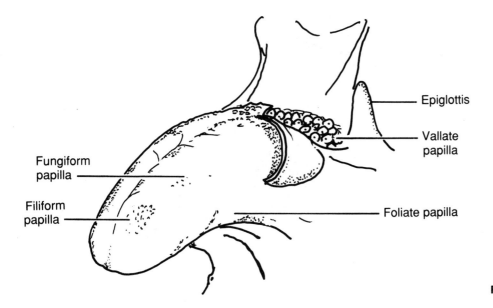

Fungiform papilla

Filiform papilla

Epiglottis

Vallate papilla

Foliate papilla

Figure 2–7. The tongue (dorsal surface).

ducts located beneath the tongue in the anterior portion of the mouth (Fig. 2–6).

The sublingual glands are the smallest salivary glands and are located under the tongue. Their secretions enter the oral cavity by the ducts of Rivinus. The secretions of the salivary glands are under control of the autonomic nervous system.

THE TONGUE

The tongue functions in speech and in mastication. It is also the major organ of taste.

The surface of the tongue contains several types of papillae, which contribute to its texture. Taste buds are located along the surface of the tongue and are found in large numbers in the papillae. Four basic taste senses are experienced: salty, sour, sweet, and bitter (Fig. 2–7).

THE MAJOR MUSCLES

Muscles of mastication function in the movement of the mandible. Each side of the face has four major muscles: the temporal muscle, the medial (internal) pterygoid muscle, the lateral (external) pterygoid muscle, and the masseter (Fig. 2–8).

The temporal muscle closes and retracts the mandible. It originates in the temporal fossa and inserts onto the coronoid process and anterior border of the ramus of the mandible.

The internal (medial) pterygoid muscle closes the jaw. It originates on the pterygoid plate and inserts onto the inner (medial) surface of the angle of the mandible.

The external (lateral) pterygoid muscle opens the jaw and moves it both forward and laterally. It originates on the sphenoid bone and on the pterygoid plate and inserts

onto the neck of the condyle and into the articular disc of the temporomandibular joint.

The masseter muscle closes the jaw. It originates from the zygomatic arch, and it inserts onto the lateral surface of the angle of the mandible.

The blood for these muscles is from the maxillary artery, a branch of the external carotid artery. All the muscles of mastication are innervated by the trigeminal nerve (the fifth cranial nerve).

Secondary muscles assist the masticatory process as well. These include the buccinator, the mylohyoid, the geniohyoid, and the anterior belly of the digastric muscle.

Muscles of facial expression are superficial muscles that have a tendency to relate to other nearby muscles and are grouped by the areas they affect. These basic groups affect the scalp, ears, nose, eyelids, and mouth. They enable expression and influence nonverbal communication. Blood is supplied by the external carotid artery, and innervation is supplied by the facial nerve.

ORAL EMBRYOLOGY

Teeth begin their development at approximately the sixth week in utero. The surface tissue of the oral cavity along the future dental arch thickens. This thickening tissue is called the *dental lamina.* Ten areas along the upper and lower arches possess further growth, causing the appearance of 10 swellings or buds, which are precursors of the future primary and later *succedaneous (succeeding) teeth.* The proliferating lamina leads to the formation of the shallow invagination of each bud into the oral tissue. From this, three distinct areas for each tooth develop. The first is the *enamel organ,* which is responsible for the formation of enamel. The second is the *dental papillae,* which is responsible for the development of dentin and pulp. The third is the *dental sac,* from which the cemen-

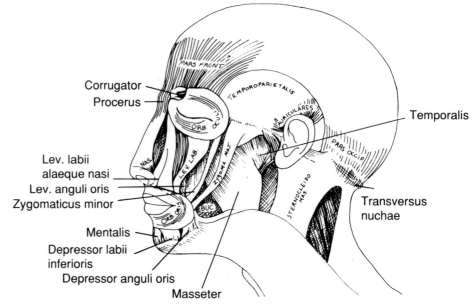

Corrugator
Procerus

Temporalis

Lev. labii
alaeque nasi
Lev. anguli oris
Zygomaticus minor

Mentalis
Depressor labii
inferioris
Depressor anguli oris

Transversus
nuchae

Masseter

Figure 2–8. Muscles of the head and face.

tum and periodontal ligament are developed. As growth continues, the teeth undergo a stage during which they all look identical to each other. This process continues until each tooth bud begins to differentiate into its final shape (eg, incisor, canine, molar). A period of *apposition* and *calcification* follows, during which enamel, dentin, and cementum are allowed to mature fully. As each tooth matures, it begins to erupt in its appropriate place in the mouth.

Each person has two complete sets of teeth during a lifetime. The primary dentition begins to erupt around 6 months of age and usually is complete by the time a child is 2 years of age. This dentition is composed of 20 teeth: a central incisor, a lateral incisor, a canine, and a first and second molar in each quadrant. Primary teeth begin to exfoliate at approximately 6 years of age, when succedaneous teeth begin to erupt. This process continues until the child is approximately 11 years of age, when the exfoliation of the primary dentition is complete. Functions of primary teeth include the maintenance of space for permanent teeth, stimulation of growth of the jaws, mastication, and speech development. Primary teeth are different in size and in external and internal design from permanent teeth.

Succedaneous teeth continue to erupt until the child is approximately 13 years of age. With the exception of the third molars, the secondary dentition is complete. Third molars erupt between the ages of 17 and 21 years. Each quadrant in the permanent dentition is composed of a central and lateral incisor, a canine, two premolars, and three molars. In total, there are 32 teeth.

TOOTH MORPHOLOGY

Teeth function primarily in the cutting and grinding of food. The shape of each tooth is determined by its function.

Incisors are used for biting, canines for tearing, and molars for crushing food. Teeth also maintain the integrity of the dental arch, protect the supporting periodontal tissue, function in producing speech sounds, and are a component in each person's facial esthetics.

The teeth of the permanent dentition are divided into four general types: incisors, canines, premolars, and molars (Fig. 2–9). A description of each permanent tooth in the human dentition is presented for review.

Incisors

Incisors act to shear or cut food and affect esthetics and speech. In the adult dentition, there are eight incisors, four in the maxilla and four in the mandible.

Maxillary Central Incisors. The permanent central incisors erupt at 7 to 8 years of age and form the midline of the maxilla. The average central incisor is a single-rooted tooth that has a crown length of 10 mm, a root length of 12 mm, and a mesiodistal length of 9 mm at its widest point. This tooth is the widest anterior mesiodistal tooth. The labial surface is convex but less convex than that of the maxillary lateral incisor. From a facial view, the crown of the tooth appears trapezoidal.

Maxillary Lateral Incisors. The maxillary lateral incisors erupt at approximately 8 to 9 years of age. The average lateral incisor is a single-rooted tooth that has a crown length of 8.8 mm, a root length of 13 mm, and a mesiodistal width of 6.4 mm at the incisal edge. The maxillary lateral incisor complements the function of the central incisor and resembles that tooth, except crown size and root bulk are smaller. Maxillary lateral incisors can exhibit more variation in tooth form than any other tooth except the third molar.

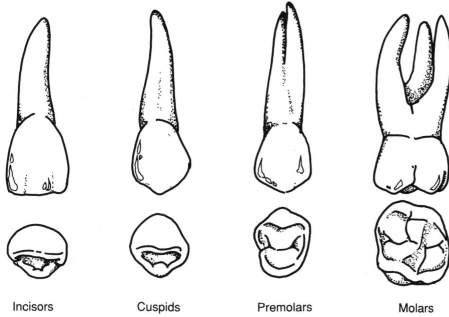

| Incisors | Cuspids | Premolars | Molars |

Figure 2–9. Tooth morphology.

Mandibular Central Incisors. The mandibular central incisors erupt at approximately 6 to 7 years of age. The average crown length is 8.8 mm, root length is 11.8 mm, and the mesiodistal diameter is 5.4 mm at the incisal edge. These single-rooted teeth usually are the smallest permanent teeth and the most symmetrical teeth in the mouth.

Mandibular Lateral Incisors. The mandibular lateral incisors erupt at 7 to 8 years of age. The average crown length is 9.6 mm, root length is 12.7 mm, and the mesiodistal diameter is 5.9 mm at the incisal edge. These single-rooted teeth resemble the mandibular central incisors but are slightly larger in all dimensions.

Canines

Canines are the longest teeth in the mouth. Like incisors, the function of these single-rooted teeth is to cut and tear food. There are four canines in the succedaneous dentition, one located in each quadrant between the lateral incisor and the first premolar. Since these teeth appear at the corners of the mouth when viewed facially, they have a great effect on appearance and esthetics.

Maxillary Canines. The maxillary canines erupt at 11 to 12 years of age. The average crown length is 9.5 mm, root length is 17.3 mm, and the mesiodistal width is 7.6 mm.

Mandibular Canines. The mandibular canines erupt at 9 to 10 years of age. The average crown length is 10.3 mm, and the root length is 15.3 mm. The mesiodistal width is 7.0 mm.

Premolars

The adult mouth contains eight premolars, four in the upper jaw and four in the lower jaw. These teeth tear food and begin the grinding process and are located between the canines and molars. They succeed the deciduous molars.

Maxillary First Premolars. The maxillary first premolars erupt at 10 to 11 years of age. The average crown length is 8.2 mm, root length is 12.4 mm, and mesiodistal width is 6.9 mm at the incisal edge. The maxillary first premolars have well-defined buccal and lingual cusps. The buccal cusps are about 1.0 mm longer than the lingual cusps. The crowns are shorter than the canines but, from the buccal aspect, look like canines. The mesial surfaces of the teeth at the junction of the crown and root have a concavity. These are the only premolars with two roots.

Maxillary Second Premolars. The maxillary second premolars erupt at 10 to 12 years of age. The average crown length is 7.5 mm, root length is 14.0 mm, and mesiodistal width is 6.8 mm at the incisal edge. The maxillary second premolars act in concert with the maxillary first premolars, and the two teeth resemble each other. The maxillary second premolars have one root as compared with the two roots of the maxillary first premolars, and the cusps of the second maxillary premolars are shorter than those of the first.

Mandibular First Premolars. The mandibular first premolars erupt at approximately 10 to 12 years of age. The average crown length is 7.8 mm, root length is

14.0 mm, and the mesiodistal width is 6.9 mm. These teeth closely resemble the mandibular canines, since the buccal cusps are long and sharp, and the lingual cusps are not pronounced. They also resemble the anatomic shape of the mandibular second premolars.

Mandibular Second Premolars. These teeth erupt at age 11 to 12 years. The average crown length is 7.9 mm, root length is 14.4 mm, and the mesiodistal length is 7.1 mm. These teeth appear with a buccal cusp and two smaller lingual cusps.

Molars

Molars perform the grinding job of mastication and reduce food to an appropriate size to swallow. They are the largest teeth in the mouth in terms of bulk. There are 12 molars in the secondary dentition. Each quadrant contains three molars located posterior to the premolars.

Maxillary First Molars. Average crown length of the maxillary first molars is 7.7 mm. These teeth have three roots, two buccal roots of approximately 12 mm length and a palatal root of about 13 mm length. These teeth are wider buccolingually than mesiodistal and are rhomboidal when viewed from the occlusal. There are usually four cusps, although there is sometimes a fifth cusp, located on the lingual surface, called the *cusp of Carabelli*. The occlusal surface is separated by a transverse ridge from the mesiolingual to the distobuccal cusps.

Maxillary Second and Third Molars. The teeth supplement the action of the first molars. Second molars are very similar to first molars. The main difference is the lack of development of the distolingual cusps. Third molars often appear as a developmental anomaly, with considerable size variation. They usually are not as well developed as second molars, and, as a rule, the crowns are smaller and the roots may be fused.

Mandibular First Molars. The average crown length of mandibular first molars is 7.7 mm. There are two roots, one mesial and one distal. Each is approximately 13.5 mm in length. In contrast to maxillary first molars, these are wider mesiodistally than buccolingual. Mandibular first molars usually have five cusps, three buccal and two lingual.

Mandibular Second and Third Molars. The mandibular second and third molars supplement the function of the first molars. Second molars usually are smaller than first molars and have only four cusps. Mandibular third molars vary considerably and usually are not as well developed as second molars. Their crowns generally follow the occlusal pattern of the other mandibular molars, but the roots often are small and not well formed.

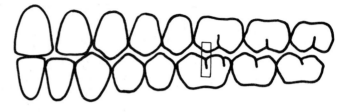

Figure 2–10. Class I neutrocclusion. Classification based on relationship of the first permanent molars.

OCCLUSION

Occlusion is the study of how the masticatory system operates. This includes the placement of teeth in the arch, articulation, and the action of the supporting joints and muscles. The goal of oral health care is to maintain or restore the structural and functional harmony consistent with good health and comfort.

Common measurements used to describe occlusion include centric occlusion, centric relation, overjet, and overbite. *Centric occlusion* occurs at maximum intercuspation (tooth-to-tooth contact). *Centric relation* is a point determined when the mandible is in its most retruded position. This measurement is important when centric occlusion cannot be determined accurately as a result of missing tooth structure. *Overjet* is the horizontal distance and *overbite* is the vertical distance between upper and lower anterior teeth when teeth are in centric occlusion.

Determining proper occlusion is important in fabricating any dental restoration, since improper occlusion, or malocclusion, can lead to the unbalanced distribution of the forces of mastication and subsequently to more severe dental problems (Fig. 2–10).

THE PERIODONTIUM

The periodontium consists of those hard and soft tissues that support tooth function. It includes the gingiva, the alveolar bone, the periodontal ligament, and the cementum. The last three function to attach the tooth to the underlying maxilla or mandible.

The gingiva is the soft tissue that covers the cervical portions of the teeth and surrounding alveolar bone. It is composed of free gingiva and attached gingiva. The free gingiva extends from the gingival margin of the tooth to the bottom of the gingival sulcus and can be separated from the tooth. When measured with a periodontal probe, a healthy gingival sulcus will have a depth of 3 mm or less. The attached gingiva extends from the bottom of the gingival sulcus to the mucogingival junction.

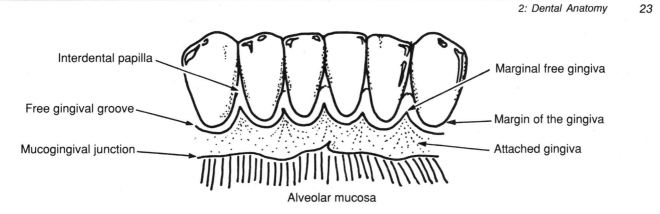

Figure 2–11. Periodontium: gingival tissues.

At the base of the mucogingival junction, an alveolar lining mucosa that extends to the cheeks, floor of the mouth, and the lips continues. The alveolar lining mucosa is thin vascular mucosa and loosely attached.

The original margin appears as a wavy path from tooth to tooth, with the gingiva being highest in the interdental spaces. This tissue, which appears interproximally, is the interdental papilla (Fig. 2–11).

The tissue covering the free and attached gingiva is toughened through the process of keratinization and appears stippled. The covering of the alveolar tissue and sulcular tissue is not keratinized and can be damaged more easily.

Each tooth is connected to the underlying alveolar bone through an attachment apparatus. The attachment apparatus consists of the alveolar bone, the periodontal ligament, and the tooth cementum. It supports each tooth by suspending it in a sling mechanism. The periodontal ligament is the tissue enclosing each tooth and connecting the alveolar bone to the cementum. Cementum is a hard material similar to enamel, covering the root surfaces of each tooth. Alveolar bone is similar to bone found elsewhere in the body. However, the condition of this bone is dependent on the function of the tooth it surrounds. If the tooth is under high stress, the alveolar bone tends to become denser, whereas if the tooth is missing, the bone has a tendency to be resorbed by the body (Fig. 2–12).

A healthy periodontium is essential for the maintenance of oral health. It has become increasingly clear that most tooth loss during the middle and later years is caused by poor periodontal health and a general weakening of the periodontium.

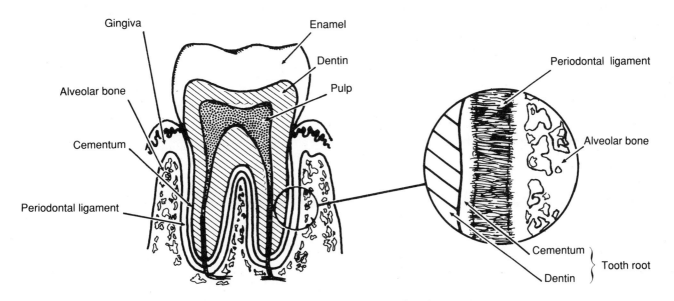

Figure 2–12. Periodontium: individual tooth and structures.

Questions

DIRECTIONS (Questions 1 through 12): Each of the questions or incomplete statements in this section is followed by four suggested answers or completions. Select the ONE lettered answer or completion that is BEST in each case. Check your answers with the correct answers at the end of the chapter.

1. The type of bone supporting the teeth is called

   (A) cortical bone
   (B) periodontal bone
   (C) alveolar bone
   (D) epiphyseal bone

2. The mandible is formed by two bones fusing at the

   (A) symphysis
   (B) condyles
   (C) ramus
   (D) coronoid notch

3. Which is the most prominent bone making up the skeletal structure of the cheek?

   (A) vomer
   (B) hyoid
   (C) ethmoid
   (D) zygomatic

4. Foramina are

   (A) protuberances in bones
   (B) openings in bone
   (C) fossae
   (D) smooth depressions in bones

5. The outer portion of the mandible is composed of

   (A) spongy bone
   (B) medullary bone
   (C) cortical bone
   (D) cartilage

6. The maxilla does not contact the

   (A) frontal bone
   (B) nasal bone

   (C) zygomatic bone
   (D) temporal bone

7. The maxillary tuberosity is located

   (A) anterior to the maxillary sinus
   (B) posterior to the maxillary third molar
   (C) lateral to the masseter muscle
   (D) posterior to the mandibular third molar

8. The maxillary sinus is

   (A) an air-filled cavity
   (B) a fluid-filled pocket
   (C) an immovable joint
   (D) filled with cartilage

9. Which tooth is most often located under the maxillary sinus?

   (A) maxillary central incisor
   (B) maxillary cuspid
   (C) maxillary first molar
   (D) maxillary third molar

10. The incisive foramen is located

    (A) behind the mandibular central incisors
    (B) behind the maxillary central incisors on the hard palate
    (C) below the mandibular second premolar
    (D) behind the maxillary second molar on the hard palate

11. The mental foramen is located

    (A) posterior to the mandibular third molar
    (B) below the mandibular central incisors
    (C) below the mandibular second premolar
    (D) behind the maxillary central incisors

12. The articular disc is part of the

    (A) orbit
    (B) frontal process
    (C) hyoid bone
    (D) temporomandibular joint

Anterior

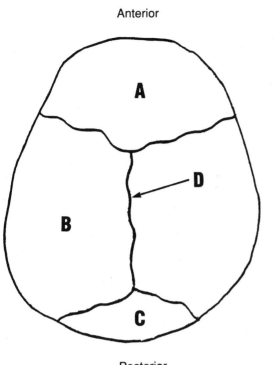

Posterior

Figure 2–13.

DIRECTIONS: Refer to Figure 2–13 to answer Questions 13 through 16. Select the letter from the figure that correctly illustrates the anatomic landmarks listed.

13. Frontal bone

14. Sagittal suture

15. Parietal bone

16. Occipital bone

DIRECTIONS: Refer to Figure 2–14 to answer Questions 17 through 20. Select the letter from the figure that correctly illustrates the anatomic landmarks listed.

17. Maxillary bone

18. Nasal bone

19. Mental foramen

20. Infraorbital foramen

DIRECTIONS: Refer to Figure 2–15 to answer Questions 21 through 25. Select the letter from the figure that correctly illustrates the anatomic landmarks listed.

21. Temporal bone

22. Coronoid process

23. Zygomatic bone

24. Sphenoid bone

25. Condylar process

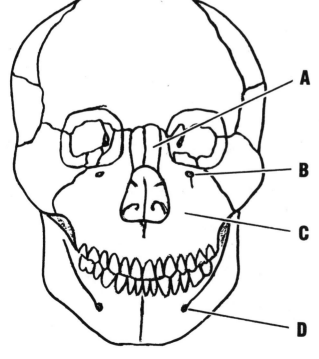

Figure 2–14.

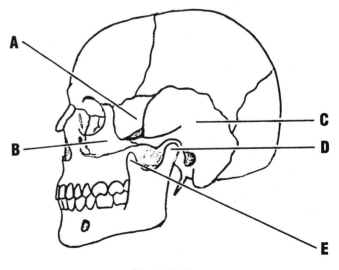

Figure 2–15.

DIRECTIONS (Questions 26 through 35): Each of the questions or incomplete statements in this section is followed by four suggested answers or completions. Select the ONE lettered answer or completion that is BEST in each case. Check your answers with the correct answers at the end of the chapter.

26. Which of the following is not known as a muscle of mastication?

    (A) mylohyoid
    (B) temporal
    (C) masseter
    (D) lateral pterygoid

27. Which muscle inserts into the coronoid process?

    (A) temporal
    (B) masseter
    (C) medial pterygoid
    (D) lateral pterygoid

28. The muscle forming the cheek is the

    (A) masseter
    (B) orbicularis oris
    (C) buccinator
    (D) superior constrictor

29. The muscle surrounding the opening of the mouth is the

    (A) mylohyoid
    (B) medial pterygoid
    (C) buccinator
    (D) orbicularis oris

30. The function of the inferior alveolar nerve is

    (A) sensory
    (B) motor
    (C) sympathetic
    (D) parasympathetic

31. The sensory innervation of the maxillary first molar mesiobuccal root is supplied by the

    (A) anterior superior alveolar nerve
    (B) middle superior alveolar nerve
    (C) posterior superior alveolar nerve
    (D) inferior alveolar nerve

32. The muscles of mastication are innervated by the

    (A) facial nerve
    (B) trigeminal nerve
    (C) lingual nerve
    (D) vagus nerve

33. The muscles of facial expression are innervated by the

    (A) fifth cranial nerve
    (B) sixth cranial nerve
    (C) seventh cranial nerve
    (D) ninth cranial nerve

34. The blood vessel(s) supplying the head with blood is/are the

    (A) common carotid arteries
    (B) subclavian arteries
    (C) pulmonary arteries
    (D) inferior vena cava

35. The arteries supplying blood to the mandibular and maxillary teeth are the branches of the

    (A) common carotid artery
    (B) external carotid artery
    (C) internal carotid artery
    (D) maxillary artery

DIRECTIONS (Questions 36 through 42): For each of the items in this section, ONE or MORE of the numbered options is correct. Choose answer

    A   if only 1, 2, and 3 are correct
    B   if only 1 and 3 are correct
    C   if only 2 and 4 are correct
    D   if only 4 is correct
    E   if all are correct

36. The maxilla helps form the

    (1) orbit
    (2) palate
    (3) zygomatic arch
    (4) ethmoid sinuses

37. The following structures pass through the mandibular canal.

    (1) lingual artery
    (2) incisive nerve
    (3) mental nerve
    (4) inferior alveolar nerve

38. The ramus of the mandible contains which structures?

    (1) glenoid fossa
    (2) mandibular foramen
    (3) mental foramen
    (4) coronoid process

39. A frenum is a fold of mucous membrane. Frena are located

   (1) in the maxillary labial vestibule
   (2) at the junction of the hard and soft palate
   (3) in the mandibular labial vestibule
   (4) distal to the last mandibular molar

40. The periodontium consists of the

   (1) gingiva
   (2) alveolar process
   (3) cementum
   (4) periodontal ligament

41. The interdental papillae is

   (1) pink
   (2) triangular
   (3) located between the teeth
   (4) stippled

42. Pulpal tissue consists of

   (1) enamel cells
   (2) connective tissue
   (3) ligaments
   (4) blood vessels

DIRECTIONS (Questions 43 through 84): Each of the questions or incomplete statements in this section is followed by four suggested answers or completions. Select the ONE lettered answer or completion that is BEST in each case. Check your answers with the correct answers at the end of the chapter.

43. Palatal rugae are

   (A) folds of the palatal mucosa
   (B) flaps covering the taste buds
   (C) bony palatal ridges
   (D) junctions between the hard and soft palate

44. The uvula is located along the posterior border of the

   (A) hard palate
   (B) lingual tonsil
   (C) soft palate
   (D) dorsum of the tongue

45. The retromolar pad is located

   (A) posterior to the maxillary third molar
   (B) distal to the last mandibular molar
   (C) between the maxillary central incisors
   (D) over the mental foramen

46. The palatine tonsils are located

   (A) on the soft palate
   (B) under the tongue
   (C) on the side of the fauces
   (D) adjoining the buccal fat pad

47. The tongue is composed of

   (A) adipose tissue
   (B) smooth muscle
   (C) lymphatic tissue
   (D) striated muscle

48. The vestibule lies between the

   (A) buccal gingiva and the cheek
   (B) coronoid process and condyle
   (C) tongue and the mandible
   (D) maxillary teeth and the hard palate

49. Filiform papillae are located on the

   (A) buccal mucosa
   (B) tongue
   (C) floor of the mouth
   (D) hard palate

50. The major salivary glands include all of the following EXCEPT the

   (A) sublingual gland
   (B) parotid gland
   (C) submandibular gland
   (D) lacrimal gland

51. The parotid gland is located

   (A) under the tongue
   (B) along the inferior border of the mandible
   (C) below and in front of the ear
   (D) adjacent to the thyroid gland

52. The submandibular gland is located

   (A) under the anterior third of the tongue
   (B) on the medial surface of the angle of the posterior portion of the mandible
   (C) opposite the maxillary second molar
   (D) in the anterior third of the hard palate

53. The submandibular ducts open

   (A) adjacent to the maxillary second molars
   (B) next to the palatine tonsils
   (C) on both sides of the lingual frenum
   (D) at the junction of the hard and soft palate

54. The parotid ducts open

   (A) on the buccal mucosa opposite the maxillary second molars
   (B) adjacent to the palatine tonsils
   (C) on the lateral border of the soft palate
   (D) on both sides of the lingual frenum

55. Teeth begin to develop

    (A) during the sixth week of intrauterine life
    (B) at birth
    (C) 6 weeks after birth
    (D) 6 months after birth

56. During which stage of development are dentin and enamel formed?

    (A) cap stage
    (B) bell stage
    (C) proliferation stage
    (D) apposition stage

57. Which part of the tooth forms first?

    (A) pulp
    (B) root
    (C) crown
    (D) dentin

58. The dental sac produces

    (A) enamel
    (B) cementum
    (C) dentin
    (D) pulp

59. The structure that becomes the succedaneous tooth is the

    (A) deciduous pulp
    (B) permanent tooth anlage
    (C) deciduous root
    (D) deciduous crown

60. Each developmental lobe on molars is represented by a

    (A) fissure
    (B) marginal ridge
    (C) cusp
    (D) groove

61. The most abundant tissue of the permanent tooth structure is

    (A) dentin
    (B) enamel
    (C) cementum
    (D) pulp

62. Secondary dentin

    (A) is only in the roots
    (B) adjoins the cementum
    (C) is a protective mechanism of the tooth
    (D) is the first dentin calcified

63. The hardest tissue of the body is

    (A) cartilage
    (B) bone
    (C) cementum
    (D) enamel

64. Nutrients for the pulp enter and leave the tooth through the

    (A) apical foramen
    (B) foramen ovale
    (C) mental foramen
    (D) genial tubercles

65. The periodontal ligament lies between the

    (A) enamel and dentin
    (B) alveolar bone and cementum
    (C) enamel and cementum
    (D) cementum and dentin

66. Keratinization of gingival cells is for

    (A) color
    (B) stippling
    (C) protection
    (D) frenum attachment

67. The gingiva is covered with

    (A) adipose tissue
    (B) alveolar tissue
    (C) fibrous tissue
    (D) stratified squamous epithelium

68. The unattached edge of the gingiva is the

    (A) free gingiva
    (B) connected gingiva
    (C) alveolar mucosa
    (D) buccal mucosa

69. The gingival sulcus

    (A) lies between the free and attached gingiva
    (B) is on the labial surface of anterior teeth
    (C) lies between the tooth and the internal surface of the free gingiva
    (D) is on the lingual surface of posterior teeth

70. In a mouth free from periodontal disease, the attached gingiva would appear

    (A) stippled
    (B) mottled
    (C) denuded
    (D) eroded

71. Exfoliation is the

    (A) internal absorption of succedaneous teeth
    (B) removal of permanent tooth follicles
    (C) shedding of primary teeth
    (D) technique used to remove cysts

72. At what age is the last deciduous tooth normally shed?

   (A) 9 years
   (B) 15 years
   (C) 6 years
   (D) 12 years

73. A pit is a

   (A) sharp protusion
   (B) sharp, small depression
   (C) circular elevation
   (D) elongated depression

74. Mamelons are

   (A) grooves in posterior teeth
   (B) three small elevations of enamel on anterior teeth
   (C) teeth of all mammals
   (D) small fractures in permanent teeth

75. A bifurcation exists in which tooth?

   (A) central incisor
   (B) mandibular second premolar
   (C) maxillary first molar
   (D) mandibular first molar

76. A trifurcation exists in which tooth?

   (A) maxillary first molar
   (B) maxillary second premolar
   (C) mandibular first molar
   (D) mandibular second molar

77. A diastema is

   (A) a supplemental groove
   (B) a space between adjacent teeth
   (C) anterior overlapping
   (D) an enlarged tuberosity

78. The surface of the tooth facing the midline of the mouth is the

   (A) mesial
   (B) distal
   (C) lingual
   (D) incisal

79. The surface of the anterior teeth facing the lips is the

   (A) buccal
   (B) labial
   (C) palatal
   (D) lingual

80. The lingual lobe of an anterior tooth is called a(n)

   (A) cusp
   (B) lingual depression
   (C) anterior elevation
   (D) cingulum

81. The longest tooth in the mouth is the

   (A) central incisor
   (B) lateral incisor
   (C) second premolar
   (D) canine

82. How many root canals does the maxillary first premolar have?

   (A) one
   (B) two
   (C) three
   (D) four

83. The cusp of Carabelli is sometimes found on what tooth?

   (A) maxillary first premolar
   (B) maxillary second premolar
   (C) maxillary first molar
   (D) mandibular second molar

84. Which tooth most often has fused roots?

   (A) maxillary first molar
   (B) maxillary first premolar
   (C) mandibular first molar
   (D) maxillary third molar

Answers and Explanations

1. **(C)** The bone that supports the teeth is called the alveolar bone. Other names for alveolar bone are cancellous or medullary bone. Fibers of the periodontal membrane are inserted into the part of the alveolar bone known as the lamina dura.

2. **(A)** The mandible is formed by two bones that fuse shortly after birth at the symphysis, a slight elevation between the mandibular central incisors.

3. **(D)** The zygomatic bone is the most prominent facial bone and is also called the cheekbone.

4. **(B)** Foramina are openings or holes in bone. They permit the entrance and exit of blood vessels and nerves.

5. **(C)** The outer part of the mandible is composed of cortical bone. This bone is extremely dense and hard and accounts for the strength of the mandible. The cortical bone will not permit the infiltration of anesthetics, and, therefore, block anesthesia must be used in the mandibular arch.

6. **(D)** The maxilla does not contact the temporal bone. The maxilla has four processes: the frontal, zygomatic, palatine, and alveolar.

7. **(B)** The maxillary tuberosity is a bony structure located posterior to the maxillary third molar. It is the distal extension of the alveolar ridge.

8. **(A)** The maxillary sinus is an air-filled cavity, the functions of which are to lighten the skull, warm and moisten the inhaled air, filter the inspired air, and add resonance to the voice.

9. **(C)** The teeth most often found below the maxillary sinus are the maxillary second premolars, first molars, and second molars. Inflammation of the maxillary sinus (sinusitis) can result when these teeth are percussed.

10. **(B)** The incisive foramen is located just behind the maxillary central incisors. Through this opening pass the nerves that transmit the sensory innervation of the anterior palate.

11. **(C)** The mental foramen is located below the mandibular second premolar. The vessels and nerves that enter and leave the foramen supply the vasculature and innervation to the soft tissue in the anterior portion of the mandible.

12. **(D)** Components of the temporomandibular joint are the glenoid fossa, a depression in the temporal bone, the glenoid tubercle, an anterior protuberance of the glenoid fossa that helps limit the anterior movement of the mandible, the articular disc, fibrocartilage between the glenoid fossa and the mandibular condyle, the bony protuberance in the posterior superior part of the mandibular ramus, and capsular and temporomandibular ligaments.

13. **(A)**

14. **(D)**

15. **(B)**

16. **(C)**

17. **(C)**

18. **(A)**

19. **(D)**

20. **(B)**

21. **(C)**

22. **(E)**

23. **(B)**

24. **(A)**

25. **(D)**

26. **(A)** The mylohyoid is not considered a muscle of mastication. The muscles of mastication are the masseter, medial pterygoid, lateral pterygoid, and temporal.

27. **(A)** The temporal muscle is a broad, fan-shaped muscle that originates in the temporal fossa.

28. **(C)** The buccinator muscle forms the cheek. It functions during mastication to place and hold food between the teeth.

29. **(D)** the orbicularis oris is the muscle that surrounds the mouth. It functions to close the lips, press the lips against the teeth, and protrude the lips.

30. **(A)** The inferior alveolar nerve is a branch of the mandibular nerve and is sensory to the lower teeth, lower lip, chin, and some gingival tissue. It enters the mandible canal and divides at the mental foramen into the mental and incisive nerves.

31. **(B)** The innervation of the maxillary first molar is the middle superior alveolar nerve for the mesiobuccal root and the posterior superior alveolar nerve for the palatal and distal buccal root.

32. **(B)** The muscles of mastication are all innervated by the mandibular branch of the trigeminal nerve.

33. **(C)** The muscles of facial expression are innervated by the seventh cranial nerve, the facial nerve. This nerve passes through the parotid gland. A misplaced inferior alveolar block injection into the parotid gland might anesthetize this nerve and cause temporary facial paralysis.

34. **(A)** The blood vessels that supply blood to the head are the right and left common carotid arteries.

35. **(D)** The maxillary artery supplies blood to the maxillary and mandibular teeth by branching into the inferior alveolar artery, the posterior superior alveolar artery, and the infraorbital artery. The last branches into the middle alveolar artery and the anterior superior alveolar artery.

36. **(A)** The maxilla helps form the orbit, palate, zygomatic arch, and nose.

37. **(D)** The mandibular canal contains the inferior alveolar artery, vein, and nerve. These structures supply the needs of the mandibular teeth, bone, and the anterior gingiva.

38. **(C)** The ramus of the mandible contains the coronoid process, mandibular foramen, mandibular condyle, sigmoid notch, and oblique ridges.

39. **(B)** Frena are located between the upper mucous membrane and the gingiva located between the upper central incisors, the lower mucous membrane and the gingiva located between the lower central incisors, and the mucous membrane on the floor of the mouth and the underside of the tongue. If the lingual frenum is short, the tongue is limited in movement, and the patient is known as tongue tied.

40. **(E)** The periodontium consists of the periodontal membrane, the alveolar bone, the gingiva, and cementum.

41. **(A)** The interdental papilla is pink, triangular, and located between the teeth. The interdental papilla is free gingiva, not attached gingiva, thus it would not appear stippled.

42. **(C)** The pulpal tissue consists of cells (odontoblast and fibroblast), connective tissue (fibers and intercellular material), blood vessels, lymphatic vessels, and nerve fibers.

43. **(A)** Palatal rugae are composed of folds of palatal mucosa. They extend from the suture line laterally in the anterior third of the hard palate.

44. **(C)** The uvula is the small projection located along the posterior border of the soft palate. It is muscular in composition and functions to close off the nasopharynx in swallowing.

45. **(B)** The retromolar pad is an oval soft tissue elevation located on the mandibular ridge posterior to the last molar. This is a landmark when deciding the distal extension of a removable prosthesis.

46. **(C)** The palatine tonsils are located on the side of the fauces. Children have larger tonsils than adults. This tissue is examined readily during a routine oral survey. The most common pathologic condition of tonsils makes them appear swollen and spotted with small abscesses.

47. **(D)** The tongue is composed of striated, or voluntary, muscle. The musculature is divided into intrinsic muscles, concerned with the shape of the tongue, and extrinsic muscles, concerned with moving the tongue to different areas of the mouth.

48. **(A)** The vestibule is a potential space located between the labial mucosa of the cheek and lips and the buccal and labial gingiva. Removable prostheses often extend into the vestibule.

49. **(B)** The mucous membrane of the dorsum of the tongue contains the following papillae: fungiform, filiform, foliate, and vallate.

50. **(D)** The sublingual, parotid, and submandibular glands are the major salivary glands.

51. **(C)** The parotid glands, are located below and in front of the ears. The glands become enlarged when a person has the mumps.

52. **(B)** The submandibular gland is located on the medial surface of the mandible at the angle of the mandible. The third major salivary gland is the sublingual gland, which is located under the tongue.

53. **(C)** The submandibular ducts (Wharton's) open in small elevations on both sides of the lingual frenum.

54. **(A)** The parotid ducts (Stensen's) open on the buccal mucosa opposite the maxillary second molars. To decrease salivary flow, a cotton roll may be placed in the maxillary fold to press against the orifice of the duct.

55. **(A)** Teeth begin to develop at 6 weeks of intrauterine life. The initial stage is the formation of tooth buds by the downward proliferation of cells from the dental lamina.

56. **(B)** It is during the bell stage that cells of the developing tooth differentiate into ameloblasts and odontoblasts and begin to deposit the enamel and dentin matrices, respectively.

57. **(C)** The first part of the tooth to be formed is the crown. It is not until the enamel and dentin have reached the future cementoenamel junction that root formation begins.

58. **(B)** The dental sac becomes the periodontal membrane and the cementum.

59. **(B)** The structure that becomes the succedaneous tooth is the permanent tooth germ anlage. This structure begins to form during the cap stage and is located lingual to the developing tooth buds derived directly from the dental lamina.

60. **(C)** The developmental lobe on molars is represented by a cusp. The mandibular first molar is formed by the fusion of five developmental lobes, whereas the mandibular second molar is formed by the fusion of four developmental lobes.

61. **(A)** The most abundant tooth tissue is dentin. Dentin is a living tissue maintained by the pulp. The tooth is capable of forming additional dentin by odontoblastic activity.

62. **(C)** Secondary dentin is slowly and continuously deposited throughout the vital life of the tooth. If an irritant is present, the odontoblasts respond by quickly depositing secondary dentin, known as reparative secondary dentin, to protect the tooth.

63. **(D)** The hardest and most brittle tissue of the body is enamel.

64. **(A)** Nutrients for the pulp enter and leave the tooth through the apical foramen. The apical foramen is most often located near, but not at, the anatomic apex of the root.

65. **(B)** The periodontal ligament lies between the cementum and the alveolar bone. It is made up of collagenous fibers, some of which are embedded in the cementum and some of which are embedded in the alveolar bone.

66. **(C)** Keratinization of the attached gingiva and the mucosa of the palate provides protection to the underlying tissue from the trauma of mastication.

67. **(D)** The gingiva is covered with stratified squamous epithelium.

68. **(A)** The edge or cuff of the gingiva not attached to the tooth is the free gingiva. The gingival papilla is the interdental extension of the free gingiva.

69. **(C)** The gingival sulcus is bordered by the tooth, the internal surface of the free gingiva, the gingival attachment, and the oral cavity.

70. **(A)** Healthy attached gingiva has an orange peel or stippled effect.

71. **(C)** Exfoliation is the shedding of primary teeth. This is an active process that occurs between the ages of 6 and 12 years and is caused by the resorption of the roots of the primary teeth.

72. **(D)** The last deciduous teeth to be shed are the deciduous second molars. This usually occurs between 11 and 12 years of age.

73. **(B)** A pit is a sharp, small depression usually found at the junction of two fissures. A fissure is a developmental defect caused by the incomplete fusion of developing lobes.

74. **(B)** Mamelons are three small elevations of enamel on the incisal edge of anterior teeth. Each elevation represents part of a developmental lobe. Mamelons are quickly worn away by use shortly after the tooth erupts.

75. **(D)** A bifurcation is the space between roots of teeth that have two roots. Teeth that have bifurcations are the mandibular first and second molars and the maxillary first premolars.

76. **(A)** A trifurcation is the space between the roots of teeth that have three roots. The maxillary molars are teeth with three roots.

77. **(B)** A diastema is a space between adjacent teeth. It most frequently exists between the maxillary central incisors. A diastema can be created by the movement or drifting of teeth, caused by the lack of supporting bone.

78. **(A)** The surface of the tooth that faces the midline is the mesial surface. The surface that is the farthest from the midline is the distal surface.

79. **(B)** Anteriorly, the surface of the teeth facing the lips is the labial surface. Posteriorly, the surface of the teeth facing the cheek is the buccal surface. The surface of the upper teeth facing the palate is the palatal surface. The surface of the lower teeth facing the tongue is the lingual surface.

80. **(D)** Anterior teeth are formed by the fusion of four developmental lobes. Three form the labial portion of the tooth, and one forms the lingual lobe known as the cingulum.

81. **(D)** The longest tooth in the mouth is the canine. The great length accounts for the stability of the tooth, which makes it an excellent abutment for prosthetic appliances. The canine often is referred to as the cornerstone of the mouth.

82. **(B)** The maxillary first premolar usually has two roots, buccal and palatal, as well as two root canals.

83. **(C)** The cusp of Carabelli is the fifth cusp sometimes present on the palatal surface of the mesiolingual cusp of the maxillary first molar. The cusp is nonfunctional.

84. **(D)** Third molars often have fused roots.

BIBLIOGRAPHY

Dahlberg A. *Dental Morphology and Evolution.* Chicago: University of Chicago Press, 1971.

Fuller JL, Denehy GE. *Concise Dental Anatomy and Morphology.* Chicago: Year Book Medical Publishers, Inc, 1977.

Goss CM. *Gray's Anatomy,* 30th ed. Philadelphia: Lea & Febiger Publishers, 1985.

Graber, TM. *Orthodontics,* 3rd ed. Philadelphia: WB Saunders Co, 1972.

Greep RO, Weiss L. *Histology,* 3rd ed. New York: McGraw-Hill Inc, 1973.

Kraus BS, Jordan RE, Abrams L. *Dental Anatomy and Occlusion.* Baltimore: Williams & Wilkins Co, 1969.

Orban B. *Oral Histology and Embryology,* 9th ed. St. Louis: CV Mosby Co, 1980.

Sicher H. *Sicher's Oral Anatomy,* 7th ed. St. Louis: CV Mosby Co, 1980.

Torres H, Ehrlich A. *Modern Dental Assisting,* 4th ed. Philadelphia: WB Saunders Co, 1990.

Wheeler S. *An Atlas of Tooth Form,* 5th ed. Philadelphia: WB Saunders Co, 1984.

Wheeler S. *Dental Anatomy, Physiology and Occlusion,* 6th ed. Philadelphia: WB Saunders Co, 1984.

CHAPTER 3

Preventive Dentistry

INTRODUCTION

Knowledge of disease prevention concepts and patient education skills is becoming mandatory for dental auxiliaries. The dental assistant must learn how to effectively motivate and train dental patients to assume greater responsibility in their own preventive treatment. Properly designed plaque control programs will assist patients in changing poor dental habits by providing new strategies for achieving dental health success. This chapter addresses the basic skills and concepts for preventing dental disease, including oral physiotherapy techniques, plaque etiology, nutritional counseling, plaque control programs, fluoride therapy, and the application of dental sealants.

SOFT DEPOSITS

Bacterial plaque is a soft, sticky, dense gelatinous layer of bacteria that adheres to the teeth and gingival tissues. Dental plaque is classified as a soft deposit and may be removed by proper toothbrushing methods and the use of dental floss, if accessible.

In the early stages of bacterial plaque formation, the pellicle layer is colorless and difficult to detect with the human eye. Later stages of plaque formation take on a thicker whitish appearance. Bacterial plaque is composed primarily of organized bacteria and salivary microorganisms held together in a sticky matrix.

The formation of bacterial plaque occurs rapidly in the oral cavity, and within 12 to 24 hours of removal, a thin film of bacterial plaque will begin to cover the teeth and gingival tissues again. Fermentable carbohydrates and sucrose in the diet increase the production of harmful bacterial plaque irritants (acids), which demineralize the tooth enamel, leading to dental caries. The irritants (acids) in dental plaque create gingival inflammation of the gums, causing gingival tissues to bleed and become swollen.

Materia Alba

Materia alba is a white or grayish mass of bacterial and oral cellular debris that accumulates around the gingival margins and on the surfaces of teeth. Materia alba is a loosely attached soft deposit that may be removed by vigorous rinsing or by water irrigating devices. The appearance of materia alba in the oral cavity is unesthetic and is associated with poor oral hygiene habits.

Dental Stains

Extrinsic stains often come from food, tobacco, coffee, or tea. The stains coat the outer surfaces of the teeth and can be removed through coronal polishing techniques. Extrinsic stains range in color. Yellow and brown stains often are associated with food pigments and poor oral hygiene. Green stains may be caused by the remnants of Nasmyth's membrane around the newly erupted teeth of children. Orange and red stains are caused by certain types of chromogenic bacteria in the oral cavity as are black line stains, which occur around the cervical one-third of the tooth surface.

Intrinsic stains can occur during tooth formation and are caused more often by medication or systemic diseases. Intrinsic stains cannot be removed by coronal polishing techniques. The discoloration of the teeth may range from gray to black due to metallic materials coming in contact with the teeth. An intrinsic brown stain of the teeth, often referred to as dental fluorosis or mottled enamel, will occur if there is an excess of 2 parts per million of fluoride in the drinking water ingested during the mineralization stage of tooth formation. A common form of intrinsic stain is a result of ingestion of tetracycline during the calcification stage of tooth development. The discoloration may range from light yellow or gray to a characteristic darker gray banding around the cervical area of the teeth.

HARD DEPOSITS

If dental plaque is not removed, it may calcify. A mineralized mass called calculus results. Calculus is classified as a hard deposit and can be removed only by the use of dental instruments, such as scalers and curettes.

The accumulation of calculus above the gingival margin is known as *supragingival* calculus. This type of calculus is visible to the human eye. Supragingival calculus usually collects just above the gingival margin of the teeth near the ducts of the sublingual salivary glands of the anterior mandibular teeth and on the buccal surfaces of the maxillary second molars adjacent to Stenson's (parotid) salivary duct.

The formation of calculus below the gingival margin of teeth is known as subgingival calculus. Subgingival calculus is irritating to the gingival tissues and may lead to further gingival diseases due to plaque on and within the caculus matrix.

TOOTHBRUSHES AND BRUSHING TECHNIQUES

The proper toothbrush should be approximately ½-inch wide and contain two, three, or four rows of evenly spaced soft bristles. The tip of each bristle should be rounded, polished, and approximately 0.007 inches or less in diameter. The handle should be aligned on the same plane as the head of the toothbrush and provide a comfortable grasp to enable easy access to all areas of the mouth. Most common methods of brushing are the Bass, Charters, modified Stillman, and rolling stoke techniques.

The *Bass technique* emphasizes sulcular brushing and is the most effective method of brushing for removal of dental plaque deposits from beneath the gingival margin. The bristles of the toothbrush are placed at a 45-degree angle to the long axis of the tooth and gently placed into the sulcus. The brush is then vibrated back and forth with very short stokes for 10 to 15 seconds in each area (Fig. 3–1).

The *Charters technique* was designed to stimulate the gingival margin around each tooth. It is most effective when interdental spaces are open. The bristles are pointed toward the occlusal or incisal surfaces at a 45-degree angle to the tooth. The bristles are pressed lightly in order to flex and force the bristle tips between the teeth. A firm but gentle vibrating motion is used. The bristle ends do not enter the sulcus.

The *modified Stillman technique* is used to remove plaque from the cervical and interdental areas. The bristles of the brush are placed at a 45-degree angle to the apex of the tooth. The brush, lying firmly against the gingiva, is vibrated in a rotary motion. The wrist is turned slightly so that the brush slowly rolls down over the gingiva and teeth. A modified Stillman approach to brushing incorporates a rolling stroke after the vibratory stroke to ensure better plaque removal. With this technique, the bristles do not enter the sulcus.

The *rolling stroke technique* is the simplest. Bristles are placed at the gingival margin of the teeth, with the side of the bristles pressing against the gingiva. The gingival tissues will be slightly blanched. The brush is then rolled following the contours of the teeth onto the occlusal surfaces, and the process is repeated approximately 10 times on each tooth surface. Occlusal surfaces are cleaned with a back-and-forth motion. A drawback of this technique is that the sulcus is not cleaned.

DENTAL FLOSS AND FLOSSING TECHNIQUE

An important oral physiotherapy device for the removal of interproximal plaque is dental floss. Dental floss must be manipulated properly to avoid damaging tooth structure or gingiva. The interproximal areas of the teeth are the most frequent sites of dental caries and gingival inflammation, and toothbrushing alone is not an effective method of cleaning these areas. Flossing correctly can be difficult for the patient to learn. Each patient must be given sufficient support to ensure that the method is learned properly (Fig. 3–2).

A piece of floss that is either waxed or unwaxed, approximately 18 inches long, should be wrapped around the middle finger of each hand until the fingers are about 2 inches apart. The floss is then guided interproximally

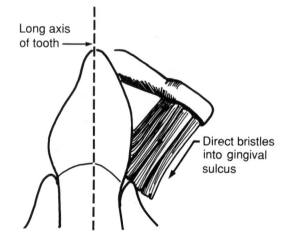

Figure 3–1. Toothbrush positioned for sulcular brushing.

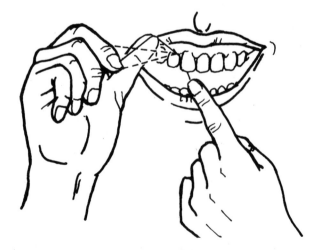

Figure 3–2. Flossing technique.

with the thumb or index finger through the contact area with a short gentle seesawing motion. The dental floss must not be forced or snapped through the contact areas. Once through the contact area, the dental floss is pressed against the tooth and slightly curved to slide beneath the gingival margin until resistance is felt. While sliding the dental floss against the tooth surface, a scraping motion is used to remove the sticky plaque away from the gums and off the teeth. Various types of specialty dental floss are available for cleaning fixed bridgework and dental implants and require specific adaptation techniques for effective plaque removal.

ORAL PHYSIOTHERAPY DEVICES

Several oral physiotherapy products are available to the dental patient for special dental health needs. Additional devices and products that can be used by the patient to clean the teeth and gums may include toothpaste, mouth rinses, disclosing agents, periodontal brushes, dental floss holders and threaders, wooden aids, and water irrigating devices. Specialty products for cleaning removable dental appliances and dentures also are available. These devices may include harder bristle toothbrushes, partial clasp brushes, denture toothpaste, and immersion agents used for cleansing and soaking removable partials and dentures.

Toothpaste and dentifrices serve several functions. In addition to polishing teeth and decreasing mouth odors, they provide therapeutic benefits through the addition of fluorides to reduce the incidence of dental caries and desensitizing agents to reduce tooth sensitivity. Ingredients of toothpaste include water, which acts as a solvent, abrasives, which clean and polish, detergents, which provide foaming action, humectants, which prevent dehydration, binders, which join the solid and liquid ingredients, and flavorings.

Mouthwashes can be classified into two categories: cosmetic and therapeutic. Cosmetic rinses have no dental value that has been scientifically substantiated. Therapeutic rinses include the addition of fluoride for caries control and the addition of antibacterial plaque agents to promote healthier gingival tissues by reducing the oral microbacterial count.

Disclosing tablets and solutions are nontoxic, nonirritating, inexpensive dyes that identify plaque by coloring the deposits. Many deposits on teeth are not visible, and the tablets or solutions help the patient visualize these areas before or after brushing and flossing.

Interproximal brushes are cone-shaped nylon brushes used to remove plaque in open interproximal and bifurcated and trifurcated root areas. The brush is slightly moistened before insertion, and an in-and-out motion is used for cleansing. The plastic-coated interproximal brush is also an adjunct to hygiene maintenance of dental implants.

Perio aids/piks are used to cleanse under the gingival margins and exposed furcation areas. Concave interdental surfaces also are best reached with the aid of the perio pik. The device consists of a plastic handle with a hole located at either end to insert the toothpick. The tip is angled and traced around the gingival margin to remove sulcular plaque deposits.

A rubber tip is a cone-shaped piece of rubber used to stimulate the gingiva. The side of the tip is pressed against the gingiva with sufficient pressure to cause some blanching of the tissue and is then moved in circular motions. A rubber tip is useful in reshaping the gingiva after periodontal surgery, improving keratinization of tissue, and reducing the severity of interproximal inflammation.

Wooden interdental devices are triangular-shaped wedges made of balsawood. They are used for cleaning the interproximal areas where there are exposed tooth surfaces due to gingival recession. Care must be taken to use this device properly because gingival tissue may be traumatized if the adjoining teeth are forced apart.

A floss holder is a device made for those patients who have difficulty grasping or manipulating the dental floss between their fingers. The floss holder is also a beneficial oral physiotherapy supplement for handicapped patients with limited dexterity. Care must be taken to avoid cutting the gingival tissues during application.

Floss threaders are plastic or metal devices used to thread floss under and between the pontics of fixed bridges and splinted teeth. These devices are important, since these areas are difficult to reach and are susceptible to plaque retention.

Water irrigation devices remove loose food debris around teeth. They are an adjunct to toothbrushing but are not a substitute for it, since these instruments do not remove plaque. They are useful for patients with orthodontic and fixed prosthetic appliances. Proper attention must be given to the direction of the pulsing water jet so as not to cause injury to the delicate gingival tissues. The pressure of the water jet stream should never be set on high. Medications may be added to the water jet reservoir to enhance therapeutic results after mechanical debridement with the floss and toothbrush.

FLUORIDES

The most efficient and economical method of decreasing the prevalence of dental caries is by the use of fluorides. Fluorides can be administered systemically through addition to the water supply and vitamin supplements or applied topically (directly onto the exposed surfaces of erupted teeth). Fluoride itself is a mineral nutrient essential in the formation of sound teeth and bones. However, if too much fluoride is absorbed during tooth developmental periods, the teeth can appear mottled.

Systemic Fluorides

Many people receive fluoride in their drinking water in the amount of 1 part per million (ppm). If a community's central water supply is not fluoridated, individual community organizations, such as a school, can supplement their water supplies. In addition, fluoride supplements come in the form of chewable tablets or liquids that can be added to a child's daily diet. Vitamins also may contain trace amounts of fluoride.

Topical Fluorides

Topical fluoride is applied directly to the surfaces of teeth and may be either an adjunct to fluoridated water or the sole source of fluoride for a child. Common topical fluoride agents include sodium fluoride, acidulated phosphate fluoride, and stannous fluoride.

Sodium fluoride is available in a 2% aqueous solution. A series of four treatments is given, with intervals of several days to 1 week apart.

Acidulated phosphate fluoride has proved more effective than sodium fluoride alone and is applied topically every 6 months.

Stannous fluoride is used in a .04% gel. Applications for root desensitization, caries control, or periodontal antimicrobial therapy may be prescribed.

Methods of application for topical fluoride gels may include disposable trays or trays that can be sterilized. Topical fluoride gels or solutions may be painted on the teeth with a cotton tip applicator. A summary of fluoride characteristics is outlined in Table 3–1.

Dental personnel must be aware of the potential dangers of fluoride toxicity. Failure to administer the correct dosage of prescribed fluoride agents may result in acciden-

tal overdose and serious injury. Recommended amounts and methods of delivery for application of the fluoride agent must always be strictly adhered to. Dental auxiliaries should always keep patients in an upright position when administering a topical fluoride in a tray form. The patient should be instructed to keep a saliva ejector in the mouth to pick up excess flow of fluoride. Always caution the patient not to swallow immediately after the removal of the fluoride trays. The patient should be instructed to expectorate for several minutes after removal of the fluoride trays and then given proper home care instructions. Children should never be left unattended during the application of fluoride agents.

DENTAL SEALANTS

Caries preventive treatment also includes the application of resin sealants. Pit and fissure sealants are caries-reducing agents that are applied directly to caries-free tooth surfaces to seal anatomic faults in the enamel of primary and permanent teeth. The most prevalent sites for caries are occlusal surfaces, where lesions usually begin in the deep pits and narrow fissures.

The tooth surface being treated is etched with phosphoric acid, and a resin sealant that mechanically bonds to enamel is applied and polymerized. This process results in the formation of a physical barrier, decreasing the possibility of caries formation.

NUTRITION AND DIET ANALYSIS

Nutrition is the process that includes use of food in growth, repair, and maintenance of body tissues, digestion and absorption of food, and transport of food to the cells.

Good nutrition is a combination of basic food elements and chemical substances called nutrients. Nutrients are essential for providing the nourishment necessary for the body to function properly. Six general classes of nutrients can be identified: proteins, carbohydrates, fats, minerals, vitamins, and water.

Proteins, made up of amino acids, are either structural, serving as building blocks (eg, collagen fibers, the major constituents in skin, bone, and cartilage), or functional, including enzymes and hormones. Primary sources of protein include meat, poultry, fish, eggs, legumes, vegetables, nuts, cheese, and milk.

Carbohydrates provide sources of energy and include sugars (glucose, sucrose, lactose), starches (rice, potatoes, grains), and polysaccharides (cellulose, roughage). Carbohydrates are the principal energy source for most living systems and are the basic materials from which other molecules are built. Excess carbohydrates are stored in the liver.

Fat serves a role both as a structural material and as an energy reserve. It is important to the nervous system in providing insulation for nerves. Fats are found in meats, poultry, fish, oils, and dairy products.

TABLE 3–1. COMPARISON OF TOPICAL FLUORIDE CHARACTERISTICS

Fluoride Agent	Advantages	Disadvantages
Sodium fluoride (NaF) 2%	Does not stain teeth Stable solution when stored in polyethylene bottle Less objectionable taste Gingival irritation does not occur	Success of treatment dependent on series of several appointments
Acidulated phosphate fluoride (APF) 1.23% NaF with 0.1 M orthophosphoric acid	Does not stain teeth Stable when stored in polyethylene bottle Pleasant taste may be flavored Requires single application	Can irritate inflamed gingival tissues May cause etching effects on resin restoration or porcelain
Stannous flouride (SnF₂) .4%	Available in liquid solution May be incorporated in dentifrice for caries control Brush-on gel form available for patient home use	Taste is objectionable May cause staining of teeth Short shelf-life May be irritating to inflamed gingival tissues

Minerals are important in assisting enzymes in biochemical reactions. Essential minerals include calcium, sulfur, sodium, potassium, magnesium, iron, iodine, chlorine, and copper. Very small amounts of these minerals are needed to maintain adequate nutrition.

Vitamins are organic compounds not synthesized by the body but necessary for good health. Essential vitamins include A, B, C, D, E, and K.

Water is essential for all organisms and constitutes 50% to 70% of total body weight. Without water, we become dehydrated—a minor problem initially but one that can lead to serious complications and possibly death.

Good nutrition is essential for the maintenance of oral hygiene. Dietary counseling is given to patients to provide them with the knowledge necessary to maintain a dietary balance. Four basic food groups provide the sources for a balanced diet. The four food groups recommended for daily intake are the milk group, meat group, fruits and vegetable group, and bread and cereal group.

The *milk group* includes dairy products consisting of different types of milk, yogurt, cheese, ice cream, custards, and puddings that are an excellent source of protein, riboflavin, and calcium. The recommended daily allowance (RDA) for adults is two servings per day and for children three or more servings per day. For pregnant women, this amount is increased to four or more servings daily.

The *meat group* includes meat, poultry, fish, eggs, nuts, dried peas and beans, and lentils. Meats, poultry, and fish provide high-quality iron and B vitamins. The RDA is two or more servings daily.

The *fruit and vegetable group* provides vitamins that are eliminated by the body and must be replenished daily. This food group also provides minerals essential to good health and fiber. Citrus fruits are good food sources for vitamin C, a water-soluble vitamin, and dark leafy green vegetables provide a rich source of vitamin A, a fat-soluble vitamin. Four or more servings a day should be derived from this food group.

Breads and cereals provide vitamin B, protein, and iron. Sources include rice, pasta, whole grains, and enriched cereals. Nutrients often are lost during processing and added later to compensate for this loss. Four or more servings a day are recommended from this group.

Suggested snack foods that aid in the maintenance of good oral health include fresh fruits and vegetables, cheese, eggs, nuts, lunch meats, fish, fowl, plain yogurt, milk, unsweetened juices, potato chips, popcorn, and sugar-free soft drinks.

Table 3–2 indicates the function and sources of key nutrients and disorders that can arise from nutritional deficiencies.

PLAQUE-CONTROL PROGRAMS

Prevention and interception of dental disease occur only when patients have the knowledge and skills that enable them to participate in these processes. Educating and motivating patients to make a commitment to prevention is accomplished in a plaque-control program. Information is presented to patients to change their behavior in an effort to make them primarily responsible for maintaining good oral hygiene. A sample program follows.

Visit 1. Patients are made aware of how dental plaque forms. Basic instruction in brushing and flossing is provided, and disclosing agents are used to permit patients to see and remove soft deposits from their teeth. The relationship of dental plaque and dental disease is discussed.

Visit 2. Techniques of brushing and flossing are reviewed and reinforced. Adjunct oral physiotherapy techniques are introduced based on individual patient need. Patients are provided with basic nutritional guidelines and a self-administered diet history review sheet. Emphasis should be placed on a low sugar and carbohydrate intake.

Visit 3. Diet history is reviewed, and constructive behavioral strategies helpful in changing poor eating habits are suggested. Home care is reviewed and evaluated. Corrections are made at this time regarding technique. Positive reinforcement is stressed to reward good behavior. Motivational strategies are emphasized and applied.

Visit 4. All previous sessions are reviewed for positive reinforcement. During this visit, patients are asked to describe or exhibit their individual strategies for prevention and to assess their own success. This visit can be repeated if necessary until success is achieved. The importance of future dental recall visits for preventive maintenance is reinforced. Long-term appointments may be set up at this visit also.

TABLE 3–2. KEY NUTRIENTS

Nutrient	Functions	Sources	Deficiency
Proteins	Build and maintain body tissues; help body carry on normal processes	Meat, poultry, fish, milk, cheese, eggs, plants (soybean)	Kwashiorkor, marasmus
Carbohydrates	Supply energy	Sugars, syrups, cereals, grains, bread, jam and jelly, pasta, crackers, pretzels, dried fruits	None specifically, but excessive intake can lead to dental caries
Fats	Provide insulation and support for internal body organs	Oils, butter, egg yolks, nuts, meats	None, but excessive fat intake can lead to coronary disease
Minerals	Assist in the formation and maintenance of body structures and metabolism	Milk, meat, fish, nuts, whole grains, shellfish	Bone deformities, muscle tremors, anemia
Water	Essential for maintaining normal body processes and stable body temperature	Drinking water and other liquids	Dehydration, shock, death
Vitamins			
Fat soluble			
A	Assists in proper maintenance of epithelial cells, plays role in vision	Fish, liver, oils, vegetables, yellow fruits	Night blindness, severe drying of skin
D	Builds and maintains bones and teeth, regulates calcium and phosphorus metabolism	Milk, fish, eggs, liver, butter, sunshine	Rickets, poor tooth development
E	Essential for normal reproduction	Wheat germ, vegetable oil, green vegetables	Unknown
K	Contributes to normal blood clotting	Green vegetables, cabbage, cauliflower, soybean oil	Defective clotting
Water soluble			
C	Aids in resisting infections, healing, and maintaining a healthy gingiva, strengthens blood vessels	Citrus, fruits, broccoli, parsley, green vegetables, melons, tomatoes, berries	Scurvy
B_1 (thiamine)	Helps normal body function growth, assists in carbohydrate metabolism	Yeast, wheat germ, whole grains, pork, liver	Growth retardation, nerve disorders, beriberi
B_2	Contributes to normal function of body cells	Fish, eggs, whole grains, liver, meat, greens	Glossitis, cheilosis, dermatitis
B_6	Contributes to normal function of body cells	Meat, liver, vegetables, whole grain cereals	Anemia, skin lesions
B_{12}	Contributes to blood regeneration	Liver, milk, cheese	Pernicious anemia, neurologic disturbances
Niacin	Helps other cells use nutrients	Yeast, eggs, milk, green vegetables	Pellagra
Pantothenic acid	Assists in proper metabolism	Yeast, liver, kidney, eggs	Lack of proper metabolism
Folacin (folic acid)	Contributes to normal function of cells	Plant foods, greens, liver	Unknown
Biotin	Helps body use proteins, carbohydrates, and fats	Kidney, liver	Epithelial sensitivity, muscular pains

Questions

DIRECTIONS (Questions 1 through 45): Each of the questions or incomplete statements in this section is followed by four suggested answers or completions. Select the ONE lettered answer or completion that is BEST in each case. Check your answers with the correct answers at the end of the chapter.

1. What is considered to be the primary cause of dental disease?

   (A) sugar
   (B) plaque
   (C) saliva
   (D) materia alba

2. The first step in the formation of plaque is

   (A) pellicle
   (B) bacterial colonization
   (C) materia alba
   (D) food debris

3. The oral hygiene devices most commonly used in daily plaque removal are?

   (A) rubber bands and a toothbrush
   (B) a toothbrush and dental floss
   (C) an ultrasonic scaler and a toothbrush
   (D) water irrigators and dental floss

4. Nutrition is

   (A) ingested food
   (B) proper diet
   (C) the intake of nutrients
   (D) the process by which the body assimilates and uses food

5. The main role of the assistant in preventive dentistry is

   (A) dispensing fluoride rinses
   (B) taking x-rays
   (C) patient education
   (D) recording vital signs

6. What oral hygiene device should the auxiliary recommend to patients who have a fixed partial bridge?

   (A) floss holder
   (B) partial clasp brush
   (C) mouth rinse
   (D) bridge cleaners

7. A water irrigator is used

   (A) to remove plaque
   (B) as a substitute for a toothbrush
   (C) to remove loose food debris
   (D) as a substitute for dental floss

8. Which of the following nutrients has been found to be an overwhelming cause of the development of plaque and dental caries?

   (A) proteins
   (B) carbohydrates
   (C) minerals
   (D) vitamins

9. The preferred toothbrush is

   (A) soft, natural bristled
   (B) soft, nylon bristled
   (C) medium, natural bristled
   (D) medium, nylon bristled

10. How often should a patient be recalled?

    (A) every 8 months
    (B) each year
    (C) whenever the patient decides
    (D) the time varies with the oral condition of the individual patients

11. Using the heel or toe of the brush is helpful for cleaning which tooth surfaces?

    (A) buccal surfaces of molars
    (B) lingual surfaces of molars
    (C) lingual surfaces of anterior teeth
    (D) facial surfaces of anterior teeth

12. The best means of massage for the interdental papilla is the use of a

(A) perio aid
(B) water irrigating device
(C) balsawood wedge
(D) rubber tip

13. Abrasion of the teeth may occur from using a

(A) hard toothbrush
(B) extra fine dental floss
(C) medium bristle brushes
(D) water irrigating devices

14. When is an occlusal sealant contraindicated?

(A) on primary teeth
(B) when there are deep pits and fissures
(C) on severely decayed teeth
(D) on occlusal surfaces of posterior teeth

15. The sunshine vitamin is

(A) vitamin A
(B) vitamin D
(C) vitamin E
(D) vitamin K

16. Disclosing agents identify

(A) plaque
(B) carious lesions
(C) gingival recession
(D) calculus

17. Which oral physiotherapy aid most appropriately is used to clean interdental areas when large interproximal spaces or open contacts exist?

(A) dental floss
(B) regular toothbrush
(C) perio aid
(D) interproximal brush

18. Which of the following toothbrushing methods is the most effective method of removing plaque from the sulcus?

(A) rolling stroke method
(B) Bass method
(C) Charters method
(D) modified Stillman method

19. The most common stain found on adult teeth is

(A) tobacco stain
(B) yellow stain
(C) green stain
(D) black line stain

20. The process of demineralization will occur with

(A) caries
(B) calculus
(C) green stain
(D) black stain

21. If the fluoride ion combines with enamel, a more perfect crystal is formed called

(A) hydroxyapatite
(B) fluorapatite
(C) fluoridation
(D) ionization

22. How can one best motivate a patient when educating in the dental preventive philosophy?

(A) present as much information as possible on the first visit
(B) provide a dental prophylaxis and fluoride treatment
(C) present information to the patient in a manner that will stimulate personal interest
(D) motivation is not a part of the auxiliary's responsibilities

23. Good sources of protein may include

(A) milk, meat, fish, eggs
(B) bread, cereal, sugar, starch
(C) margarine, ice cream, apples, pecan pie
(D) water, nuts, popcorn, pasta

24. A hard deposit commonly found on the lingual surfaces of lower anterior teeth is

(A) dental plaque
(B) subgingival calculus
(C) supragingival calculus
(D) materia alba

25. In the majority of mouths, plaque will reform after brushing within what period of time?

(A) 1 minute
(B) 5 minutes
(C) 1 hour
(D) 12 to 24 hours

26. Stains that can be removed by coronal polishing procedures are called

(A) extrinsic
(B) intrinsic
(C) supragingival
(D) exogenous

27. Nutrients are essential to the daily diet. Which of these is NOT a nutrient?

(A) water
(B) lipids and fats
(C) amino acids
(D) baking soda

28. Teeth most likely to benefit from the application of pit and fissure sealants are

(A) anterior teeth only
(B) posterior teeth with deep pits and fissures
(C) posterior teeth with small carious occlusal pits
(D) partially erupted 6-year molars

29. Teeth should be disclosed

(A) before polishing
(B) only after polishing
(C) before and after coronal polishing
(D) at patient's request

30. Green stains on children's teeth can be the result of

(A) intrinsic staining
(B) excess topical fluoride
(C) trauma
(D) chromogenic bacteria

31. Before applying a topical fluoride gel to the teeth, the auxiliary must

(A) set up a recall appointment
(B) dry the teeth thoroughly
(C) review the x-rays
(D) provide plaque control instructions

32. Periodontal disease may cause

(A) dental decay
(B) gums to be stippled
(C) gums to recede
(D) TMJ problems

33. A deficiency of vitamin A may result in

(A) scurvy
(B) problems in enamel formation
(C) deafness
(D) pulpal necrosis

34. The vitamin responsible for proper blood clotting is

(A) vitamin K
(B) vitamin C
(C) vitamin D
(D) vitamin E

35. A riboflavin deficiency results in

(A) a malformation of dentin
(B) caries-prone teenage years

(C) cheilitis
(D) a herpetic lesion

36. What is the purpose of a low carbohydrate diet in the control of dental caries?

(A) decrease acid exposures
(B) decrease need for flossing
(C) provide a good nutritional analysis
(D) provide adequate nutrient value for a basic food group

37. What effect does a vitamin C deficiency have on the oral structures?

(A) causes gums to be firm and stippled
(B) causes bleeding and inflammation of the gingiva
(C) may cause intrinsic staining of the teeth
(D) no effect because vitamin C is a fat-soluble vitamin

38. When planning a diet for 1 day using foods from each of the four main food groups, an adult should have as recommended servings

(A) 4 servings from the meat group
(B) 4 servings from the milk group
(C) 4 servings from the fruit and vegetable group
(D) 2 servings from the bread and cereal group

39. Which of the following foods has the most nutrient value?

(A) popcorn
(B) sugarless chewing gum
(C) soda pop
(D) peanut butter

40. In plaque control instruction, what is the first decision stage the patient must go through before habits can be changed?

(A) action
(B) involvement
(C) awareness
(D) motivation

41. When using dental floss, it is necessary to clear the contact between two teeth by

(A) using an up and down motion with the floss
(B) using a gentle back-and-forth seesaw motion
(C) snapping the floss through as quickly as possible
(D) wrapping the floss around the tooth

42. A dilute sodium hypochlorite solution is recommended for cleaning

    (A) partial dentures with metal clasps
    (B) full dentures
    (C) orthodontic bands
    (D) mouths with heavy plaque accumulation

43. What is the major characteristic of gingivitis?

    (A) bone loss
    (B) inflammation
    (C) missing teeth
    (D) bad breath

44. The best time to present oral hygiene instruction is

    (A) at the beginning of the appointment
    (B) at the end of the appointment
    (C) when the patient is relaxed and receptive
    (D) after the doctor has administered the local anesthetic

45. Dental plaque may cause which of the following conditions?

    (A) caries and periodontal disease
    (B) periodontal disease and calculus
    (C) stains of the teeth only
    (D) caries only

DIRECTIONS (Questions 46 through 50): Match the oral physiotherapy devices in Column A with their functions in Column B.

COLUMN A
46. Floss holder
47. Disclosing agent
48. Perio aid
49. Balsawood cleaner
50. Interdental brush

COLUMN B
A. effective for large interproximal areas and fixed bridges
B. cleanses under gingival margins and root furcations
C. recommended for teeth with gingival recession
D. effective in identifying plaque
E. assists patients with limited dexterity

DIRECTIONS (Questions 51 through 54): Each of the questions or incomplete statements in this section is followed by four suggested answers or completions. Select the ONE lettered answer or completion that is BEST in each case. Check your answers with the correct answers at the end of the chapter.

51. The clinical appearance of materia alba is

    (A) hard and calcified
    (B) soft, white, and thick
    (C) dark brown and calcified
    (D) soft, white, and thin textured

52. When cleaning a removable partial denture, which of the following methods is NOT suitable?

    (A) brushing with a partial clasp brush
    (B) brushing with soap and water
    (C) polishing with laboratory pumice
    (D) soaking in diluted bleach for 24 hours

53. What oral hygiene device is best suited for patients who are having difficulty removing plaque from the distal surfaces of the maxillary wisdom teeth?

    (A) dental floss
    (B) bridge cleaners
    (C) toothpicks
    (D) interdental brush

54. To be of maximum benefit to the teeth, the optimum fluoride concentration is

    (A) 1 ppm
    (B) 2 ppm
    (C) 100 ppm
    (D) 1000 ppm

DIRECTIONS (Questions 55 through 68): For each of the items in this section, ONE or MORE of the numbered options is correct. Choose answer

    A   if only 1, 2, and 3 are correct
    B   if only 1 and 3 are correct
    C   if only 2 and 4 are correct
    D   if only 4 is correct
    E   if all are correct

55. Fluoride compounds most commonly used for topical application may include

    (1) sodium fluoride
    (2) stannous fluoride
    (3) acidulated phosphate fluoride
    (4) prescription fluoride chewable tablets

56. Plaque formation begins at the

    (1) midline of the lower arch
    (2) gingival margin of the tooth
    (3) occlusal surface of the tooth
    (4) proximal surface of the tooth

57. Calculus (tartar) has the ability to irritate the gingival tissue because it is

    (1) calcified
    (2) subgingival
    (3) covered with plaque
    (4) rough and irregular in texture

58. Improper toothbrushing can cause

    (1) gingival recession
    (2) periodontal disease
    (3) tooth abrasion
    (4) toothbrush attrition

59. Dentifrices

(1) remove calculus
(2) remove extrinsic stains
(3) remove intrinsic stains
(4) leave your mouth feeling fresh

60. An acquired pellicle

(1) is the first sign of periodontal disease
(2) is very susceptible to extrinsic stain
(3) is removed by irrigation or rinsing
(4) forms within minutes after brushing

61. Fluoride is used most effectively

(1) if ingested in a water supply during the time of tooth development
(2) if ingested in a water supply after teeth have erupted
(3) if present in a municipal water supply in the ratio of 1 ppm
(4) if present only in school water supplies for children

62. When handing out visual aid material, such as dental pamphlets, it is best to

(1) give the patient all the handout materials on the first visit
(2) reserve all such materials for the very last visit
(3) make the handout as detailed as possible using clinical terminology
(4) review the material with the patient before they leave the office

63. Subgingival calculus differs from supragingival calculus in

(1) color
(2) method of attachment
(3) location
(4) method of formation

64. Foods that are high caries producers include

(1) fruits and vegetables
(2) natural honey, raisins, syrup
(3) nuts, cereals, grains
(4) soft drinks, breath mints

65. Which of the following are considered detergent foods?

(1) apples, pears, water
(2) raisins, cheese, crackers
(3) lettuce, celery, carrots
(4) marshmallows, peanut butter, bananas

66. Under what circumstances are there differences in the recommended daily allowances of food?

(1) child vs adult
(2) male vs female
(3) small person vs large person
(4) pregnant vs nonpregnant

67. Mouthrinses are

(1) therapeutic
(2) cosmetic
(3) effective for removal of loose food debris
(4) breath fresheners only

68. Which type of patient should be on a yearly recall system?

(1) a patient with 2 mm to 3 mm sulcus depths
(2) a caries-free patient
(3) a patient who brushes and flosses daily
(4) an edentulous patient with dentures

Answers and Explanations

1. **(B)** Bacterial plaque is the primary cause of dental disease. Microorganisms found in plaque produce harmful exotoxins that are acidogenic and lead to the demineralization of enamel and dental caries. Other microorganisms in bacterial plaque lead to the degeneration and irritation of the gingival tissues, causing gum disease.

2. **(A)** An acquired pellicle is the first step in plaque formation. Plaque requires 24 hours to mature, but a pellicle or film takes only minutes to form.

3. **(B)** The oral hygiene devices most commonly used in daily plaque removal are the toothbrush and dental floss. The toothbrush removes the plaque and debris from the occlusal, facial, and lingual surfaces of the tooth. Dental floss is used to remove plaque from the proximal (mesial and distal) surfaces of the teeth. Other oral hygiene devices, such as toothpicks, can be substituted for dental floss if the particular condition dictates.

4. **(D)** Food is used by the body for fuel, growth, repair, and regulation of body functions. Nutrition is the process in which ingested food is assimilated and used by the body. Metabolism is the sum of all anabolic and catabolic chemical changes that food undergoes in the process of nutrition.

5. **(C)** The main role of the assistant in preventive dentistry is to educate and motivate patients. The information offered usually includes material about plaque control and proper nutrition.

6. **(D)** A bridge cleaner is the best oral hygiene device to use for fixed partial bridgework. The bridge cleaner is threaded with dental floss, which can be inserted easily under the pontic of the fixed bridge.

7. **(C)** Water irrigators are used to remove loose debris. They will not remove plaque or calculus.

8. **(B)** Foods containing high levels of sugars are most responsible for producing caries. Carbohydrates have been found to be the most influential nutrient in causing caries. All carbohydrates are broken down to produce sugars, which interact with oral bacteria to form acids that can cause decay.

9. **(B)** The toothbrush most effective in removing tooth accumulated material is soft and nylon. Softness is preferred to decrease the possibility of damage to hard and soft tissues, and nylon has been accepted as a material of consistent quality that is superior to natural bristles.

10. **(D)** The time between recall visits, examination, and oral prophylaxis varies according to the needs of the individual patient. Patients with a high caries index or those who are susceptible to periodontal disease are recalled more often than are patients who are less susceptible to oral disease. The usual time between recall visits is 6 months.

11. **(C)** The heel and toe of a toothbrush are most effective in cleaning lingual surfaces of anterior teeth, since these areas are narrow and curved.

12. **(D)** Rubber tips are best used to stimulate interdental papilla. This process helps keratinize the gingiva and decrease inflammation. Balsawood wedges are used primarily to clean large interproximal tooth surfaces and secondarily to massage the papilla. Wedges are not as effective as rubber tips because they are stiffer and more difficult to manipulate.

13. **(A)** In general, hard toothbrushes are not recommended because they can cause abrasion of the gingiva or enamel.

14. **(C)** Occlusal sealants are used primarily on undecayed tooth surfaces in order to prevent decay from forming. They are not used on severely decayed surfaces.

15. **(B)** Vitamin D, which is largely derived from sunshine, is instrumental in balancing the calcium and phosphorus ratio in the body. It is essential for bone and tooth formation.

16. **(A)** Disclosing agents stain invisible plaque and, consequently, let the patient visualize this material. Carious lesions, gingival recession, and calculus can be identified only through clinical examination.

17. **(D)** An interproximal brush is most effectively used when interdental spaces are sufficiently large. Dental floss is most effective in cases of tight contacts.

18. **(B)** The Bass technique is the most effective method of removing plaque from the sulcus because the bristles of the brush actually enter the sulcus. The Bass technique requires the bristles of a soft nylon brush to be placed at a 45-degree angle into the gingival sulcus. The brush is then rotated in small circular motions.

19. **(B)** The most common stain found on adult teeth is yellow stain. Yellow stain is an extrinsic stain that is caused by poor oral hygiene.

20. **(A)** The process of demineralization will occur with caries. When foods high in sucrose come in contact with bacterial plaque, they produce an acid that causes the tooth enamel to demineralize.

Sucrose + plaque = acid formation → dental decay (demineralization of enamel)

21. **(B)** Fluorapatite is formed when the fluoride ions combine with hydroxyapatite, resulting in stronger enamel that is less soluble to acid attacks. Fluoride ions are incorporated throughout the tooth calcification cycle if fluoride is administered systemically during that time period.

22. **(C)** Patient motivation is an important facet of the preventive dentistry philosophy. Patient education information should be presented in a manner that will stimulate the patient's specific dental health needs for best results and patient compliance.

23. **(A)** Good sources of protein include milk, meat, fish, and eggs. Proteins are made up of amino acids. There are about 20 amino acids that act as building blocks for proteins. Proteins are used by the body as building structures, enzymes, hormones, and a source of energy if needed.

24. **(C)** Supragingival calculus is found commonly on the lingual surfaces of the lower anterior teeth just above the gingival margin. The salivary gland located in the anterior part of the floor of the mouth contributes to the rapid formation of this hard deposit.

25. **(D)** Bacterial plaque forms daily. To avoid deleterious effects of plaque, it should be thoroughly removed every day.

26. **(A)** Stains that can be removed by coronal polishing procedures are classified as extrinsic stains. Extrinsic stains occur on the external surfaces of teeth. Common extrinsic stains are yellow stain caused by poor oral hygiene and food pigments, tobacco stain caused by byproducts of tar and tobacco, brown stain, and green stain, which occurs in children.

27. **(D)** Baking soda is not an essential daily nutrient. Key nutrients include water, lipids or fats, carbohydrates, proteins, minerals, and vitamins.

28. **(B)** Teeth most likely to benefit from the application of pit and fissure sealants include posterior teeth with deep pits and fissures. Posterior teeth with carious lesions and partially erupted teeth are contraindicated for sealants. Carious teeth must be restored with a permanent type of restoration, such as amalgam. Partially erupted teeth are not good candidates for sealants because the tooth surface has not fully developed. The importance of recalls and periodic examinations for sealant evaluations by the dentist must be emphasized to the patient.

29. **(C)** Teeth should be disclosed before and after coronal polishing. Disclosing agents may be used to identify the soft deposits before coronal polishing for the benefit of the operator and the patient to aid in patient education.

30. **(D)** Green stains on children's teeth are often the result of chromogenic bacteria. This is due to poor oral hygiene. It is an extrinsic stain and can be removed during oral prophylaxis.

31. **(B)** Before applying a topical fluoride gel, the auxiliary must dry the teeth thoroughly. Penetration of the fluoride ions is more effective when applied to a clean (plaque-free) dry tooth surface. Special attention to drying occlusal surfaces is recommended, since these areas are most susceptible to dental caries.

32. **(C)** Periodontal disease may cause gums to recede. Recession of the gingival tissue is due to the apical migration of the junctional epithelium along the tooth surface, leading to apparent exposure of the root surface.

33. **(B)** A deficiency of vitamin A affects structure and function of ameloblasts and causes faulty enamel formation. Vitamin A also affects vision, growth, keratinization, and resistance to infection.

34. **(A)** Vitamin K, found in green vegetables and egg yolks, is essential for formation of prothrombin, an agent necessary to promote proper blood clotting.

35. (C) Oral manifestations of riboflavin deficiency are cheilitis (lips become swollen and crack easily, especially at the corners of the mouth) and glossitis (tongue is red and swollen).

36. (A) The purpose of a low carbohydrate diet in the control of dental caries is to decrease the number of acid exposures per day for the dental patient. All carbohydrates are broken down to produce sugars, which interact with oral bacteria to form acids that can cause decay. Each acid exposure contributes to the demineralization process of enamel, leading to dental caries.

37. (B) Vitamin C has an important role in wound healing. Oral manifestations of a deficiency of vitamin C are poor wound healing, friable bleeding gingiva, and tooth mobility.

38. (C) The recommended daily servings for an adult are as follows. Fruit and vegetable group—4 servings, bread and cereal group—4 servings, meat group—2 servings, and milk group—2 servings. Balancing foods from the four basic food groups assists in fulfilling the minimum amount of nutrients required for maintaining a healthy body.

39. (D) Peanut butter has the highest nutrient value, and is a good source of protein. Nuts may be classified under the meat group and fulfill the daily food requirements for nutritional value from that food group.

40. (D) The patient must be motivated first in order to begin change. Old habits cannot be changed unless the individual recognizes an inner desire to change. Theories of motivation stress that a human being's basic primary needs must be met and satisfied before actual learning and motivation can begin.

41. (B) When using dental floss, the contact area is cleared by using a gentle back-and-forth seesaw motion.

42. (B) A dilute sodium hypochlorite solution, such as household bleach, is recommended for cleaning dentures. The technique is known as *immersion*. The solution is effective in removing light stains and dental plaque and serves as an antimicrobial agent for denture disinfection in the dental laboratory. Over-the-counter denture products, such as powders or tablets, also may be used. When cleaning partial dentures with metal framework, care must be taken to avoid tarnish or discoloration of the metals with certain immersion agents.

43. (B) Gingivitis is simply an inflammation of the gingiva that does not include involvement of underlying supporting structures.

44. (C) The best time to present oral hygiene instruction is when the patient is relaxed and receptive to the auxiliary's instructions. Giving oral hygiene instruction at the end of the appointment is not suggested, since the patient may be tired or numb and unable to feel the placement of the toothbrush bristles or the dental floss against the teeth and gingiva.

45. (A) Dental plaque is directly related to caries etiology and the initiation of periodontal disease.

46. (E)

47. (D)

48. (B)

49. (C)

50. (A)

51. (B) Materia alba is food debris that can be removed by irrigation. Materia alba is soft and white and has a texture similar to cottage cheese.

52. (D) When cleaning a removable partial denture, soaking in diluted bleach for 24 hours is not recommended because the solution may tarnish the metal framework and cause an unpleasant odor and surface pitting of the resin material.

53. (D) The interdental or interproximal brush often is recommended for patients who have limited access to the distal surfaces of wisdom teeth.

54. (A) The optimum amount of fluoride in drinking water is 1 ppm. Excessive amounts of fluoride (more than 2 ppm) may cause alteration in the calcification of enamel, resulting in a condition known as mottled enamel. The process of adding fluoride to the drinking water is called fluoridation.

55. (A) Fluoride compounds most commonly used for topical application include sodium fluoride, stannous fluoride, and acidulated phosphate fluoride gel.

56. (C) Plaque forms at the gingival margin and on the proximal surfaces of teeth because these areas are not as likely to be exposed to the self-cleansing process that occurs during normal mastication. Plaque is an invisible, soft, gelatinous mass of bacteria and pellicles adhering to tooth surfaces. Plaque is an organized bacterial mat. As plaque matures, there are alterations in the number and type of bacteria. If the bacterial mat is not disrupted, it will calcify and become calculus.

57. (E) Calculus is a hardened or calcified material that can be removed only through mechanical means.

Calculus has a rough and irregular texture that tends to harbor plaque easily, leading to further gingival irritation and destruction. Calculus may be found subgingivally and supragingivally depending on location and severity of gingival disease.

58. **(B)** Improper toothbrushing (ie, scrubbing the gingiva and tooth surfaces too hard) causes gingival recession and tooth abrasion.

59. **(C)** A dentifrice or toothpaste is an abrasive material that removes extrinsic stain. Dentifrices contain pleasant flavorings that result in a feeling of cleanliness when used.

60. **(D)** An acquired pellicle is the first step in plaque formation. Plaque requires 24 hours to mature, but a pellicle or film takes only minutes to form.

61. **(B)** Fluoride is used most effectively if ingested during the period of tooth development. Through a complex process, fluoride hardens the tooth matrix, making it more impervious to the decay process. The optimum ratio in municipal water supplies is 1 ppm.

62. **(D)** When handing out visual aid material, such as dental pamphlets, it is best to review the material with the patient before he or she leaves the dental office to make sure that the patient understands the material and to answer any questions the patient may have about the dental information.

63. **(B)** Subgingival calculus is darker and not as thick as supragingival calculus. Subgingival calculus is located below the gumline, and supragingival calculus is located above the gumline. The methods of attachment and formation are similar and begin with the maturation of bacterial plaque.

64. **(C)** Foods that contain high levels of sugars are most responsible for producing caries. Such foods as honey and syrups are especially harmful because they stick or cling to the tooth surface for long periods of time, causing acid exposures. Soft drinks and candy mints also are recognized as high caries producers due to their high sucrose content.

65. **(B)** Detergent foods include fresh fruits and vegetables. Their textures actually help perform a cleansing action during the mastication process.

66. **(E)** Recommended daily allowances of foods differ among patients on the basis of such factors as age, sex, body size, and pregnancy.

67. **(A)** Mouthrinses may be classified as therapeutic or cosmetic and are helpful in removing loose soft deposits, such as food debris and materia alba. A mouthrinse may be used in the dental office before a dental procedure to reduce aerosol contamination when working with the high-speed handpiece and refresh the mouth after a dental procedure. Mouthrinses with astringent properties are used before impressions to keep the mouth dry.

68. **(D)** All patients should be seen on a regular recall basis. Edentulous patients should be regularly recalled at least once a year to examine the soft tissues and occlusion and to repair dentures.

BIBLIOGRAPHY

Bernier JL, Muhler JC. *Improving Dental Practice Through Preventive Measures,* 3rd ed. St. Louis: CV Mosby Co, 1975.

Caldwell RC, Stallard RE. *A Textbook of Preventive Dentistry.* Philadelphia: WB Saunders Co, 1977.

Carlos JP. *Prevention and Oral Health.* Baltimore: DHEW Publication No. (NIH) 74-707, 1973.

Guthrie HA. *Introductory Nutrition,* 7th ed. St. Louis: CV Mosby Co, 1989.

Harris NO, Christen AG. *Primary Preventive Dentistry,* 3rd ed. Norwalk, Conn: Appleton & Lange, 1990.

Hefferson JJ, Ayer WA, Koehler HM, eds. *Foods, Nutrition and Dental Health.* South, Ill: Pathodox Publishers, 1980.

Newman HN. *Dental Plaque.* Springfield, Ill: Charles C Thomas Publishers, 1980.

Randolph PM, Dennison CI. *Diet, Nutrition, and Dentistry.* St. Louis: CV Mosby Co, 1981.

Section on Instructional System Design, Department of Pediodontology, School of Dentistry, University of California, San Francisco. *Developing a Plaque Control Program,* Berkley, Calif: Praxis Publishing Co, 1972.

Section on Instructional System Design, Department of Pediodontology, School of Dentistry, University of California, San Francisco. *Plaque Control Instruction.* Berkley, Calif: Praxis Publishing Co, 1978.

Silverstone LH. *Preventive Dentistry.* Fort Lee, NJ: Update Publishing International Inc, 1978.

Torres H, Ehrlich A. *Modern Dental Assisting,* 4th ed. Philadelphia: WB Saunders Co, 1990.

CHAPTER 4

Biomedical Sciences

INTRODUCTION

The dental auxiliary plays an integral role within the dental environment by implementing appropriate measures for effective infection control. A basic understanding of the biomedical sciences is necessary to facilitate the prevention of disease transmission. This chapter presents a synopsis of microbiology, oral pathology, and pharmacology. Each of the sciences play an important role in the critical cycle of infection control and in the recognition of normal and abnormal conditions of the oral cavity.

MICROBIOLOGY

The oral cavity harbors numerous types of microorganisms that can be transmitted easily during routine dental procedures. The importance of recognizing potential dangers form pathogenic microorganisms is the responsibility of all dental staff.

Microbiology is the study of biologic microorganisms seen only with the aid of a microscope. These organisms are either single celled or multicelled, some beneficial and others potential pathogens to humans. The three major classifications of microorganisms are viruses, fungi, and bacteria.

Viruses are the smallest infectious agents, containing a strand molecule of nucleic acid encased in a protein shell. Viruses are parasites that replicate only in living cells. There are animal viruses, plant viruses, and bacterial viruses, known as bacteriophages. Examples of pathologic conditions caused by viruses include herpes simplex, influenza, infectious hepatitis, serum hepatitis, HIV, rabies, and poliomyelitis. Antibiotic drug therapy usually is ineffective for the treatment of viral infections.

Fungi include yeasts and molds. They are widely distributed microorganisms that grow as a mass of branching, interlacing filaments containing nuclei and organelles. A common intraoral disease caused by fungi is candidiasis or thrush. Antifungicide drugs, such as nystatin, effectively fight some fungal infections.

Bacteria are microorganisms that appear in three basic shapes: rodlike, spherical, and spiral. Rod-shaped bacteria are called bacilli, spherical bacteria are called cocci, and spiral bacteria are called spirilla. Bacteria have nuclei and are enclosed in cell walls. They have the ability to replicate themselves, and some are motile. Common pathologic conditions caused by bacteria are dental caries, periodontal disease, pneumonia, and rheumatic fever. Antibiotic drug therapy generally is used to fight systemic bacterial infections.

Normal microbial constituents of the mouth include fungi, such as *Candida albicans*, and bacteria, such as *Streptococcus mutans* and *Staphylococcus*. These microorganisms are not harmful in normal amounts. It is only when they proliferate and disrupt homeostasis that pathologic conditions occur.

Immunity

Infection is the process during which a microorganism enters into a relationship with the host, establishes itself, and multiplies within the host. The tissue environment controls susceptibility or resistance to given microorganisms. If the host lacks sufficient resistance, infection occurs.

Immunity is the property of a host to resist specific infections. *Acquired immunity* can be produced by an injection of antibodies of one person into another or by the formation of antibodies in a person as a result of previous exposure to a microorganism. Measles and poliovirus immunizations are examples of injected immunity. An acquired immunity to mumps or another disease results from a previous episode of the disease. The host may be born with natural antibodies against specific microorganisms, which is termed *natural immunity*.

Modes of Disease Transmission

Infectious microorganisms may be transferred in various ways, including, direct contact, indirect contact, inhalation (aerosol droplets), contaminated food or water, and through cuts or breaks in the skin from an infectious vehicle source. The highest risk of infection transmission in the dental office is from the dental patient. Through direct contact with the dental patient during routine dental procedures, the dental team may be exposed to a variety of microorganisms from the patient's saliva, blood, and aerosol droplets inhaled at close proximity during treatment. Accidental needlesticks, sharp instrument injuries, or spatters of blood and saliva on the skin or in the eye are examples of how a contaminated vehicle can be a source of infectious disease transmission.

Cross-contamination can occur if inappropriate methods of sterilization, disinfection, and waste disposal are not practiced by all staff members. The spread of infectious microorganisms via the indirect contact mode of transmission occurs when dental staff touch other inanimate objects with soiled gloves or hands or by way of another contaminated vehicle. Common examples of objects frequently touched in the dental operatory include dental unit light switch, operator's chair, operatory telephone, dental x-rays, dental charts, pens, and pencils. Each of these objects is a potential source of cross-contamination and serves to transmit infectious microorganisms to other dental staff members or to other patients if inappropriate sterilization, disinfection, or waste disposal methods are not practiced.

Protective Barrier Techniques

In order to reduce the risk of infectious disease transmission in the dental environment, protective barrier techniques must be used by all staff members during patient treatment (Fig. 4-1).

Protective barrier techniques include the use of a disposable face mask, protective eyewear or face shield, and disposable gloves. Face masks should be changed for each patient and replaced if they become wet or soiled. Before placing gloves, the auxiliary should secure the surgical mask in place. The face mask should cover the

nose and mouth and protect against inhalation of pathogens during patient treatment.

Protective eyewear with sideguards should be wide enough to protect the eye, easily disinfected, and worn at all times during clinical procedures to protect eyes from flying debris and contamination. Protective face shields should be used during clinical procedures that produce aerosol sprays. Use of the high-speed handpiece and ultrasonic scaling procedures produce aerosol sprays and release potential pathogenic microorganisms that can be inhaled.

Protective barriers for the hands include gloves and proper handwashing techniques. Before placing gloves, hands should be scrubbed thoroughly with a liquid soap. All jewelry should be removed, since microorganisms may harbor under rings and watches. A nailbrush should be used to clean under fingernails. Surgical procedures require the use of a standard surgical scrub that is performed in a sequential order. Initial surgical hand scrubs take anywhere from 5 to 10 minutes. Hands, wrists, and arms up to the elbow are scrubbed with overlapping circular strokes and sufficient soap lather. A sterile towel is used to dry the hands before gloving.

Gloves must be worn by all staff members performing clinical patient care. The gloves serve as protective barriers for the dental staff and reduce the potential of cross-contamination in the dental office. Gloves that are torn or punctured should be discarded and replaced with a new pair of gloves. Gloves must be changed between patients whether worn for treatment or for examination. Sterile

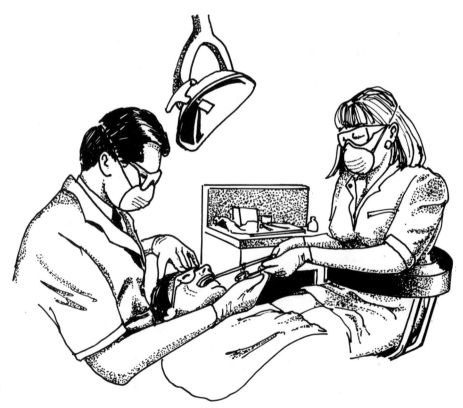

Figure 4-1. Protective barrier techniques reduce the risk of disease transmission.

surgical gloves are recommended for oral surgery and surgical periodontal procedures. Before removing gloves, rinse the gloved hands with soap and water to prevent transmission of infections microorganisms to the hands during removal of the soiled gloves. Always wash the hands thoroughly after removal of gloves.

Sterilization and Disinfection

Asepsis is the term used to describe freedom from pathologic microorganisms (pathogens). Conversely, sepsis refers to the existence of disease-producing organisms. Sterilization and disinfection are methods used, respectively, to destroy pathologic microorganisms completely or partially. Sterilization destroys all forms of life, including bacterial spores and viruses by chemical or physical agents. All instruments that will penetrate tissue or will come in contact with the mucosa and skin should be appropriately sterilized. Disinfection destroys most microorganisms by either physical or chemical agents. A disinfectant is used on environmental surfaces (counter tops) and other inanimate fixtures, such as the dental unit and dental chair. High level disinfectants are recommended for items that are used intraorally and cannot be sterilized by other approved methods.

Recognized methods of sterilization include dry heat, steam autoclave (moist heat), chemical vapor under pressure, immersion in a high level disinfectant, and ethylene oxide.

Dry heat ovens use heat alone to sterilize instruments and material. Sterilization cycles may last from 1 to 2 hours. The dry heat method of sterilization is effective for instruments that tend to rust or dull easily under other approved methods of sterilization.

Steam autoclaves (moist heat) use high temperatures to achieve sufficient pressure that will generate steam. The steam under pressure method of autoclaving is preferred by most dental offices because of the shorter sterilization time cycles and the autoclave's effectiveness in destroying infectious microorganisms, including spores and viruses.

Chemical vapor sterilizers use such agents as formaldehyde, alcohol mixtures, water and acetone, or other related chemicals. Under heat, the sterilizer creates sufficient pressure to generate a gas that is an effective, recognized method of sterilization. The use of chemical vapor sterilizers requires adequate ventilation because of the release of potentially harmful vapors.

Immersion methods of chemical sterilization are used when other approved methods of heat sterilization cannot be applied. Dental instruments or materials that have been contaminated by the penetration of soft tissues or come in contact with the skin must be immersed for long exposure time cycles of up to 10 hours. Only products approved and registered by the Environmental Protection Agency (EPA) can be effectively used.

Ethylene oxide sterilization methods involve the use of special gas sterilizers. Large health clinics and institutions commonly use this form of sterilization. Ethylene oxide is an effective method of sterilization for most dental materials, such as plastic, cloth, and nitrous oxide armamentarium, including rubber hoses and nondisposable rubber masks. The sterilization time cycle is long, averaging a minimum of 12 hours, with an adequate aeration time period following removal from the sterilizer. Appropriate ventilation is required when working with the ethylene oxide gas sterilizer.

Asepsis must be adhered to after appropriate sterilization methods have been employed to prevent contamination of the sterile armamentarium and maintain the chain of sterility.

Recognized methods of disinfection include the use of EPA and ADA-approved chemical disinfectants. Only broad-spectrum antimicrobial disinfectant products should be used. Chemical agents commonly employed in the dental office include glutaraldehyde, sodium hypochlorite, iodophors, and synthetic phenol compounds. Manufacturer's directions should be followed for

1. Appropriate dilutions of concentrated agents for environmental surface disinfection and instrument immersion
2. Preparation of instruments before immersion for sterilization
3. Proper exposure time for effective sterilization
4. Storage and handling specifications
5. Contraindications to certain metals and vinyl materials
6. Expiration dates

Adequate ventilation is required with the use of the disinfectant chemical agents because of possible eye irritation and toxicity from inhaled fumes. Chemical disinfection agents may be used in the dental laboratory to disinfect contaminated impressions, dental prosthesis, and wax bites.

Pre-treatment Infection Control

Prepare the operatory by using approved surface disinfectants on all environmental surfaces and inanimate objects. Allow adequate time for surface disinfectants to dry, then prepare the dental unit and chair with appropriate disposable barriers. Place plastic or foil covers on light handles and triplex syringe. Cover bracket table. Preset trays with bagged sterile instruments can be arranged in the operatory but left unopened until ready for use.

During the dental procedure, a separate disposable bag should be used to dispose of contaminated soiled materials, such as bloody gauze or cotton rolls. A clean disposable bag for each patient should be attached close to the working area before treatment.

Post-treatment Infection Control

The auxiliary is required to use appropriate protective barrier techniques during cleanup procedures. Heavy duty utility gloves are used when wiping down contaminated environmental surfaces and when scrubbing soiled instruments.

All contaminated waste is to be discarded in a separate plastic bag indicated for that purpose. Disposable needles and other sharp disposable items, such as scalpel blades, must be disposed of in an impermeable container indicated for that specific purpose only. The auxiliary must take special precautions when handling sharp instruments for disposal to avoid accidental injuries with the infectious waste.

Soiled instrument trays are taken to the sterilization area for decontamination and preparation. Scrub instruments or place in holding solutions until ready to be scrubbed. An ultrasonic cleaner may be used to effectively remove debris from the instruments and minimize the potential of accidental injury from a contaminated instrument during hand scrubbing cleanup procedures.

Rinse and dry instruments before sterilization. Instruments may be wrapped or unwrapped for sterilization. If wrapping instruments in cloth, paper, or plastic, the material must be porous to allow penetration of the steam autoclave. Indicator tapes are recommended for sealing the wrapped instrument kits to allow the operator to assess the effectiveness of the sterilization cycle. Indicator tapes change in color if adequate contact time has been established and the proper temperature was reached. Indicator tapes also may be placed inside the instrument bag. Sterilization methods should be monitored closely on a weekly basis to ensure the effectiveness of the sterilization equipment, and periodic spore test or chemical monitor testing should be performed.

After sterilization, asepsis must be maintained, or instruments and materials will again become contaminated. Instruments should be removed from the sterilizing unit with sterile tongs and should be stored in areas that will maintain sterility.

ORAL PATHOLOGY

Oral pathology is a recognized dental specialty concerned with the disease processes of the oral cavity. A wide range of pathologic conditions may affect the oral and maxillofacial structures. These oral manifestations may appear as a variety of surface lesions and can occur on hard or soft tissues of the oral cavity and surrounding extraoral structures of the head and neck. Oral diseases often occur due to developmental disturbances, such as cleft lip or palate abnormalities. Other oral pathologic conditions can be caused by infectious diseases, nutritional deficiencies, systemic body dysfunctions, and abnormal growths that are cancer related. Oral diseases may appear as ulcerated lesions, cysts, vesicles, or tumors and are classified according to color, size, texture, and location.

The dental auxiliary's role includes collection and recording of clinical data, which may include a description of any abnormal findings in the head and neck region. A basic knowledge of pathology is necessary to differentiate between normal oral structures and abnormal findings in the oral cavity. Recognition of abnormal conditions in the oral cavity is vitally important for the auxiliary in order to protect oneself from infectious diseases that may be transmitted during routine dental procedures. Strict ad-

herence to proper barrier techniques, including gloves, masks, and eyewear, is indicated whenever direct patient contact is made in the oral cavity.

Pathology Tests

Specific pathology tests are performed by the doctor to distinguish benign (nonmalignant) lesions from malignant lesions. These tests may include a biopsy, which requires a minor surgical procedure to remove a small specimen of the abnormal tissue for further diagnosis. Exfoliative cytology is a nonsurgical procedure that is performed by scraping the surface of the lesion with a moistened wooden tongue blade and transferring the specimen to a prepared slide for further definitive study under the microscope (Fig. 4–2). Both tests require the expertise of the oral pathologist for final diagnosis and appropriate treatment. All laboratory reports from the oral pathologist documenting the diagnosis of the oral lesion become part of the patient's permanent dental record.

DISEASES OF THE PERIODONTIUM

Gingivitis and Periodontitis

Periodontal disease, or pyorrhea, is one of the most widespread of all oral diseases. The most common periodontal disease is gingivitis, which is an inflammation of the gingiva, believed to be caused by products of microorganisms in plaque. Gingivitis is characterized by red, edematous, tender gingiva that may bleed easily. Gingivitis can be localized, involving only a small area, or generalized, involving the entire mouth. It can be acute or chronic. This disease is prevented by eliminating plaque through daily brushing and flossing.

When periodontal disease affects the alveolar bone, it is called periodontitis. It is usually painless and can result from untreated chronic gingivitis. Periodontitis may be characterized by inflamed gingival tissues that bleed easily, periodontal pocket formation, loss of alveolar bone, furcation involvement in multirooted teeth, gingival recession, and tooth mobility (Fig. 4–3). Advanced cases of periodontal disease may reveal abscess formation and exudate on gentle probing. Treatment of periodontal disease involves scaling and root planing and surgical procedures.

Acute Necrotizing Ulcerative Gingivitis

Acute necrotizing ulcerative gingivitis (ANUG), also known as trench mouth or Vincent's infection, is characterized by ulcerations on the gingiva and a gray pseudomembrane. The diseased tissue may be localized or generalized. The characteristics of ANUG are pain, acute inflammation, bleeding, and sloughing of tissue between the teeth. In some patients, temperature is elevated and regional lymphadenopathy is present. The precise etiology of ANUG is unclear, but it appears to be related to physical and mental stress, smoking, and inadequate oral hygiene, which lowers overall resistance to bacterial infections. This disease is treated by thoroughly scaling and rootplaning the affected gingival area and instructing the patient in proper oral hygiene home care.

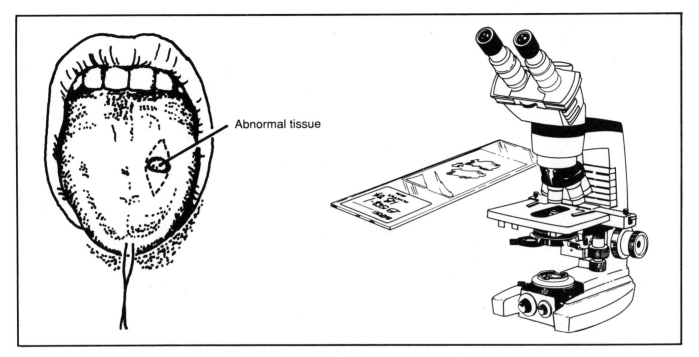

Figure 4–2. Biopsy techniques.

Pregnancy Gingivitis

Pregnancy gingivitis is characterized by enlarged swollen gingival tissues that bleed easily. The condition is exaggerated by local irritants, such as plaque and calculus. The hormonal changes taking place within the body also are contributing factors to the gingival enlargement. Small benign growths, known as pregnancy tumors or pyogenic granulomas, can occur on the gingival tissues. The most frequent site of occurrence is the anterior incisor area of the oral cavity. Pregnancy gingivitis is treated by removing the local irritants through scaling and good oral hygiene. Most gingival tissues return to normal after delivery, but if there is no resolution, an excisional biopsy may be necessary.

DENTAL CARIES

Dental caries is a disease involving the hard structures of the teeth. Dental caries is responsible for the destruction and demineralization process that affects the enamel, dentin, and cementum. All age groups are susceptible hosts to dental decay.

There are several theories about the etiology of caries. A popular theory is called the acidogenic theory. It suggests that caries is the result of the activity of acid-producing bacteria. The process occurs as follows. Easily broken down carbohydrates adhere to teeth along with acid-producing bacteria in the form of plaque. The microorganisms cause the breakdown of the carbohydrates, re-

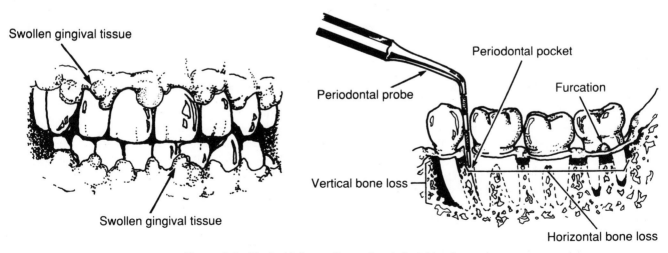

Figure 4–3. Gingival inflammation and periodontal involvement.

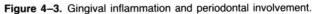

sulting in the production of acids. When acidity in a given area exceeds a certain level, the inorganic tooth matrix is demineralized, and the organic matrix is destroyed.

A major cause of caries appears to be the refined foods present in daily diets. Refined softened foods tend to be cariogenic. Other contributing factors to host resistance include tooth shape, position, and composition, as well as the chemical composition of the saliva. Saliva is a complex fluid, the composition of which varies widely from person to person. Even within the same person, daily fluctuation is great. The pH level (ie, acidity) and the amount of saliva production also are important factors. A decreasing pH level below 7 or amount of saliva or both are associated with a tendency toward increased caries.

Treatment of caries is mechanical removal of the diseased tissue and appropriate restoration. If caries are left untreated, it will dissolve the hard enamel and subsequently affect the softer dentin of the tooth. Here, the caries spreads more quickly because the dentin has a higher organic content, which is easier to attack. Left unchecked, the process continues until the pulp is affected.

DISEASES OF THE PULP

The dental pulp is a highly vascular structure, the primary function of which is the development of dentin during formation. Once matured, the pulp serves as a thermal sensor, a pain receptor and transmitter, and a supplier of nutrients. There are several causes of pulpal disease, including untreated decay, trauma, dental iatrogenic treatment, and exposure to chemical irritants. Pulpal diseases include pulpitis, pulpstones or denticles, and hyperemia. Pulpal infections also may include periapical abscesses.

DEVELOPMENTAL PATHOLOGIC CONDITIONS

In addition to those diseases that affect healthy tooth structure, there are a number of developmental anomalies. *Anodontia*, lack of development of teeth, can be either partial or complete. A person also can develop an excess number of teeth, which are called *supernumerary teeth*. Teeth that are too small (*microdontia*) or too large (*macrodontia*) can develop. Additional disturbances that affect the shape of teeth include gemination, fusion, concrescence, and dilaceration. *Gemination* occurs during the attempted division of the tooth bud. Instead of the formation of one complete tooth, two incomplete teeth develop. *Fusion* occurs when two teeth partially or completely join or fuse, resulting in a single large tooth. If this process occurs after root formation and the cementum of two teeth is joined, it is termed *concrescence*. *Dilaceration* refers to the formation of roots with sharp bends or angles. *Amelogenesis imperfecta* refers to anomalies that occur during the formation of enamel, and correspondingly, *dentinogenesis imperfecta* refers to disturbances occurring during the formation of dentin.

The most common developmental pathologic state affecting the lips or palate or both is a cleft, which appears as a result of lack of fusion. This condition occurs in approximately 1 in 800 births. If a cleft significantly interferes with the function of the oral or nasal cavity, surgical correction might be necessary.

LESIONS OF THE TONGUE

The tongue also is affected by developmental pathologic conditions, including cleft tongue, fissure tongue, geographic tongue, and hairy tongue. A *cleft tongue* results when fusion of the two halves of the tongue is incomplete. When an abnormal number of grooves or fissures appears on the dorsal side of the tongue, it is called *fissured tongue*. Benign migratory glossitis occurs when papillae on the tongue lose their surface epithelium. This also is known as *geographic tongue* because it may appear on different parts of the tongue at different times. A *hairy tongue* is characterized by an overgrowth (hypertrophy) of the filiform papillae. The tongue appears matted and may discolor, having a yellow, brown, or possibly black cast. Most of the developmental anomalies of the tongue are not clinically significant and are left untreated.

Nutritional disorders also may affect the tongue. Deficiency of vitamin B often results in a condition known as *pellagra*, where the tongue appears a bright scarlet red color, and there is a burning sensation. *Glossitis* is an inflammatory condition of the tongue with varied clinical changes in color and texture.

COMMON ORAL PATHOLOGIC CONDITIONS

Fordyce granules are a developmental anomaly characterized by elevated sebaceous glands that appear in various sites in the oral cavity. They are small, multiple, yellowish spots, usually found on the buccal mucosa. Treatment is not necessary, since the granules are not pathologically significant.

Tori are bony protrusions appearing on the palate or mandible. They grow slowly and have no clinical significance unless they interfere with the placement of an oral prosthesis. If there is interference, tori are surgically removed. *Torus palatinus* most frequently occurs along the midline of the palate, and *torus mandibularis* occurs along the lingual aspect of the mandible in the cuspid and premolar regions.

Abrasion is the pathologic wearing away of tooth structure. This condition usually occurs in the cervical area of a single tooth or of several teeth. Abrasion occurs from excessive or improper toothbrushing or from the use of abrasive toothpastes. This condition is irreversible. Further damage can be prevented through patient education.

Attrition is the normal wearing away of the functional biting surfaces of the teeth by mastication. This normal process of tooth wear may be excessive because of particular personal habits, such as bruxism and the consumption of gritty foods. *Bruxism* is the unconscious grinding or clenching of teeth during sleep, often referred to as night grinding. Severe cases of bruxism can contribute to temporomandibular joint difficulties.

Erosion is the loss of tooth structure through a chemical process. This pathologic condition usually occurs on labial or buccal surfaces of teeth and can be related to the degree of acidity of saliva. Teeth may become hypersensitive. Clinical signs of erosion may be associated with nutritional and eating disorders, such as anorexia nervosa and bulimia. Stomach acids from repeated vomiting affect the enamel of the teeth, causing a decalcification effect similar to caries formation.

AUTOIMMUNE DISORDERS

Recurrent aphthous ulcers are referred to commonly as canker sores. In their early stages, aphthous ulcers are extremely painful and uncomfortable. Clinically, the lesions look like small ulcers and may occur anywhere in the oral cavity (eg, mucous membrane of lip, cheek, tongue, and floor of the mouth). They are sometimes associated with trauma or irritation, as from an ill-fitting appliance or denture. The exact etiology is unknown, although recurrent episodes of aphthous ulcers may be indicative of an altered autoimmune response of the oral epithelium or physical trauma.

LESIONS ASSOCIATED WITH INFECTIOUS DISEASES

Herpes simplex, commonly known as herpes or simply as cold sores, is a contagious viral infection characterized by blisterlike lesions that usually appear on the lips, but they are found intraorally as well. Herpes is associated with severe sunburn, trauma, emotional stress, fever, and allergy. The disease is usually left untreated and runs its course in 7 to 14 days.

Varicella, commonly known as chickenpox, is a disease of viral origin in which fluid-filled lesions appear on the body. Occasionally, these small lesions occur intraorally.

Mumps, or parotitis, involves unilateral or bilateral swelling of the parotid and other salivary glands. Mumps is contagious and is found usually in children, although adults have been reported to contract the disease.

Moniliasis, also called candidiasis or thrush, is an infection caused by the fungus, *Candida albicans.* It is characterized by an elevated soft white plaque on the tongue or other oral tissues. Thrush appears in infants and debilitated persons. It has become more common in adults as a side effect of antibiotic medication, which tends to decrease other flora normally found in the oral cavity, allowing the fungal infection to dominate. Candidiasis frequently is associated with patients who have HIV infection. The lesions commonly occur on the palate and buccal mucosa and dorsal surface of the tongue. The

appearance is white to yellow and is curdlike in texture which when scraped off leaves a raw, bleeding area. Treatment may include application of an antifungal agent.

Acquired immunodeficiency syndrome (AIDS) is an infectious disease that attacks the human immune system. Patients who have been infected with the human immunodeficiency virus (HIV), which causes AIDS, are susceptible to various types of oral lesions and other opportunistic infections. Oral lesions frequently associated with AIDS include candidiasis, ANUG, hairy leukoplakia of the tongue, herpes simplex, and Kaposi's sarcoma.

Syphilis is a highly contagious disease, usually transmitted through sexual contact. However, the disease can be contracted through direct contact with the oral cavity of a person who is in an infectious stage. During the primary stage, chancres appear primarily on the genitalia but also can arise on the soft tissues of the oral cavity. During the secondary stage, highly infectious oral lesions called mucous patches appear on the tongue, gingiva, or buccal mucosa. Tertiary syphilis is characterized by centrally necrotized oral lesions called gumma.

TUMORS OF THE ORAL CAVITY

Tumors are areas of swollen tissue often found in the oral cavity. It should be noted that the word tumor does not imply a cancerous or carcinogenic lesion.

Benign Tumors

Papillomas are benign outward growths of surface epithelium commonly found on tongue, lips, buccal mucosa, gingiva, and palate. Papillomas are surgically removed only if they become uncomfortable to the patient or if they appear in areas that are easily traumatized.

Pigmented nevi, or moles, occur most commonly on the skin, but they also are seen in the oral cavity. Moles are congenital anomalies characterized by brown pigmentation. Removal is recommended if they appear in easily irritated areas or if an observable change in color, size, or shape occurs.

A *fibroma,* or epulis, is an overgrowth of connective tissue that can result from infection or irritation. Fibromas grow slowly and are characterized by a change in color. They can occur anywhere in the oral cavity and usually are surgically removed.

Hemangiomas are tumors characterized by a proliferation of blood vessels. They vary widely in size and appear red or blue in color. Hemangiomas usually occur on the skin, lips, or buccal mucosa. They are clinically significant because they can hemorrhage if punctured.

Pyogenic granulomas are inflammatory overgrowths of unknown etiology. They frequently are seen on the gingiva and appear deep red or purple in color. They grow quickly and then remain static. Although painless, most are surgically removed. Tumors that are similar in composition often appear during the third month of pregnancy.

Leukoplakia appears as white patches or plaque occurring on mucosal surfaces. Unless infected, it is usually painless. The cause of leukoplakia is unclear, but factors related to its development appear to include tobacco, alcohol, irritations, vitamin deficiencies, and hormonal imbalances. Early diagnosis and histologic examination are important because leukoplakia can precede a malignant condition in 10% of cases. Treatment includes elimination of the irritating factors and surgical removal.

Malignant Tumors

Basal cell carcinoma occurs on exposed areas of the face and scalp, usually superior to the lower lip. Characterized by small elevated areas that become ulcerated, it is more prevalent in fair-skinned people. The most likely cause of basal cell carcinoma is overexposure to the sun. This tumor grows slowly and usually does not metastasize (spread). Treatment is surgical removal, with histologic examination of the removed tissue. Prognosis for patients treated for this condition is usually good because of the lack of metastasis.

Epidermoid or *squamous cell carcinoma* is the most common form of cancer of the oral cavity. It can occur anywhere in the oral cavity and can have a different appearance in different areas. Possible causes of this disease include smoking, alcohol, nutritional deficiencies, syphilis, exposure to the sun, and viruses. Treatment for epidermoid or squamous cell carcinoma includes surgical removal, radiation therapy, and chemotherapy. Treatment may include any of the proposed modalities either alone or in any combination.

Melanomas are often fatal neoplasms that usually occur on the skin and oral mucosa. Their appearance is similar to that of pigmented nevi, or moles, except that they have irregular borders and may have a history of rapid growth. Melanomas are uncommon and appear to be caused by trauma or irritation. Treatment is usually radical surgical removal followed by radiation, chemotherapy or both.

PHARMACOLOGY

Pharmacology is the scientific body of knowledge concerned with the properties of drugs and the interactions of chemical compounds within living systems. Drugs are classified as either proprietary (brand name), which are protected by a trademark, or generic (nonbrand), which reflects the products' chemical composition.

Drugs can be used as a means of sustaining and maintaining health. Examples of commonly used drugs in dentistry include antibiotics, sedatives, and analgesics. Antibiotics aid in the defense mechanisms of the body by inhibiting growth or destroying invading bacteria. Sedatives and hypnotics are examples of central nervous system depressants that can be useful by producing a calming effect for anxious dental patients. Pain-relieving drugs, such as nonnarcotic analgesics, assist in alleviating mild to moderate pain after dental procedures. Aspirin is an especially useful analgesic because it exhibits properties that are antipyretic (fever reducing) and anti-inflammatory.

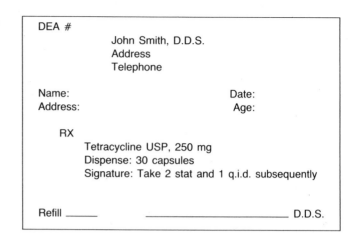

Figure 4–4. Sample prescription order.

The interaction of one drug with another might result in a deleterious effect on the patient. It is particularly important for an auxiliary who has taken a medical history to alert the doctor if the patient is currently taking medication in order to prevent future problems with additionally prescribed medications. For example, aspirin should not be prescribed for a patient taking an anticoagulant drug because these two drugs enhance each other's effect, and the patient could develop difficulties controlling bleeding as a result.

Prescription Writing

A prescription is a written order to a pharmacist directing him or her to dispense a certain drug with specific instructions to a patient. The dentist is the only member of the oral health care delivery team who is legally allowed to prescribe drugs.

A prescription contains the doctor's name, address, telephone number, and Drug Enforcement Agency (DEA) number. The patient's name, address, age, and the date of the prescription also are listed in the heading portion of the prescription order. The body of the prescription includes the superscription, or Rx symbol, which is an abbreviation literally meaning "take thou." The body of the prescription also contains the name of the drug to be dispensed, the strength, and the amount. Directions for the patient regarding information on how to take the drug are listed in the body of the prescription. At the bottom of the prescription order is information indicating whether a substitution for a generic brand drug is permissible. Refill information also is listed on the prescription form. The prescription must include the doctor's written signature. All prescriptions must be written in ink, and a duplicate copy or written documentation of the prescription must be recorded in the patient's dental chart for legal purposes. Figure 4–4 shows a sample prescription.

A number of abbreviated Latin words and phrases are used when writing prescriptions. Commonly used Latin terms and abbreviations follow.

ac	before meals
bid	twice a day
c	with
disp	dispense
h	hour
pc	after meals
prn	as needed
qid	four times daily
tid	three times daily
stat	immediately
per os	by mouth

Methods of Administration

Drugs are administered in a variety of ways, including topically (on the surface), orally, sublingually (under the tongue), rectally, by inhalation, and by injection. Injections can be given intravenously (into a vein), intramuscularly (into a muscle), intradermally (just breaking the skin surface), and subcutaneously (somewhat deeper than intradermally, into subcutaneous tissue). Parenteral administration refers to the introduction of medication in locations of the body other than the gastrointestinal tract.

Drugs most commonly are administered orally because of the relative ease of administration and low cost. A major disadvantage of drugs given orally, however, is that their potency can be diminished or eliminated by interaction with stomach enzymes, such as insulin. Sublingual administration produces rapid onset through the rich vascular network located beneath the tongue. Rectal administration of drugs is advantageous for patients with stomach disorders or for those who are unable to take a drug orally. Drugs administered by inhalation have a very quick onset. Parenteral administration has an almost immediate onset, but it can be extremely dangerous if the drug is toxic to a given patient.

Proper Handling of Drugs in the Dental Office

Ordering and Inventory. Careful records must be kept of all prescription drugs ordered for the dental office. This responsibility often is delegated to the dental auxiliary. Accurate inventory is required on a periodic basis to monitor and control the potential abuse of prescription drugs. All narcotic drugs ordered for the dental office must be ordered through the Bureau of Narcotics on special duplicate supply order forms. Narcotic drugs must be stored in a locked cabinet. When a narcotic drug is dispensed to a patient, the exact amount, date, and name of the patient must be recorded in the drug log book. Each entry must be initialed by the auxiliary. This information must be documented also in the patient's dental chart.

Storage. Drugs should be stored according to the manufacturer's directions. Certain drugs, such as nitroglycerin, often stored in the office emergency kit must be monitored and replaced every 6 months, since they have a short shelf-life. Other drugs and medications must be kept out of direct sunlight and extreme temperature changes.

Overexposure to air may cause a change in the consistency of the drug, consequently affecting the potency of the medication. Prevention of moisture contamination also must be considered. All caps or lids must be tightly applied, and well-fitted stoppers must be secured in bottled medications. Drugs that show changes in color or consistency and have reached their expiration dates must be discarded. All narcotic drugs that are discarded must be recorded on the drug log sheet. For security purposes, this procedure should be witnessed by two staff members and the doctor.

Telephone Procedures. Prescription drugs often are requested by patients over the telephone. The dental assistant is not authorized by law to phone in a prescription for a patient. Inquiries related to prescriptions, such as dosage and refill questions, often are phoned into the dental office directly from the pharmacy. In these special cases, the dental assistant may provide this information to the pharmacist under direct verbal instruction from the dentist. Prescription refills conducted by phone must be followed up by careful and complete documentation in the patient's dental record.

Categories of Medications

Analgesics (nonnarcotic) are administered to relieve mild to moderate pain. Mild analgesics include aspirin, acetaminophen (Tylenol), and propoxyphene hydrochloride (Darvon). Aspirin, in addition to being an analgesic, has antipyretic (fever-reducing) and anti-inflammatory properties.

More potent analgesics are available only by prescription and include codeine, opiate, and synthetic opiate compounds. These drugs are sometimes prescribed for patients who have experienced painful procedures, such as extractions or complicated surgical procedures.

Local anesthesia, administered by injection, causes a short-term reversible loss of sensation in a specific area of the body. Common local anesthetics include procaine (Novocain), lidocaine (Xylocaine), and mepivacaine (Carbocaine). Some local anesthetics contain vasoconstrictors, such as epinephrine, that prevent systemic absorption, thereby making the anesthetic longer acting in the specific area. Epinephrine, which dilates bronchial muscles and increases activity of the heart, is administered to patients who show evidence of severe allergic reaction or anaphylactic shock.

Anesthetics are either general or local. General anesthetics induce sleep, eliminate noxious reflexes, and relax muscles. General anesthetics are administered intravenously or by inhalation methods. Intravenous drugs used for surgical procedures include methohexital sodium (Brevital) and thiopental sodium (Pentothal). Inhalation agents used for general anesthesia may include Halothane, and Enflurane. A thorough explanation of preoperative instructions is required for dental patients undergoing general anesthesia. Postoperative responsibilities include close monitoring of vital signs and an adequate recovery period, with close supervision of the patient by the dental auxiliary.

Analgesia is the first stage of anesthesia, during which a patient remains conscious, has an increased threshold for pain, and might experience some amnesia. Drugs commonly used for intravenous conscious sedation include diazepam (Valium) and meperidine hydrochloride (Demerol). Nitrous oxide and oxygen analgesia are administered by inhalation methods and are used commonly for various types of dental procedures.

Nitrous oxide may be used in conjunction with intravenous sedation and is beneficial for patients who are anxious or apprehensive. Hypertensive and cardiac patients may also benefit from nitrous oxide administration because it reduces stress and produces a higher concentration of oxygen.

Precautions and contraindications must be considered when administering any type of drug. Avoidance of prolonged nitrous oxide administration or high intake of the gas will reduce the potential of nausea and dizziness. Contraindications for nitrous oxide administration include nasal obstructions, pregnancy, and patients who will have difficulty communicating their reflex and mood changes during the induction phase of nitrous oxide administration.

Nitrous oxide is effective primarily through the replacement of nitrogen in the bloodstream and must be administered with oxygen. Effective sedation may be reached with concentrations of nitrous oxide as low as 15% or as high as 50% depending on the patient and type of dental procedure performed. Nitrous oxide is a sweet-smelling gas that is nonflammable.

Antibiotics are organic substances that destroy or inhibit the growth of bacteria. These drugs are used to prevent or alleviate bacterial infections and prophylactically prevent them. Penicillin is a bactericidal antibiotic that kills a wide range of microorganisms. It is currently the most frequently prescribed antibiotic in dentistry for use in both local and systemic infections. Penicillin often is used prophylactically to prevent infection after surgery.

Some patients may have existing medical conditions that require antibiotics to be given prophylactically to prevent dangerous infections that could prove fatal. The patient's physician should be consulted before dental treatment in all questionable cases. Erythromycin and tetracycline are bacteriostatic antibiotics often prescribed for patients who are allergic to penicillin.

Antifungal agents are administered for treatment of fungal infections of the oral cavity. Nystatin is commonly used as an oral suspension to treat *Candia albicans* in cases of thrush.

Antihistamines are effective in cases of severe allergic reactions. These drugs may produce several side effects, including drowsiness and xerostomia.

Central nervous system depressants include barbiturates, which are sedative hypnotics principally used to induce sleep, reduce anxiety, and alleviate convulsions. Common barbiturates are phenobarbital, secobarbital, and pentobarbital. Barbiturates should be dispensed with caution, however, since abuse can lead to respiratory depression, resulting in coma or death. Patients should be told that mixing alcohol with barbiturates is particularly dangerous. Antianxiety drugs, such as diazepam (Valium) and chlordiazepoxide (Librium), are similar in action to barbiturates but are less potent.

Central nervous system stimulants include caffeine, epinephrine, and amphetamines. Caffeine contained in coffee, tea, and chocolate affects the cerebral cortex and causes restlessness and alertness. Epinephrine is contained in many local anesthetics because of its vasoconstrictive properties. Amphetamines are psychomotor stimulants and mood elevators, the disadvantages of which include a mild to moderate letdown after the initial stimulation. Central nervous system stimulants are prescribed rarely by dentists.

Narcotics are potent analgesics (pain-relieving drugs) derived from natural opiates or synthetic compounds. Common narcotics include codeine, meperidine (Demerol), and morphine. These drugs greatly elevate the pain threshold and are prescribed for moderate to severe pain. Toxic doses of narcotics can cause marked respiratory depression. Furthermore, if abused, dependency can occur. Other types of narcotic drugs may cause aggressiveness or rapid speech. The dental staff should observe each patient for possible signs and symptoms of drug abuse. Patients under the influence of drugs may exhibit irrational or unusual behavior patterns that must be handled appropriately to avoid injury to the patient or dental staff.

Questions

1. Which are the smallest microbes?

   (A) viruses
   (B) fungi
   (C) bacteria
   (D) algae

2. Bactericidal refers to

   (A) inhibiting bacterial growth
   (B) bacteria in the bloodstream
   (C) killing bacteria
   (D) the effect of bacteria on people

3. What becomes contaminated in the operatory with each operation?

   (A) dental charts
   (B) reception area
   (C) floor
   (D) all surfaces that come in contact with any microbes from the patient's mouth

4. A protective nongrowing form of a microorganism is referred to as a

   (A) spore
   (B) fungus
   (C) cell
   (D) virus

5. The ultrasonic cleaner is used to

   (A) sterilize handpieces
   (B) clean instruments
   (C) sterilize instruments
   (D) pasteurize fluids

6. Instruments are washed before being autoclaved

   (A) to prevent rusting
   (B) to prevent debris from harboring microbes
   (C) to kill any spores
   (D) to kill any viruses

7. A surgical mask is used during a dental operation to

   (A) avoid odors of various dental materials
   (B) protect the patient from inhaling the aerosol created by the high-speed handpiece
   (C) protect the operator and auxiliary from inhaling the aerosol created by the high-speed handpiece
   (D) protect the patient from inhaling the aerosol created by the low-speed handpiece

8. Carbon steel instruments are best sterilized by

   (A) dry heat
   (B) autoclaving
   (C) disinfectants
   (D) flaming

9. The most effective way to kill microbes is

   (A) cold sterilization
   (B) boiling water
   (C) autoclaving
   (D) ultraviolet light

10. How can you tell whether a package of instruments has been autoclaved?

    (A) temperature-sensitive tape will turn color
    (B) instruments are a different color after being autoclaved
    (C) the autoclave bags are left open
    (D) instruments feel warm

11. The effectiveness of a disinfectant solution is altered by the

(A) number of instruments
(B) dilution with water
(C) room temperature
(D) number of bacteria on the instruments

12. A person who harbors a disease without feeling its effect is called a

(A) retainer
(B) transmitter
(C) carrier
(D) neophyte

13. The passage of an infectious microbe from one patient to another is called

(A) plague
(B) rehosting
(C) microbe transfer
(D) cross-infection

14. Dental laboratory infection control includes disinfection of all of the following EXCEPT

(A) rubber bite blocks
(B) impressions
(C) gypsum casts
(D) wax registration records

15. Dental prosthesis should be disinfected

(A) with soap and water
(B) daily with an immersion agent
(C) before sending to the laboratory
(D) never disinfect a dental prosthesis

DIRECTIONS (Questions 16 through 22): For each of the items in this section, ONE or MORE of the numbered options is correct. Choose answer

A   **if only 1, 2, and 3 are correct**
B   **if only 1 and 3 are correct**
C   **if only 2 and 4 are correct**
D   **if only 4 is correct**
E   **if all are correct**

16. Hands should be washed

(1) before and after using gloves
(2) with an antimicrobial soap
(3) for a full 15 seconds between each patient
(4) for a full 5 minutes if part of a surgical dental team

17. The term *universal precautions* implies

(1) every patient must complete a medical history before treatment
(2) all patients are apprehensive

(3) use gloves and face masks when treating infectious patients only
(4) infection control procedures should be implemented for all patients

18. Protective barriers for the dental staff may include

(1) disposable gowns
(2) protective eyewear/faceshield
(3) disposable gloves and face mask
(4) lead lined aprons

19. Chairside infection control includes the use of

(1) a high-velocity evacuation system
(2) preset trays
(3) rubber dam whenever possible
(4) proper waste disposal methods

20. Radiographic infection control includes

(1) use of barriers for x-ray equipment
(2) using sterilized film
(3) placing exposed films in isolation paper cups
(4) changing processing solutions weekly

21. Dental handpieces should be

(1) autoclaved after each use
(2) oiled weekly with sterile solutions
(3) disinfected only with an approved disinfectant spray
(4) sterilized according to manufacturer's directions

22. Disposal of infectious waste includes

(1) the use of sturdy leakproof bags
(2) labeling bags as hazardous waste
(3) disposing according to state and local regulations
(4) a sealed, puncture-resistant container for needles, blades, and broken glass

DIRECTIONS (Questions 23 through 85): Each of the questions or incomplete statements in this section is followed by four suggested answers or completions. Select the ONE lettered answer or completion that is BEST in each case. Check your answers with the correct answers at the end of the chapter.

23. A written direction to a pharmacist to prepare a drug is called

(A) a prescription
(B) an order blank
(C) a slip
(D) a label

24. Which member of the dental team is responsible for writing drug orders?

   (A) assistant
   (B) receptionist
   (C) hygienist
   (D) dentist

25. Before prescribing any drug

   (A) an accurate medical history must be taken
   (B) a Snyder test should be performed
   (C) a complete blood count should be performed
   (D) a urinalysis should be performed

26. The type of administration that allows the drug the fastest onset of action is

   (A) intramuscular
   (B) subcutaneous
   (C) intravenous
   (D) sublingual

27. When determining the dosage of a drug, an important consideration is the patient's

   (A) height
   (B) age and weight
   (C) appetite
   (D) headsize

28. Some drugs cannot be taken orally because

   (A) they are in liquid form
   (B) saliva will dilute them
   (C) the enamel will corrode
   (D) the digestive system will alter the drug

29. The abbreviation q4h means

   (A) every 4 days
   (B) 4 times a day
   (C) every 4 hours
   (D) for 4 days

30. Prescription fluoride may include all of the following EXCEPT

   (A) stannous fluoride gel
   (B) sodium fluoride liquid
   (C) acidulated phosphate fluoride gel
   (D) fluoride toothpaste

31. Which federal agency ensures public safety in relation to drugs?

   (A) Federal Safety Commission
   (B) Food and Drug Administration
   (C) American Dental Association
   (D) American Medical Association

32. Antihistamines are used to

   (A) delay the effects of a narcotic
   (B) premedicate and allay fears
   (C) enhance the effects of antibiotics
   (D) counteract allergic reactions

33. Tranquilizers are

   (A) used in dentistry before root canal therapy
   (B) used in dentistry after any surgical procedure
   (C) used in dentistry whenever antibiotics are used
   (D) almost never used in dentistry

34. The most commonly used analgesic is

   (A) codeine
   (B) aspirin
   (C) meperidine
   (D) morphine

35. Some patients cannot take aspirin because of

   (A) a previous heart attack
   (B) the gastrointestinal irritation
   (C) the production of gas pains
   (D) the severe headaches it causes

36. Lidocaine is a

   (A) local anesthetic
   (B) general anesthetic
   (C) narcotic
   (D) barbiturate

37. A drug used to prevent epileptic attacks is

   (A) ampicillin
   (B) a tranquilizer
   (C) Dilantin
   (D) monoamine oxidase

38. Addictive analgesic drugs are known as

   (A) narcotics
   (B) antihistamines
   (C) tranquilizers
   (D) stimulants

39. The condition that exists when a drug becomes necessary and its discontinuance would cause mental or physical changes is termed

   (A) summation
   (B) addiction
   (C) addition
   (D) accumulation

40. Hydrogen peroxide can be used as a (an)

(A) hemostatic agent
(B) anodyne
(C) oxidizing mouthwash
(D) treatment for herpetic lesions

41. The function of a hemostatic agent is to

(A) thicken the blood
(B) thin the blood
(C) stop bleeding
(D) increase the number of blood platelets in the circulating blood

42. The most commonly used local anesthetic is

(A) epinephrine
(B) lidocaine (Xylocaine)
(C) Carbocaine
(D) nitrous oxide

43. Epinephrine in local anesthesia causes

(A) increased uptake of the anesthetic by blood vessels
(B) hyperventilation
(C) prolonged effects of the anesthetic
(D) tissue irritation

44. Ethyl chloride can be used as a (an)

(A) topical anesthetic
(B) general anesthetic
(C) inhalant
(D) local anesthetic

45. Which antibiotic can cause staining of a child's primary teeth if it is taken by a pregnant woman during her last trimester of pregnancy?

(A) tetracycline
(B) penicillin
(C) erythromycin
(D) streptomycin

46. An antibiotic is a drug

(A) that inhibits viruses
(B) used only for pulmonary infections
(C) that increases circulation
(D) produced by a microorganism that destroys other microorganisms

47. The use of drugs in cancer therapy is called

(A) radiotherapy
(B) electrocautery
(C) chemotherapy
(D) psychotherapy

48. Which of the following drugs is applied topically?

(A) nitrous oxide
(B) fluoride
(C) penicillin
(D) epinephrine

49. The type of drug used for prophylactic premedication for valvular heart disease is

(A) narcotic
(B) antihistamine
(C) antibiotics
(D) tranquilizer

50. A common drug used in the dental office to decrease anxiety is

(A) nitrous oxide
(B) caffeine
(C) aspirin
(D) benzocaine

51. Nitrous oxide should NOT be used on patients who have

(A) dental caries
(B) gingival infections
(C) high pain threshold
(D) nasal obstructions

52. Following each use, the nitrous oxide rubber tubing and mask must be

(A) disinfected only
(B) sterilized
(C) washed with soap and hot water only
(D) thrown away

53. Abrasion is the

(A) chemical erosion of the dentinoenamel junction
(B) fracture of cusps of a molar
(C) wearing away of tooth structure by mechanical means
(D) result of defective enamel

54. Mottled enamel is the result of

(A) tetracycline taken by the mother during pregnancy
(B) oral secretions
(C) ingestion of too much fluoride
(D) incorrect tooth brushing

55. A cleft lip is caused by a lack of fusion between the

(A) frontonasal process and median nasal process
(B) maxillary process and median nasal process

(C) maxillary process
(D) soft palate and hard palate

56. A supernumerary tooth located between the maxillary central incisors is called a (an)

(A) odontoma
(B) incisive cyst
(C) ectopic eruption
(D) mesiodens

57. Tori are

(A) lymphatic tissues
(B) bony protuberances
(C) fibrotic tissues
(D) adipose tissues

58. The physiologic wearing away of teeth is called

(A) abrasion
(B) erosion
(C) decalcification
(D) attrition

59. Which of these terms denotes a congenital absence of teeth?

(A) microdontia
(B) macrodontia
(C) supernumerary
(D) anodontia

60. Which of these terms describes cellular death?

(A) necrosis
(B) atrophy
(C) hyperemia
(D) xerostomia

61. All of these are signs of inflammation EXCEPT

(A) heat
(B) pain
(C) swelling
(D) regeneration

62. Which disease causes swelling of the parotid glands?

(A) measles
(B) ANUG
(C) mumps
(D) chickenpox

63. An oral fungal infection is called

(A) leukoplakia
(B) thrush/candidiasis
(C) herpes
(D) nevi

64. White patches on the soft tissues are called

(A) leukoplakia
(B) Fordyce's granules
(C) tori
(D) fibromas

65. Erythema is

(A) a type of oral carcinoma
(B) cryotherapy
(C) redness of the skin
(D) a form of bacteria

66. Which condition is the result of defective enamel formation?

(A) hypercementosis
(B) concrescence
(C) dentinogenesis imperfecta
(D) enamel hypoplasia

67. Immunology refers to the study of

(A) resistance to disease
(B) factors that cause disease
(C) population studies
(D) fluoridation

68. Tic douloureux is a pathologic condition of which cranial nerve?

(A) I
(B) V
(C) VII
(D) X

69. The unconscious grinding of teeth is called

(A) bruxism
(B) abrasion
(C) granulation
(D) kinesiology

70. Which of these terms describes cracks or peeling at the angle of the mouth?

(A) cellulitis
(B) cheilosis
(C) keratosis
(D) exotosis

71. A salivary stone is called

(A) tartar
(B) a salivary nodule
(C) a sialograph
(D) a sialolith

72. The ability to ward off disease is known as

    (A) infection
    (B) host resistance
    (C) postponement
    (D) the autogenic ability

73. An antibody is

    (A) an autoimmune disease
    (B) part of the body's defense system
    (C) an enzyme
    (D) a catalyst

74. Bacterial invasion of the circulatory system is referred to as

    (A) hyperemia
    (B) toxemia
    (C) bacteremia
    (D) granuloma

75. A recurrent viral infection in the mouth is

    (A) pyogenic granuloma
    (B) herpes simplex
    (C) aphthous ulcer
    (D) thrush

76. Acute necrotizing ulcerative gingivitis often is referred to as

    (A) trench mouth
    (B) pregnancy tumor
    (C) gingivosis
    (D) epulis

77. Which of these dental conditions is relatively harmless and causes the patient no pain?

    (A) necrotizing ulcerative gingivitis
    (B) herpes labialis
    (C) geographic tongue
    (D) aphthous ulcer

78. Which term describes calcified areas within the pulp chamber?

    (A) pulp polyp
    (B) pulp stone (denticle)
    (C) secondary dentin
    (D) odontomas

79. Hormonal changes can affect the

    (A) periodontium
    (B) formation of a mucocele
    (C) fluoride uptake of permanent molars
    (D) pulp of the tooth

80. Cancer is definitively diagnosed by

    (A) color reagents
    (B) biopsy
    (C) tactile senses
    (D) radiographs

81. Neoplasm refers to

    (A) tissue dysplasia
    (B) a malignant growth
    (C) a new growth
    (D) an allergic reaction

82. Benign refers to

    (A) aplasia of the buccal mucosa
    (B) desquamation of the oral mucosa
    (C) a lesion composed of normal tissue
    (D) ulcerative lesions on the tongue

83. Leukemia is a disease of

    (A) nerve tissue
    (B) muscle tissue
    (C) cartilage tissue
    (D) blood tissue

84. The spreading of cancer to different sites in the body is called

    (A) metastasis
    (B) toxemia
    (C) peritonitis
    (D) carcinoma

85. HIV/AIDS is a disease of

    (A) the endocrine system
    (B) the immune system
    (C) the oral cavity
    (D) noninfectious origins

Answers and Explanations

1. **(A)** Viruses, the smallest microbes, are composed of DNA or RNA in a protein coat. Viruses are cuboidal, spherical, elongated, or tadpole-like. Some diseases caused by viruses are herpes simplex, infectious and serum hepatitis, rabies, influenza, poliomyelitis, and AIDS.

2. **(C)** Bactericidal refers to killing bacteria. Bacteriostatic refers to inhibiting bacterial growth. Bacteremia is the presence of bacteria in the bloodstream.

3. **(D)** All surfaces in the operatory that come in contact with microbes from the patient's mouth become contaminated, including instruments, equipment, and people.

4. **(A)** Spores are a protective bacterial form. Some bacteria assume this form under unfavorable conditions. When conditions are again favorable, the bacterium will emerge from its spore form and begin to grow again.

5. **(B)** Ultrasonic cleaners can be used to debride and cleanse instruments. After removing instruments from the ultrasonic bath, rinse instruments thoroughly and dry before sterilization procedures. The ultrasonic cleaner does not sterilize instruments.

6. **(B)** Instruments must be washed thoroughly before any sterilization technique is employed. Debris not removed could harbor bacteria and insulate them from the bactericidal effect of the sterilization technique.

7. **(C)** When using a high-speed handpiece, an aerosol is created that consists of water spray, saliva, microbes from the patient's mouth, and debris (eg, tooth, filling material). The aerosol could cause respiratory infections to the operator and assistant. The use of a surgical mask will avoid the inhalation of the aerosol. Protective glasses will prevent eye injuries from flying debris.

8. **(A)** Carbon steel instruments are best sterilized by dry heat. This procedure will avoid rusting and dulling of sharp edges.

9. **(C)** Autoclaving, steam under pressure, is the most effective way to kill microbes. The heat from the steam sterilizes the instruments.

10. **(A)** A thermochromatic indicator, tape, part of the sterilization package, will change color after it has been autoclaved.

11. **(B)** The effectiveness of a disinfectant solution is altered by dilution. Wet instruments placed in disinfectant solution will dilute the concentration. Therefore, the solution will not kill the organisms it is capable of killing in its correct concentration.

12. **(C)** A person who harbors a disease without feeling its effect is a carrier. The carrier might be a person who has never had symptoms of the disease or a person recovering from the disease. A carrier can transmit the disease to other people.

13. **(D)** The passage of an infectious microbe from one patient to another is called cross-infection. This is an indirect transmission of disease and may take the following route in dentistry: patient's mouth → contaminated hand instruments → another patient's mouth.

14. **(A)** The dental laboratory can harbor numerous infectious microorganisms and must follow appropriate infection control procedures to prevent disease transmission. Rubber bite blocks must be sterilized according to the manufacturer's directions either by steam autoclave or ethylene oxide methods. Impressions, wax bite registrations, and gypsum cast models (once separated from the impression) should be disinfected with an approved disinfectant agent once they have come in contact with the patient's mouth.

15. **(C)** Dental prosthesis should be disinfected before sending to the laboratory to prevent disease transmission. A dilute sodium hypochlorite solution can be used to soak and disinfect the prosthesis.

16. **(E)** Hands should be washed before placing and removing gloves with an antimicrobial soap for 10 to 15 seconds. If part of a dental surgical team, it is necessary to perform a thorough surgical scrub for 5 to 10 minutes on the hands, wrists, and arms up to 2 inches above the elbow.

17. **(D)** The term *universal precautions* is an approach established by the Centers for Disease Control (CDC) that implies that all patients should be treated as if they were infective and advocates the use of the same infection control practices for all patients.

18. **(A)** Protective barriers for the dental staff may include disposable gowns, protective eyewear, faceshields, disposable gloves, and disposable masks.

19. **(E)** Chairside infection control includes the use of a high-velocity evacuation system to reduce the amount of spatter during the use of the handpiece or ultrasonic equipment. Application of a rubber dam also is recommended to minimize the spatter of blood and saliva. Preplanning needed instruments by presetting trays eliminates reaching into instrument cabinets during chairside procedures with soiled gloves. Chairside infection control also includes the use of proper waste disposal methods.

20. **(B)** Radiographic infection control measures include the use of barriers, such as a polyethylene bag over the x-ray tube head, and the placement of exposed x-ray film in isolation paper cups to prevent cross-contamination.

21. **(D)** Dental handpieces should be sterilized according to the manufacturer's directions. Some types of handpieces can be autoclaved (steam under pressure), but others cannot and must be disinfected with an approved agent.

22. **(E)** Disposal of infectious contaminated waste must be conducted according to the laws and regulations for waste disposal in each state. Standard guidelines for infectious waste disposal include the use of leak-proof bags that are labeled appropriately as hazardous or infectious waste. A puncture-proof, sealed container should be used for all sharp items, such as needles, blades, disposable syringes, and broken glass.

23. **(A)** A prescription is a written direction to a pharmacist to prepare a drug. A prescription includes the following information: doctor's name, address, and telephone number, patient's name, address, and age, date, drug name and dosage, quantity of the drug, directions for use, and doctor's signature and DEA (narcotic registration number).

24. **(D)** The dentist is responsible for prescribing drugs and the only member of the dental team who legally can write a prescription.

25. **(A)** Before prescribing any drug, an accurate medical history must be taken. Some factors in a patient's history that can influence drug administration are a history of drug allergies, other drugs the patient might be taking, and physical and mental states.

26. **(C)** Intravenous drug administration has the fastest onset of action. An intravenous injection introduces the drug directly into the bloodstream. This method is used also to infuse a large amount of fluid into the body.

27. **(B)** When determining dosage, important considerations are the patient's age and weight, other drugs the patient is taking, route of administration, the disease entity, and past experiences the patient has had with the drug.

28. **(D)** Some drugs taken orally might not be absorbed or effective or could irritate the lining of the stomach.

29. **(C)** Some common Latin abbreviations are q4h (every 4 hours), qid (4 times a day), prn (as needed), and ac (before meals).

30. **(D)** A fluoride toothpaste may be bought over-the-counter (OTC). A prescription is not required for OTC products.

31. **(B)** The Food and Drug Administration is responsible for ensuring public safety in relationship to drugs. Manufacturers of a new drug must prove that the drug is safe and effective before it can be used by the public.

32. **(D)** Antihistamines are used to treat allergic reactions. A common side effect of these drugs is drowsiness.

33. **(D)** Tranquilizers are rarely used in dentistry. These drugs are used for their long-range sedating effects.

34. **(B)** The most commonly used analgesic is aspirin. Aspirin also functions as an antirheumatic, antipyretic, and antiinflammatory agent.

35. **(B)** Some patients claim to have adverse gastrointestinal effects after the ingestion of aspirin. Stomach ulcers have been induced in animals with salicylates.

36. **(A)** Lidocaine is the most common local anesthetic used in dentistry.

37. **(C)** A drug used to prevent epileptic attacks is diphenylhydantoin (Dilantin). A side effect of this drug is fibrous hyperplasia of the gingiva.

38. **(A)** Addictive analgesic drugs are narcotics. Care must be taken when these drugs are prescribed, since they can become physiologically habit forming.

39. **(B)** Addiction is the condition existing in a patient where a drug, after repeated use, becomes needed by the body and its cessation would cause mental or physical changes. Addiction includes developing tolerance to the drug being used.

40. **(C)** Hydrogen peroxide diluted with water can be used as an oxidizing mouthwash. It is also used as an irrigant in root canal therapy.

41. **(C)** Hemostatic agents stop bleeding by aiding the normal clotting mechanism. Examples of hemostatic agents used in dentistry are absorbable gelatin sponges, absorbable oxidized cellulose, and alum.

42. **(B)** The most commonly used local anesthetic is lidocaine (Xylocaine). Local anesthetics can be classified into four groups: para-aminobenzoic acid, meta-aminobenzoic acid, benzoic acid, and amides.

43. **(C)** Epinephrine in local anesthesia causes prolonged effects of anesthesia. Epinephrine is a vasoconstrictor. It decreases the size of the blood vessels—hence a decrease of the circulation in the area, and the anesthetic remains active for a longer period of time.

44. **(A)** Ethyl chloride can be used as a topical anesthetic. Ethyl chloride temporarily freezes the area to which it is applied.

45. **(A)** Tetracycline taken at the time of enamel formation may result in staining of the enamel. Enamel formation takes place during the last trimester of pregnancy through early childhood.

46. **(D)** An antibiotic is a drug produced by a microorganism that destroys bacteria. Commonly used antibiotics are penicillin, erythromycin, tetracycline, streptomycin, bacitracin, and chloramphenicol.

47. **(C)** The use of drugs in cancer therapy is called chemotherapy. Other modes of treatment for cancer are surgery and radiation.

48. **(B)** Fluoride is applied topically to the teeth as either a gel for a liquid. Fluoride is a prescription drug and an adjunct to preventive dentistry. Other drugs applied topically in dentistry include topical anesthetic agents and Orabase. These drugs are applied intraorally.

49. **(C)** Prophylactic means preventing disease. Examples of prophylactic measures are the use of antibiotics to prevent subacute bacterial endocarditis (SBE) or infective endocarditis. Infective endocarditis is a microbial (bacterial) infection of the heart valves that have been damaged in a previous episode of rheumatic fever or rheumatic heart disease. Antibiotic premedication also is required for patients with a history of reduced capacity to resist infection, prosthetic heart valves, mitral valve prolapse, renal transplant or dialysis, and prosthetic joint replacements of the body.

50. **(A)** Nitrous oxide-oxygen often is used as a sedative in the dental office. It is applied to a patient through a nose mask. The sedative effects are eliminated at the end of the procedure by giving the patient pure oxygen.

51. **(D)** Nitrous oxide should not be used on patients with nasal obstructions, since the drug is an inhalation agent and is ineffective if not inhaled sufficiently. Patients with other nasal complication, such as sinusitis or nasal injuries, preventing proper inhalation methods are not good candidates for the administration of nitrous oxide.

52. **(B)** The nitrous oxide rubber tubing and mask must be sterilized after each use. Appropriate methods of sterilization must be used according to manufacturer's recommendations. Most rubber items can be sterilized safely in a gas sterilizer using ethylene oxide. Proper time and temperature for adequate sterilization and aeration after the cycle are important. Some rubber nitrous oxide nasal nose pieces are disposable. Most rubber tubing is not disposable. Before sterilization, it is best to wash the rubber nosepiece with soap and water.

53. **(C)** Abrasion is the mechanical wearing away of tooth structure by a foreign body. The most common cause is toothbrushing with a stiff bristle brush using an abrasive dentifrice. Other causes are such habits as pipe smoking and habitually holding other objects between the teeth.

54. **(C)** Mottled enamel is the result of a disturbance during tooth formation due to the ingestion of excess fluoride. The enamel has a brown opaque appearance. The treatment is usually cosmetic and may range from fillings to full coverage.

55. **(B)** A cleft lip is a defect below the ala of the nose on one or both sides. It is caused by the lack of fusion between the maxillary process and the median nasal

process. A cleft palate is the lack of fusion along the median line of the palate. It can vary from a cleft of part of the soft palate to a cleft of the entire soft and hard palate.

56. **(D)** The most common supernumerary tooth is a mesiodens, located between the maxillary central incisors. The second most common supernumerary tooth is the maxillary fourth molar.

57. **(B)** Tori are bony protuberances or exotosis. They most frequently are located on the hard palate or the lingual surface of the mandible in the premolar area. Tori become a problem if a prosthesis is to be constructed over them. If they are enlarged, they can be surgically removed.

58. **(D)** Attrition is the physiologic wearing away of the occlusal and proximal surfaces of teeth associated with aging. This process occurs in both the primary and permanent dentition. Excessive attrition can be caused by bruxing and other oral habits.

59. **(D)** Anodontia denotes a congenital absence of teeth. This lack of a developing tooth germ affects both primary and permanent dentitions. Microdontia refers to teeth that are smaller than normal, and macrodontia refers to teeth that are larger than normal. Supernumerary teeth are extra or additional teeth in a normal dentition.

60. **(A)** The term *necrosis* describes cellular death. Necrosis is the most extreme form of degeneration of a cell.

61. **(D)** Symptoms of inflammation are redness caused by the dilation of blood vessels, heat caused by dilation of blood vessels, swelling caused by fluids leaving the blood vessels and accumulating in the area, pain caused by pressure of fluids on sensory nerves, and impairment of function. Regeneration is not a sign of the inflammation process.

62. **(C)** Mumps usually causes inflammation and swelling of the parotid glands. The patient has fever and chills and might find it difficult to open the mouth.

63. **(B)** Thrush, or moniliasis, is caused by the fungus *Candida albicans*. This organism is found normally in the oral cavity. An imbalance attributable to nutritional problems or antibiotic therapy is responsible for its overgrowth and the subsequent disease state.

64. **(A)** A white patch in the oral cavity is called leukoplakia. The cause is a chronic irritant, such as smoking or rubbing by the sharp edge of a fractured tooth. Some leukoplakia areas undergo changes and become carcinomas.

65. **(C)** Erythema is an abnormal redness of the skin attributable to inflammation, x-ray treatment, or a disease process.

66. **(D)** Enamel hypoplasia is a condition that results from defective enamel formation. The enamel usually is pitted or grooved across the crown as a result of the disturbance of the ameloblasts during the enamel matrix formation.

67. **(A)** Immunology is the study of resistance to disease. Immunity can be acquired or natural. Natural immunity is obtained in utero, and acquired immunity is obtained after birth as the result of antibodies being introduced by injection or as the result of infection.

68. **(B)** Tic douloureux is a pathologic condition of the fifth cranial nerve. It is associated with trigger zones on the face that when stimulated, set off an excruciating pain, usually lasting a few seconds. The cause of this disease is unknown, but it could be related to the proximity of blood vessels to the trigeminal nerve.

69. **(A)** The unconscious grinding of teeth is called bruxism. Some possible causes are occlusal discrepancies and psychologic factors associated with tension release.

70. **(B)** Cheilosis is a condition caused by a nutritional deficiency of vitamin B (riboflavin). The condition is characterized by cracks or fissures at the angle of the mouth and a dry, cracked surface of the lips.

71. **(D)** A salivary stone is known as a sialolith. If the stone blocks the duct of a salivary gland, the gland may swell due to the backup saliva. A sialograph is the radiograph used to help diagnose the problem. The treatment is removal of the stone by manipulation or surgery.

72. **(B)** The ability to ward off disease is known as host resistance. It can be natural, such as elements in saliva that decrease the caries rate, or acquired, such as the decrease in tooth solubility caused by the incorporation of fluoride into the tooth.

73. **(B)** Antibodies are proteins that are part of the body's defense system. They are produced in response to a foreign body, an antigen. Immunity, the ability of the body to resist infection, depends on the formation of antibodies.

74. **(C)** Bacterial invasion of the circulatory system is referred to as bacteremia. This type of infection usually involves the whole body and is known as a systemic infection.

75. (B) Herpes simplex is the virus that causes recurrent sores in the oral cavity. The disease is initiated by an attack of primary herpes, which is contagious in young children. The lesions of primary herpes are widespread throughout the mouth. Subsequent attacks usually are associated with single lesions. There is no known specific treatment for the lesion, which takes about 14 days to heal.

76. (A) Another term for acute necrotizing ulcerative gingivitis (ANUG) is trench mouth or Vincent's disease. Symptoms of ANUG include ulcerations on the gingiva, bleeding gums, sloughing gingival tissues, and elevated temperature. Patients with a history of AIDS commonly exhibit gingival symptoms similar to those of ANUG.

77. (C) Geographic tongue is a harmless condition of the tongue characterized by areas on the dorsum of the tongue that appear as patches due to a loss of epithelium. The condition causes the patches to change patterns.

78. (B) The term *pulpstones* or *denticles* describes calcified masses in the pulp.

79. (A) Hormonal changes affect the periodontium. Examples of endocrine changes in the mouth are pregnancy gingivitis, increased rate of bone loss in diabetes, swelling of the gingiva during the menstrual cycle, and accelerated rate of eruption caused by hyperthyroidism.

80. (B) The definitive diagnosis of cancer is made by removing a piece of the lesion (a biopsy) and studying it under a microscope.

81. (C) Neoplasm refers to a new growth that will not disappear when the etiologic agent is removed. Neoplasms are classified as benign or malignant. Malignant tumors are life threatening and will result in the death of the host if they are not removed.

82. (C) Benign refers to tumors (neoplasms) composed of normal tissue. They are named according to their tissue of origin with the suffix *oma*. These lesions are dangerous if they are located in areas wherein their physical presence, pressure by growth, or creation of hypersecretion is damaging. This can occur in the brain, trachea, or endocrine glands, as well as other parts of the body.

83. (D) Leukemia is a disease of white blood cells. Manifestations of the disease appear in the oral cavity as spontaneous hemorrhage, poor healing, and gingival enlargement.

84. (A) Metastasis is the spreading of cancer to different sites in the body. The most frequent malignant oral tumor is squamous cell carcinoma, which metastasizes through the lymphatic system.

85. (B) AIDS is a disease of the immune system. The acquired immunodeficiency syndrome (AIDS) is a fatal condition with a variety of symptoms that affect the entire body, including the oral cavity. AIDS is caused by the human immunodeficiency virus (HIV).

BIBLIOGRAPHY

Ciancio SG, Bourgault PC. *Clinical Pharmacology for Dental Professionals*, 3rd ed. Chicago: Year Book Medical Publishers, Inc, 1989.

Facts About AIDS for the Dental Team, 2nd ed. American Dental Association Council on Dental Therapeutics, Chicago: American Dental Association, October 1988.

Giunta JL. *Oral Pathology*, 3rd ed. Philadelphia: BC Decker, Inc, 1989.

Goth A. *Medical Pharmacology*, 10th ed. St. Louis: CV Mosby Co, 1981.

Infection Control in the Dental Environment. Department of Veterans Affairs, American Dental Association, Department of Health and Human Services and Centers for Disease Control. Washington DC: Eastern Dental Education Center Learning Resources Center Veterans Administration, 1989.

Jawetz E, et al. *Review of Medical Microbiology*, 18th ed. Norwalk, Conn: Appleton & Lange, 1989.

Robbins SL, Angell M. *Basic Pathology*, 3rd ed. Philadelphia: WB Saunders Co, 1981.

Rowe AHR, Alexander AG. *Clinical Methods, Medicine, Pathology and Pharmacology—A Companion to Dental Studies*, 1st ed. Boston, Mass: Blackwell Scientific Publications, 1988, vol 2.

Scopp IW. *Oral Medicine*, 2nd ed. St. Louis: CV Mosby Co, 1973.

Seymour RA, Walton JG. *Adverse Drug Reactions in Dentistry*, 1st ed. New York: Oxford University Press, 1988.

Shafer WG, Hine MK, Levy BM. *Textbook of Oral Pathology*, 4th ed. Philadelphia: WB Saunders Co, 1983.

Shin D, Avers J. *AIDS/HIV Reference Guide for Medical Professionals*, 1st ed. West Los Angeles, Calif: CIRID/UCLA School of Medicine, Publishers, 1988.

Torres H, Ehrlich A. *Modern Dental Assisting*, 4th ed. Philadelphia: WB Saunders Co, 1990.

Tyldesley WR. *Oral Medicine*, 3rd ed. New York: Oxford University Press, 1989.

CHAPTER 5

Chairside Assisting

INTRODUCTION

As the demand for dentistry has escalated, it has been recognized that dentists must increase the efficiency of their work production in order to be effective and to maintain a minimum of psychologic and physical stress. As a result, dentists have begun to apply industrial principles of work and time management in the dental office. By delegating more chairside responsibilities to the dental auxiliary and applying the concepts of four-handed sitdown dentistry, dental procedures can be more efficiently performed, with an increase in work production and a decrease in the fatigue factor for the dentist.

Research has shown that a dentist using one full-time auxiliary can increase productivity by 33% and by using two auxiliaries can increase productivity by 90%. This chapter provides a synopsis of general chairside dental assisting principles and procedures, including four-handed sitdown dentistry concepts and methods and dental charting techniques. An overview of the recognized dental specialties is presented, with additional review material for chairside assisting in orthodontics and oral maxillofacial surgery.

PRINCIPLES OF DENTAL AUXILIARY USE

One of the most important concepts offered by industry is increased production through elimination or reduction of delaying factors. All tasks that can be *eliminated* produce the highest return (100%). For example, it has been demonstrated that every time a patient rinses his or her mouth, approximately 18% of useful chair time is wasted. If this process can be eliminated through the use of high-speed suction, approximately 11 minutes per working hour can be gained.

Tasks or instruments that cannot be eliminated can be *combined*. Production increases range from 50% to 75%. For example, double-ended instruments decrease the number of hand transfers by as much as 50%.

If elimination and combination are inappropriate, tasks and instruments can be *rearranged* to facilitate use. For example, if the three-way syringe is used more often than any other instrument, it should be located in the most accessible position.

When none of the previous three principles is applicable, tasks should be *simplified*. An example of simplification is the use of disposable, prepared materials. If elimination, combination, rearrangement, or simplification cannot be applied, procedures should be *standardized* to reduce the number of variables. For instance, each time an amalgam procedure is done, it should be done in the same manner, with the same instruments.

MINIMIZATION OF MOTION

Stress and fatigue are decreased if movement is minimized and controlled. Industrial time and motion studies have identified five classifications of motion.

Class I motions involve only the fingers, for example, transfer of most instruments. *Class II motions* involve the fingers and wrists, for example, transfer of a double-handled instrument, such as scissors. *Class III motions* involve the use of fingers, wrist, and elbows, for instance, placement of the rubber dam clamp.

The next two classifications of motion are the most physically taxing and should be eliminated if possible. *Class IV motions* involve the entire arm and shoulder, such as when reaching to adjust an overhead light. *Class V motions* involve the entire arm and torso, as in turning to reach for an instrument. Class V motions are most fatiguing because they involve refocusing the eyes (accommodation) to different light intensities and distances.

ZONES OF OPERATING ACTIVITY

A basic principle of four-handed sitdown dentistry is proper positioning of the operator, assistant, patient, and equipment. The benefits of proper positioning include minimizing physical stress of the members of the operating team while maximizing visibility and patient comfort (Fig. 5–1).

To help visualize the positioning relationship in the operatory, the face of the clock can be superimposed on the properly positioned dental team. The patient's mouth is located at the center of the clock, and 12 o'clock is located above the patient's head.

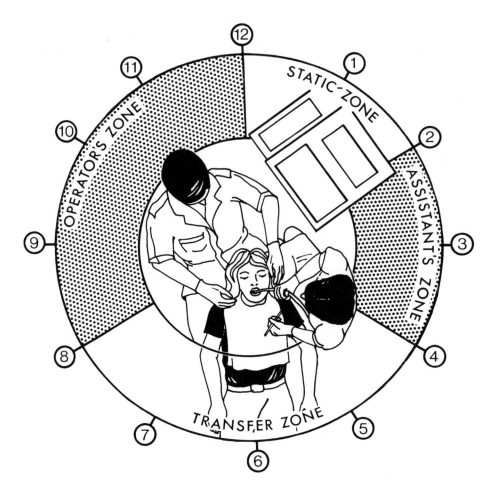

Figure 5–1. Zones of operating activity.

The following zones of operating activity can be identified for a right-handed operator (a mirror image is used for a left-handed operator). The operator's zone is at 8 to 12 o'clock depending on the quadrant and tooth surface being treated. The assistant's zone is between 2 and 4 o'clock regardless of the quadrant and tooth surface being treated. The static zone is located from 12 to 2 o'clock. This zone contains equipment that is used infrequently, such as the nitrous oxide unit. The transfer zone is at 4 to 8 o'clock, in which instrument transfers are made either at the patient's mouth or below the chin. The operator should be positioned such that his or her back touches the back rest, thighs are parallel to the floor, and feet are resting flat on the floor.

The assistant should be seated in a position as close to the patient's head as possible, with eye level 6 inches above that of the operator. The thigh nearest the patient should be resting against the patient's chair. The wrap-around arm of the stool, if there is one, should be placed beneath the ribcage. The assistant's feet rest on the base of the stool.

Seating the Patient
The manner in which an assistant introduces a patient to an operatory affects the entire procedure. The assistant should lead the patient to the operatory and, with hand motions, indicate where the patient should sit. The patient's chair should be at a comfortable height for a sitting position, and the chair arm should be raised, if possible. After the patient is seated, the patient's napkin is secured. The assistant should then slowly tilt the chair backward until the patient's calves are parallel to the floor. If the procedure to be accomplished is located in the maxilla, the patient should be supine. If the area being treated is in the mandible, the patient's back should be between a 25-degree and 45-degree angle to the floor. The patient's head should be as close to the top of the dental chair and the operator as possible. The light is positioned approximately 30 inches from the operating field, and the chair is elevated to a comfortable working height for the operator. Patients who might have difficulty in a supine position include the elderly and those with respiratory or circulatory problems or both. These patients should be treated in an upright position. Once the patient is positioned, the assistant should remain with him or her until the operator enters.

After a procedure is completed, the assistant should slowly return the patient to an upright position. The patient should remain seated until equilibrium is regained. The assistant can then dismiss the patient.

Transferring of Instruments

It is the dental assistant's responsibility to prepare and position all instruments used for a procedure. The instruments should be placed in a manner that affords accessibility and efficiency. Once placed in the appropriate position, the instruments are transferred between the assistant and the operator in a prescribed manner.

The assistant transfers instruments from the left hand (for a right-handed operator) to the operator's right hand. During transfers, it is necessary for the operator to use only Class I motions. The stages of instrument transfer are as follows.

- Signal stage. The operator makes a Class I motion, moving the instrument out of the working field while maintaining the finger rest.
- Pretransfer stage. The assistant positions the instrument to be transferred parallel to the working instrument.
- Midtransfer stage. The assistant holds the instrument to be transferred between the index finger and thumb and removes the instrument previously used from the operator's hand with the fourth finger of his or her left hand.
- Transfer stage. The instrument to be transferred is placed in the proper position into the operator's hand.
- Transfer completion stage. The assistant releases the transferred instrument, and the operator returns to the operating field. If the instrument is to be reused, it is repositioned into the pretransfer stage.

The transfer process is altered slightly when transferring a syringe or any double-handled instrument. The stages remain the same, but the operator must make a Class II motion in releasing the finger rest. With the palm facing up, the operator positions his or her hand under the patient's chin to receive the new instrument. The other steps in the transfer process remain the same.

To properly complete a transfer, both the operator and assistant must know the appropriate way in which to grasp instruments. Different instruments are held in different grasps. For example, explorers and spoon excavators are held in a pen grasp, whereas chisels and hatchets are held in a palm–thumb grasp. Double-handled instruments such as forceps and syringes, are held in palm grasps.

Efficient transfer is an integral part in increasing productivity by using the principles of motion economy and work simplification.

Suction and Retraction

In addition to proper patient positioning and efficient instrument transfers, high-speed evacuation and proper retraction are important in increasing accessibility and decreasing stress.

The primary function of high-speed suction is to provide a working field free of saliva and debris and eliminate the use of the cuspidor during a procedure. A properly positioned suction tip will decrease the size of the area of bacterial aerosol created close to the high-speed handpiece. Concurrently, the tip can be used for retraction purposes, permitting increased visibility and protection of the patient's tissues.

A number of principles are used for suction tip placement. The assistant holds the tip in his or her right hand (when working with a right-handed operator) with a reverse palm or thumb to nose grasp. When working on a posterior tooth, the tip should be positioned as close to the tooth as possible without injuring the soft tissue. The beveled tip should be held parallel with either the buccal or lingual surface of the tooth. While working on an anterior tooth, the tip should be placed opposite the surface of the tooth being treated, with beveled tip parallel to and bisecting the incisal edges of the teeth. The tip should not be placed on the back of the tongue or soft palate, to avoid gagging. If it is placed too close to the water coolant of the handpiece, the water will be evacuated before it reaches the tooth. The tip should be positioned before the operator places the handpiece and mirror.

A mirror or suction tip or both can be used to retract the cheeks and tongue. The operator using the mirror and the assistant using the suction tip retract the tissue closest to each. For example, a right-handed operator working in the lower right quadrant retracts the cheek and the assistant retracts the tongue.

Tray Setups

The use of prepared tray setups also decreases delaying factors. This system involves having trays easily accessible and containing instruments and materials needed to perform given procedures in optimum positions.

Benefits accrued by use of these tray setups include adaptability to any procedure, ease of storage, maximization of interruptions to retrieve a forgotten instrument or material, and decrease in time needed for preparing and cleaning operatories.

Trays are either plastic or metal. Plastic trays are lighter in weight and less expensive than metal trays. Moreover, they come in different colors and can be color coded for different procedures. Disadvantages of using plastic trays include their inability to be sterilized and decreased durability. Because metal trays can be autoclaved, they can be opened at the time of use to ensure asepsis. Disadvantages of their use include their cost and inability to be sterilized in small autoclaves.

The instruments and materials that are routinely placed on the trays are those that are used 90% of the time. The arrangement of instruments and materials on the tray is dependent on frequency of use. The more frequently an instrument or material is picked up and placed down, the more convenient and accessible it must be. For example, a tray setup used by an assistant working with a right-handed operator would have the hand instruments located on the left side of the trays. This placement is closest to where they will be used and in the most accessible part of the tray.

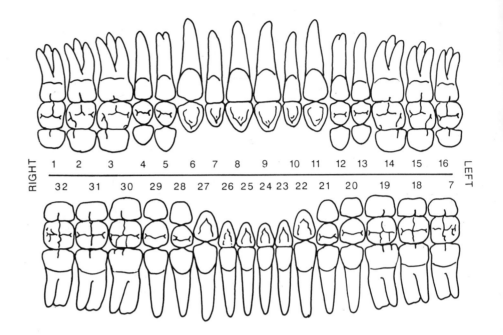

Figure 5–2. The adult dentition.

Hand instruments are placed vertically on an elevated mat to allow the assistant to see and grasp them easily. The tray must be kept orderly, and instruments are replaced in the same position from which they are taken.

CHARTING

Charting is the process of recording the present condition of the hard and soft tissues in the oral cavity. Symbols and abbreviations are used to minimize time and space on the chart. Reasons for accurate charting include facilitating treatment planning and permitting future comparisons of dental lesions. Dental charts also are used to identify persons involved in accidents and in other aspects of forensic dentistry. Accurate record keeping is critical when charting, and dental records may be used legally as evidence in a court of law involving malpractice suits.

Diagnostic tools used by the dental team to chart a patient's oral condition include radiographs, study models, health history, and clinical examination. The dentist using the diagnostic tools dictates the findings to the dental assistant, who records them on the patient's chart. Entries should be made in ink.

The location of each existing restoration and area of the oral cavity to be charted is identified in a standard manner. All tooth surfaces facing the midline are called *mesial*, and those away from the midline are termed *distal*. Surfaces of anterior teeth facing the lips are called *labial*, and those of posterior teeth facing the cheeks are termed *buccal*. All surfaces that face the tongue are called *lingual*. The biting edges of anterior teeth are called *incisal*, and the chewing surfaces of posterior teeth are called *occlusal*.

In addition to the symbols and abbreviations used to transcribe the existing conditions of the oral cavity, a tooth-identification system is used. Several tooth-identification systems can be implemented. The most popular include the Universal system, the Palmer system, and the International system.

The Universal System

The Universal system identifies the adult dentition by numbers 1 through 32. Number 1 is the maxillary right third molar. The numbering proceeds around the maxillary arch to number 16, which is the maxillary left third molar. The mandibular left third molar is number 17, and the numbering again proceeds around the mandibular arch to the mandibular right third molar designated number 32 (Fig. 5–2).

The deciduous dentition is identified by the letters A through T. The letter A is the maxillary right second primary molar, and the lettering proceeds around the maxillary arch to the letter J, which is the maxillary left second primary molar. The mandibular left second primary molar is lettered K, and the lettering proceeds around the mandibular arch to the mandibular right second primary molar, designated by the letter T (Fig. 5–3).

The Palmer System

The Palmer system divides the mouth into quadrants. Each quadrant in the adult dentition consists of the central incisor, numbered 1, to the third molar, numbered 8. For example, the maxillary right 6 represents the maxillary right first molar. The deciduous dentition also is divided into quadrants, with the teeth identified by letters A through E. For example, the maxillary right B represents the maxillary right lateral incisor.

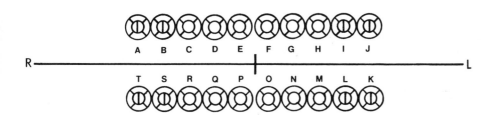

Figure 5–3. The deciduous dentition.

The adult dentition is identified as follows.

```
         8 7 6 5 4 3 2 1 | 1 2 3 4 5 6 7 8
RIGHT   ─────────────────┼─────────────────── LEFT
         8 7 6 5 4 3 2 1 | 1 2 3 4 5 6 7 8
```

The International System

The International system divides the adult and deciduous teeth into quadrants. The adult teeth in each quadrant are numbered 1 through 8, and the deciduous dentition is numbered 1 through 5. Another number placed before the tooth number indicates the quadrant in which the tooth is located. If the first number is 1, it represents the adult maxillary right quadrant, 2 is the adult maxillary left quadrant, 3 is the adult mandibular left quadrant, 4 is the adult mandibular right quadrant, 5 is the deciduous maxillary right quadrant, 6 is the deciduous maxillary left quadrant, 7 is the deciduous mandibular left quadrant, and 8 is the deciduous mandibular right quadrant. In this system, number 32 represents the adult mandibular left lateral incisor, and number 25 represents the maxillary left first molar.

The adult dentition is identified as follows.

```
        18 17 16 15 14 13 12 11 | 21 22 23 24 25 26 27 28
RIGHT  ─────────────────────────┼───────────────────────── LEFT
        48 47 46 45 44 43 42 41 | 31 32 33 34 35 36 37 38
```

Periodontal Charting

A record of periodontal probing depths, recession, tooth mobility, bleeding points, suppuration, and root furcations, indications of periodontal disease activity, is charted using special symbols and abbreviations. These symbols are transferred directly onto the charting form to correspond with the exact location on the tooth. Six separate measurements are taken of each tooth to record periodontal pocket depths (Fig. 5–4).

DENTAL SPECIALTIES

Dental specialties recognized by the dental profession include Dental Public Health, Endodontics, Oral Pathology, Oral and Maxillofacial Surgery, Orthodontics, Pedodontics, Periodontics, and Prosthodontics.

The dental specialist has advanced graduate training in a designated specialty field. More complex or difficult cases often are referred by the general dental practitioner to the dental specialist for treatment. A description of each specialty role follows.

Dental Public Health

Within the purview of public health dentistry fall the areas of community, municipal, state, and national dental health programs. The duties and responsibilities of dentists and auxiliaries depend on the scope of individual programs.

Many public health programs offer public education and prevention-oriented components, whereas others concentrate on research and direct patient care. The assistant's role in public health dentistry can vary greatly. In the direct provision of services, the assistant may perform tasks similar to those of an assistant in any private practice, whereas in public education, prevention, and research areas, he or she might assume complex roles involving the application of a variety of skills.

All clinical functions are regulated by state law, but auxiliaries in certain federal programs may be exempt from state restrictions. As state laws regarding performance of functions vary from state to state, so too do the assistant's responsibilities. Some states permit assistants to perform expanded functions, tasks traditionally performed by dentists. These expanded functions include reversible tasks, such as placing orthodontic separators, placing and removing temporary restorations, and testing pulp vitality.

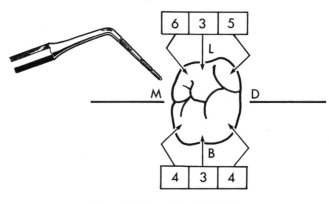

Figure 5–4. Periodontal charting.

Endodontics

Endodontics is the specialty concerned with the treatment of pulpal and periapical diseases of the teeth. Some of the treatments involve pulp capping, pulpotomy, pulpectomy, instrumentation and obturation of infected root canals, and removal of diseased periapical tissues.

All diagnostic tests and aids are designed to help the practitioner make a correct diagnosis. Some of the important tests used by endodontists are as follows. Percussion is checked by striking the crown of the tooth with the handle of an instrument to determine whether a tooth is sensitive. This is done in conjunction with the percussion of adjacent teeth in order to obtain subjective separation of symptoms by the patient. Palpation, the touching of suspected areas, can help determine whether swelling is present. The mobility test, to determine the buccolingual range of movement, in conjunction with a radiograph, helps determine whether the remaining alveolar bone is sufficient to consider restoring the tooth. A radiograph is the most common diagnostic tool because it can help determine what is happening in the periapical areas of suspected teeth. Pulp testing by the use of heat and cold or small amounts of an electric current through the application of an instrument called a vitalometer determine the vitality of a tooth.

Instrumenting the canal removes the infected pulp and prepares the canal for obturation, or filling. The instrumentation is accomplished by using reamers, broaches, and files. Reamers enlarge the canal slightly and are used to measure the length of the canal. Broaches are used to remove the affected nerve and any debris from the canal. Files are used to increase the diameter of the root canal so that it can be filled. All instrumentation is done using an irrigant, which serves to break down the soft tissue in the canal and lubricate the area. The preferred irrigant is sodium hypochlorite diluted with 1 to 2 parts water or hydrogen peroxide. The canals are dried with assorted paper points and medicated. Obturation or filling of the canal is done with gutta percha points and special endodontic condensers or spreaders. The gutta percha material can be compressed and condensed into the canal, sealing the apex. A glass bead sterilizer may be used during endodontic procedures for sterilization of the armamentarium. Once the procedure is completed and the apex of the canal is sealed, the tooth is ready to be fully restored to function.

Oral Pathology

The specialty of oral pathology deals with the abnormal conditions and diseases of the oral cavity and maxillofacial structures. A wide range of pathologic conditions and manifestations may affect the dental patient as a result of developmental disturbances, such as cleft lip or palate. Systemic dysfunctions and infectious diseases, such as AIDS, also may cause oral lesions. Nutritional deficiencies and abnormal growths or tumors are of concern for the oral pathologist.

Specialized tests, such as a biopsy that includes a minor surgical procedure to remove a specimen of the suspicious lesion for further study and analysis, require the expertise of an oral pathologist. Final diagnosis of the abnormal lesion is made by the oral pathologist and documented in a formal laboratory report to the referring general practioner. Appropriate dental treatment for the patient may be conducted by the oral pathologist and oral surgeon in conjunction with the general practioner. This specialty area is addressed in detail in Chapter 4.

Oral and Maxillofacial Surgery

Oral surgery treatment ranges from simple exodontia to the most complicated maxillofacial surgery.

All patients who are scheduled to undergo treatment must undergo assessment of general physical condition, that is, knowledge of a patient's vital signs (pulse, blood pressure, respiration rate, and body temperature), to determine whether a patient can physically sustain the rigors of surgery. More complicated procedures require additional testing.

Preparation for oral surgery also includes treatment of pain and anxiety through premedication. Administration of anesthesia is either local or general, including conscious or unconscious sedation.

During oral surgery, it is mandatory that aseptic techniques be followed to prohibit contamination of the operating field. The assistant must be aware of the proper procedures for handling instruments. This applies to the sterilization of instruments, as well as to their transfer.

The most common oral surgery procedure is the simple extraction. Teeth are removed with specifically designed forceps and elevators. Extractions of impacted teeth, retained roots, or alveolar bone and dental implants are more complicated procedures.

Even more complicated procedures involve the treatment of fractures of the mandible or maxilla and maxillofacial surgery, which may include sectioning portions of the facial area to compensate for abnormalities resulting from genetic or traumatic causes. In addition, treatment of oral cancer falls under the purview of the oral surgeon.

After treatment, a patient might suffer from pain, postoperative bleeding, and swelling. The patient must be protected against the possibility of infection, which requires specific postoperative instructions, including postoperative antibiotic therapy if indicated.

Orthodontics

Orthodontics is the study of the growth and development of the jaws and face. Also included are the position of teeth, influences on development, and prevention and correction of malocclusions.

Malocclusions develop as a result of many factors. Face form, jaw relation, and the final position of the teeth depend greatly on heredity. Anomalies must be corrected to provide proper functioning in the mouth. Additional factors affecting growth of structure are diet, metabolism, and poor habits, such as thumbsucking, mouth breathing, and poor swallowing habits. The number and size of teeth are important and can determine the ability of a person to have a properly functioning mouth.

Three basic classifications of occlusion were developed by Dr. Edward Angle. *Class I occlusion* refers to maxillary and mandibular molars in correct relationship to one another. In a Class I relationship, the mesiobuccal cusp of the maxillary permanent first molar occludes in the buccal groove of the mandibular first molar.

In *Class II occlusion,* the lower molars are in a distal relationship to the maxillary molars, and the lower jaw is retruded, giving the appearance of protruding maxillary anterior teeth. Class II occlusion is further subdivided into two categories. Division I is characterized by V-shaped arches instead of U-shaped arches and by protrusion of the maxillary incisors. Division II of the classification is characterized by maxillary arches that are wider than normal and by maxillary incisors that show a marked lingual inclination with an excessive overbite.

Class III occlusion is characterized by the mandible anterior to its normal position. Mandibular incisors might be in total crossbite in relationship to upper anterior teeth, and maxillary arches might be restricted in growth. The mandible protrudes prominently.

Diagnostic tools for classifying occlusion include clinical examination, health history, tooth relationships, and soft tissue appraisal. In addition, plaster study models, bite records, and cephalometric radiographs are necessary.

Resolution of occlusal problems usually is accomplished by tooth movement through application of measured forces in the desired direction. Teeth are either tipped or moved until they reach their new positions. Some teeth are more resistant than others. For example, molars often are more resistant than are anterior teeth.

Orthodontic treatment can be either preventive or interceptive. Careful diagnosis and early treatment for relatively minor problems can minimize future patient discomfort and expense.

Pedodontics

The area of dentistry concerned with the prevention, diagnosis, and treatment of children's dental problems is called pedodontics. This specialty recognizes that children present special problems to the dentist because of growth and behavioral factors. In addition, prevention and treatment of disease in the child permit identification of future problems in the adult.

Children must be given proper strategies to cope with subjective or objective fears of dental treatment. This area is addressed in detail in Chapter 9. Its importance should not be underestimated.

Care of the pedodontic patient requires recognition that the purpose of treatment is not simply care of the primary dentition but management of the eruption and health of the permanent dentition as well. This involves treatment in all phases of dentistry. Particular attention is paid to prevention in an attempt to prevent caries through fluoride treatments and prophylactic operative procedures.

Thumbsucking is certainly the most common oral habit exhibited by children. It is generally agreed that if this habit is not discontinued by the time the permanent teeth erupt, deleterious effects can occur. The severity of these effects is determined by the position of the finger in the mouth and the amount of force exerted. Other detrimental habits include lip sucking or biting, tongue thrusting, and mouth breathing.

The principles of general dentistry apply to the pedodontic patient, except that the situation is dynamic, since two sets of teeth are involved. It is, therefore necessary, to intercept and prevent the progress of dental disease by early and consistent treatment.

Periodontics

Periodontics is the specialty concerned with the hard and soft tissues that support the teeth. These tissues are the gingiva (free and attached), the attachment apparatus, and alveolar bone.

The primary cause of periodontal disease is bacteria in dental plaque. If plaque is not removed at least once every 24 hours, it begins to calcify and eventually will form calculus. Once the deposit reaches the calculus stage, it can no longer be removed by simple brushing.

Periodontal disease can be recognized with the help of radiographs and clinical examination. A full mouth series of radiographs shows the quantity and quality of alveolar bone loss. The approximate depth of each sulcus can be determined by use of a periodontal probe. Sulci depths in excess of 3 mm are considered a potential for periodontal disease, since the patient has reduced access for proper home care. The most important diagnostic tool, however, is visual inspection of the color, texture, and architecture of the gingiva as well as monitoring attachment loss over time.

Treatment of periodontal disease depends on the disease state. The most common treatment begins with scaling and root planing to remove calculus and plaque. Suggested treatment for disease that has progressed can include gingivectomy or gingivoplasty, periodontal flap surgery with ostectomy or osteoplasty, regenerative surgical therapy, or supportive periodontal therapy.

If after scaling or root planing, residual periodontal pockets or poorly formed gingiva remain with an absence of underlying bony defects but with a sufficient amount of attached gingiva, a gingivectomy or gingivoplasty may be performed.

Gingivectomy refers to removal of tissue, and gingivoplasty indicates reshaping. These procedures are performed only if sufficient healthy gingival tissue remains after these surgeries.

If alveolar bone is involved, a periodontal flap is made to gain access to underlying osseous tissue. An ostectomy or osteoplasty, removal or reshaping of bone, can then be performed in order to return the oral cavity to an acceptable maintainable level of health.

Regenerative surgical therapy is similar to conventional periodontal surgical techniques but incorporates the use of new periodontal materials that can be placed next to the root surface of a periodontally involved tooth to promote regeneration of new attachment fibers of gingival tissues to the surface of the tooth root. Postoperative healing may require special oral hygiene instructions and should be explained to the patient thoroughly by the dental auxiliary before dismissal.

Surgical dental implants may be performed by the periodontist to replace missing teeth. A specially treated metal, usually titanium, is used to form the implant screw or cylinder. Endosteal implants are embedded into the bone and may require more than one visit to fully complete the dental procedure. Through the process of osseointegration, the metal titanium screw integrates directly to the underlying bone, creating a firm stable bond for the insertion of the prosthetic tooth. The dental auxiliary must follow strict surgical sterility procedures throughout the entire procedure to prevent cross-contamination of presterilized implant materials. Patient postoperative instructions and special oral hygiene home care instructions should be given before dismissing the implant patient.

Prosthodontics

The replacement of missing teeth in partially or fully edentulous mouths falls under the specialty area of prosthodontics. The task of replacement is accomplished with either fixed or removable prostheses.

Fixed Prosthetic Appliances. Fixed prosthetic appliances are used to replace missing teeth in the mouth when remaining teeth are sufficiently strong to support such appliances. A fixed prosthetic appliance, when put in place, cannot be removed. This appliance is used to restore normal mastication to keep remaining teeth from moving, as well as for esthetic purposes. Often this kind of appliance is a more satisfactory solution than a removable appliance.

In fabricating a fixed appliance, strong remaining teeth are used as abutments. The cemented bridge is attached to the abutments, which can be shaped to accept different types of retainers. Retainers can be full crowns, three-quarter crowns, onlays, or inlays. The retainers are connected to pontics, which are used to span the edentulous area. In the preferred construction, bridges have two fixed ends. Under very limited circumstances, however, bridges can have single fixed ends or cantilevers.

Frameworks are sets of retainers and pontics that usually are fabricated from precious or semiprecious metals. The esthetic replacement teeth are then fabricated and attached to the framework. These replacement teeth can be made from porcelain fused to the gold or acrylic veneers.

A bridge is designed to rely on satisfactory abutments identified by radiographs and study models. The teeth selected are prepared to accept the retainer. A temporary bridge is then fabricated to judge occlusion, esthetics, and the parallelism of abutments.

Final impressions are taken to make an accurate determination of abutment shape and the relationship of one abutment to another. Materials used for this impression may include hydrocolloids, rubber base, and polyether impression materials.

Final impressions are sent to the laboratory, where cast frameworks are fabricated. These frameworks are then returned to the practitioner to determine whether the fit is correct. An esthetic cover of acrylic or porcelain usually is applied, and the restoration is temporarily and, subsequently, permanently cemented in place.

Removable Prosthetic Appliances. The number of missing teeth helps determine the size and complexity of the removable prosthetic appliance. If the mouth is completely edentulous, full dentures are required. If the remaining teeth can support the forces of mastication, a partial denture can be fabricated. Fabrications of full and of partial prosthetic appliances have some procedures in common, such as preliminary and final impressions and occlusal records. The impressions must be accurate representations of both hard and soft tissue structures. From these impressions, accurate trays for border molding and final impressions are fabricated. The final impression then represents both fixed and movable tissues.

Partial dentures rely on remaining teeth for retention and support. These teeth must be prepared to hold the components of a partial denture. Components of partial dentures include saddles, which lie on the edentulous ridges, clasps, which provide direct retention to the remaining teeth, and connectors, which connect saddles and clasps into a functioning partial denture. The success of a partial denture is a function of the design and interaction of the components (framework). By direct and indirect retention, the final prosthesis should be strong enough to resist the forces of occlusion. Once the framework is completed, bite registrations must be taken. Teeth can then be added to the framework to complete the partial denture.

Full dentures require accurate impressions for retention and comfort. An improperly fitting full denture can cause difficulty in speech, mastication, and retention. Retention depends on the surface area covered, peripheral seal, adhesion, and cohesion.

After final impressions are taken, the dentist takes accurate records of the bite (centric relation), face height (vertical dimension), face form, and tooth size in order to approximate normal structure.

Materials used in making full dentures are acrylic and porcelain. Acrylics are used for both base construction and teeth, but porcelain is used only for teeth.

Questions

DIRECTIONS (Questions 1 through 100): Each of the questions or incomplete statements in this section is followed by four suggested answers or completions. Select the ONE lettered answer or completion that is BEST in each case. Check your answers with the correct answers that follow.

1. Before rendering any type of dental treatment on a patient, the dental auxiliary must

   (A) obtain a complete medical history
   (B) explain the office policy on broken appointments
   (C) approve the patient's dental insurance
   (D) obtain a complete set of radiographs

2. Color coding prepared trays allows for

   (A) more instruments to be placed on the trays
   (B) easy identification of the procedure the tray is prepared for
   (C) quicker autoclaving
   (D) multiple use of each tray

3. Hand instruments on prepared tray setups are placed in

   (A) order of use
   (B) the order the assistant prefers
   (C) size order
   (D) random sequence

4. Which is a technique for holding the high-speed suction tip?

   (A) palm–thumb grasp
   (B) inverted modified pen grasp
   (C) thumb to nose grasp
   (D) pen grasp

5. The assistant's eye level when seated is

   (A) even with that of the dentist
   (B) 4 to 6 inches below that of the dentist
   (C) 4 to 6 inches above the patient's shoulder
   (D) 4 to 6 inches above that of the dentist

6. If a right-handed operator is preparing a mandibular right molar for a crown preparation, the assistant retracts

   (A) the tongue
   (B) the cheek
   (C) both the tongue and cheek
   (D) neither the tongue nor the cheek

7. Protective barriers are necessary when

   (A) confirming appointments
   (B) presenting toothbrush instruction
   (C) ordering supplies
   (D) sterilizing instruments

8. The best position for the instrument tray is

   (A) over the patient
   (B) over the operator's lap
   (C) over the assistant's lap
   (D) in back of the assistant

9. When working in the anterior part of the mouth, the high-speed suction tip is held

   (A) below the incisal edge of the tooth being prepared
   (B) on the opposite side of the tooth being prepared
   (C) in the retromolar area
   (D) in the vestibule

10. How often should the high-speed handpiece be cleaned and lubricated?

    (A) each day
    (B) every other day
    (C) each week
    (D) each month

11. Indirect vision refers to

    (A) looking through protective glasses
    (B) looking through a mirror
    (C) looking directly at an object
    (D) using prism lighting

12. During the administration of local anesthesia, aspiration will

(A) damage the mandibular artery
(B) be extremely painful
(C) determine if the lumen of the needle is in a blood vessel
(D) ensure profound anesthesia

13. The reading that is recorded first when taking blood pressure is the

(A) systolic measurement
(B) diastolic measurement
(C) pulse pressure
(D) respiration rate

14. The patient's clinical record must include

(A) laboratory invoices
(B) medical health questionnaire
(C) study models
(D) insurance forms

15. The assistant holds the hand instrument to be transferred between

(A) thumb and forefinger
(B) small finger and palm
(C) thumb and palm
(D) small finger and forefinger

16. The fulcrum digit used in the modified pen grasp is the

(A) thumb
(B) index finger
(C) middle finger
(D) ring finger

17. If caries is present on the lingual pit of tooth No. 10, it is classified as

(A) Class V
(B) Class IV
(C) Class I
(D) Class III

18. A contraindication to topical anesthetic is

(A) permanent anesthesia
(B) allergic reaction
(C) excess salivation
(D) length of time for it to become effective

19. The matrix band should be removed

(A) firmly with a hemostat
(B) quickly with a sliding motion
(C) slowly in an occlusal direction
(D) quickly through the contact area

20. The color of the nitrous oxide cylinder tank is always

(A) blue
(B) green
(C) yellow
(D) red

21. If a patient jumps out of the chair after being treated in the supine position

(A) he or she will feel giddy
(B) his or her mouth will feel dry
(C) he or she might feel faint
(D) nothing will happen

22. Prepared materials should be held by the assistant

(A) over a waste receptacle
(B) over the prepared tray
(C) over the operator's lap
(D) as close to the area of the operation as possible

23. A mesial occlusal cavity preparation is an example of a

(A) Class I cavity preparation
(B) Class II cavity preparation
(C) Class III cavity preparation
(D) Class IV cavity preparation

24. During the placement of a rubber dam, a blunt instrument can be used to

(A) ligate the rubber dam
(B) invert the rubber dam
(C) punch small holes for the anterior teeth in the rubber dam
(D) secure the clamp

25. The rubber dam napkin is used to

(A) place the dam
(B) secure the dam
(C) avoid irritation around the patient's face
(D) help the patient swallow

26. A lubricant can be used on the rubber dam to

(A) retard the flow of saliva
(B) help clamp the last tooth
(C) repair a torn dam
(D) make it easier for the dam to be slipped between the teeth

27. A cavity preparation that includes the mesial incisal angle of a maxillary central incisor is classified as a

(A) Class I cavity preparation
(B) Class II cavity preparation

(C) Class III cavity preparation
(D) Class IV cavity preparation

28. Debridement of the cavity preparation refers to

(A) resisting dislodgement of filling materials
(B) retaining of filling material in the cavity preparation
(C) removal of debris from the cavity preparation
(D) removal of undermined enamel

29. What is a fulcrum?

(A) the amount of amalgam flow in 24 hours
(B) the maximum amount of amalgam in a cavity preparation
(C) a type of matrix retainer
(D) the stationary point of a lever system

30. During a Class II amalgam procedure, the rubber dam is removed

(A) before checking the patient's occlusion
(B) before condensing the amalgam
(C) before removing the matrix band
(D) after the matrix band is in position

31. Which of the following is NOT used to evaluate an amalgam restoration?

(A) mirror
(B) burnisher
(C) articulating paper
(D) dental floss

32. In application of the rubber dam, which tooth should be used as the anchor tooth?

(A) the tooth being prepared
(B) the most anterior tooth in the quadrant
(C) one or two teeth distal to the tooth being prepared
(D) one or two teeth mesial to the tooth being prepared

33. Removal of the rubber dam is accomplished by

(A) cutting the septal dam before removal
(B) stretching the dam for interproximal removal
(C) a quick snap
(D) stretching the dam with rubber dam forceps

34. Which of the following pieces of equipment should be disinfected after treatment of each patient?

(A) handpieces
(B) curettes
(C) film holders
(D) light handles

35. The purpose of palpating the neck of a patient is

(A) to determine TMJ dysfunction
(B) to feel enlarged lymph nodes
(C) to determine the size of extraoral x-ray film
(D) to make the patient feel more relaxed

36. In a mouth with poor oral hygiene, the white deposit that collects around the gingival margin of the teeth is

(A) dental plaque
(B) stain
(C) calculus
(D) leukoplakia

37. Coronal polishing of the occlusal surfaces is best accomplished with a

(A) prophy brush
(B) rubber cup
(C) porte polisher
(D) toothbrush

38. Instruments used on a patient with a history of hepatitis B should be sterilized by

(A) scrubbing with alcohol
(B) a dry oven for 20 minutes
(C) a cold disinfectant method
(D) a steam sterilization (autoclave) method

39. A good method of keeping a mouth mirror from fogging is

(A) hold it in cold water
(B) sponge it with alcohol
(C) blast it with cool air
(D) rub mirror against patients buccal mucosa

40. A cavity varnish is applied to the

(A) enamel walls only
(B) dentinal tubules only
(C) walls and floor of a cavity preparation
(D) floor of the cavity preparation only

41. Calcium hydroxide is used because it

(A) seals the dentinal tubules
(B) acts as a thermal insulator under metallic restoration
(C) reduces marginal leakage around the restoration
(D) stimulates the formation of secondary dentin

42. When taking an alginate impression of the upper arch the patient should be seated in a (an)

  (A) slightly reclined position with the chin tilted downward
  (B) upright position with head tilted forward
  (C) upright position with head tilted back
  (D) supine position

43. To ensure that the set alginate impression remains firmly attached in the tray during removal from the mouth, a

  (A) water-cooled or perforated tray is used
  (B) perforated or Rim-lock tray is used
  (C) custom-made compound tray is used
  (D) styrofoam disposable tray is used

44. The reason for using a plastic spatula when mixing a composite resin is that the

  (A) material sticks more readily to metal
  (B) cold metal would adversely affect the setting time of the material
  (C) material would become discolored with a metal spatula
  (D) the plastic spatulas are disposable

45. Which of the following statements is true concerning placement of a wedge for a matrix? It should

  (A) separate the teeth slightly
  (B) be placed only when a rubber dam is used
  (C) be placed so that one edge extends below the gingiva
  (D) be placed in the smallest embrasure

46. What type of matrix band is required for molars having deep gingival preparations?

  (A) universal metal matrix bands
  (B) Mylar strips
  (C) wide gingival extension metal molar bands
  (D) Class V contour matrix bands

47. A Tofflemire matrix prepared for tooth No. 28 also can be used on teeth in which other quadrant?

  (A) maxillary left
  (B) mandibular right
  (C) maxillary right
  (D) mandibular left

48. For proper stability and control of an instrument

  (A) grasp handle tightly
  (B) use intraoral fulcrum
  (C) fulcrum where most comfortable
  (D) use modified palm grasp

49. The use of outdated films, stray radiation, or unsafe darkroom light would most likely cause a

  (A) blurred film
  (B) very light film
  (C) clear film
  (D) fogged film

50. A radiation detection badge is essential for use in the dental office to

  (A) protect the x-ray machine from damage caused by overheating
  (B) estimate the radiation absorbed by the wearer
  (C) reduce the exposure of the patient to radiation
  (D) identify the operator as a licensed x-ray technician

51. Before application of a topical anesthetic, the area should be

  (A) rinsed with water
  (B) wiped with an alcohol sponge
  (C) dried with a 2 × 2 gauze
  (D) completely numb

52. A temporary filling is best packed with

  (A) heavy pressure
  (B) a condenser
  (C) a moist cotton pellet
  (D) a ball burnisher

53. What instruments are best suited for removing excess cement from the teeth?

  (A) spatula and scalpel
  (B) a dull chisel and mallet
  (C) ball burnisher and explorer
  (D) explorer and scaler

54. When removing excess cement from teeth

  (A) rest your finger as close as possible to the intraoral site
  (B) use the soft tissue as support
  (C) support your elbow on a strong flat surface
  (D) use finishing strips interproximally

55. When placing a temporary filling, it is NOT important to

  (A) carve detailed anatomy
  (B) seal the margins completely
  (C) make sure it is in proper occlusion
  (D) contact the adjacent tooth

56. The primary use of a matrix band is to

 (A) stabilize the tooth
 (B) provide the missing wall in a proximal surface cavity
 (C) aid in restoring the anatomy to a Class I restoration
 (D) restore more than one tooth at a time in the same quadrant

57. A properly placed Tofflemire matrix band should be

 (A) mounted with the retainer on the lingual side of the arch
 (B) at least 3 mm above the occlusal and 3 mm below the gingival attachment
 (C) at least 2 mm above the occlusal margin and 1 mm below the gingival margin of the preparation
 (D) mounted with the retainer on the buccal side of the maxillary arch and on the lingual side of the mandibular arch

58. A matrix band and wedge may be stabilized with

 (A) greenstick compound
 (B) rubber dam clamp
 (C) dental floss
 (D) inlay wax

59. Which of the following is NOT a hand cutting instrument?

 (A) spoon excavator
 (B) hoe
 (C) gingival margin trimmer
 (D) beavertail burnisher

60. When using a Tofflemire matrix retainer, the diagonal slot should face

 (A) toward the occlusal surface
 (B) toward the lingual surface
 (C) toward the incisal edge
 (D) toward the gingiva

61. Flour of pumice should be moist when used to polish tooth surfaces because

 (A) wet agents abrade faster than dry agents
 (B) wet agents are more abrasive than dry agents
 (C) wet agents cause less frictional heat than do dry agents
 (D) wetting causes alteration of particle size

62. Light pressure should be used when polishing with a rubber cup so as not to cause the cup to

 (A) flange into the gingival sulcus
 (B) fray
 (C) unscrew from the prophy angle
 (D) cause any unnecessary frictional heat

63. An example of an extrinsic stain is

 (A) blackline stain
 (B) tetracycline stain
 (C) hypoplasia stain
 (D) silver nitrate stain

64. Tin oxide may be used as a polishing agent for

 (A) acrylic restorations
 (B) metallic restorations
 (C) porcelain crowns
 (D) ortho appliances

65. Tying dental floss around the rubber dam clamp

 (A) ligates it more securely to the tooth
 (B) keeps the rubber dam in place
 (C) prevents accidental swallowing of the clamp
 (D) is really never done

66. In order to provide a tight seal around the teeth and prevent saliva from leaking while using a rubber dam

 (A) coronal polish the teeth first
 (B) invaginate the rubber dam
 (C) use a No. 212 rubber dam clamp
 (D) stabilize with greenstick compound

67. The rubber dam clamp should fit

 (A) on the middle third of the tooth
 (B) about 1 mm above the gingival margin
 (C) below the rubber dam on the gingiva
 (D) loosely without causing pressure on the tooth

68. When seating the rubber dam clamp

 (A) the lingual jaws are placed first
 (B) the buccal jaws are placed first
 (C) both are placed at the same time
 (D) it makes no difference

69. The most common form of fluoride used with the rigid tray system is

 (A) sodium fluoride (NaF)
 (B) stannous fluoride paste
 (C) liquid fluoride supplements
 (D) acidulated phosphate fluoride gel

70. A porous, volcanic stone commonly used as an abrasive agent is

 (A) silicone dioxide
 (B) rouge
 (C) pumice
 (D) tripoli

71. Before pulp testing the teeth with a vitalometer, the teeth must be

    (A) polished
    (B) dried
    (C) moistened
    (D) flossed

72. A very low reading on the vitalometer (0–1) probably indicates

    (A) hyperemia
    (B) necrotic pulp
    (C) dead pulp
    (D) normal pulp

73. When testing the pulp of a tooth with an electric pulp tester, a high reading (9–10) indicates that the tooth is

    (A) hyperemic
    (B) near death
    (C) nonvital
    (D) normal

74. Before placing an x-ray film in the patient's mouth, the auxiliary must perform all of the following EXCEPT

    (A) place a lead apron on the patient
    (B) remove any appliances from the patient's mouth
    (C) perform preliminary oral inspection
    (D) chart existing restorations

75. Obtaining a measurement of the length of the root canal ensures

    (A) profound anesthesia
    (B) not irritating the periapical tissues by extending instruments beyond the apex of the root
    (C) a sterile root canal
    (D) no future pain

76. An important principle during instrumentation of a root canal is the

    (A) extension of the instrument 2 mm beyond the apex of the tooth
    (B) forcing of the instrument to the apex of the root
    (C) sequential use of instruments
    (D) rotary motion of the instrument

77. Endodontic files are used

    (A) to enlarge the root canal
    (B) to remove the contents of the pulp chamber
    (C) as drains in an endodontic abscess
    (D) to reduce the occlusal forces on an endodontically treated tooth

78. The rubber dam is used in endodontics

    (A) to prevent the patient from breathing through his or her mouth
    (B) for asepsis
    (C) to accomplish quadrant dentistry
    (D) to prevent the patient from seeing the instruments

79. Gutta percha is used to

    (A) irrigate the root canal
    (B) gain access to the root canal
    (C) fill the root canal
    (D) sterilize the root canal

80. An apicoectomy is the

    (A) chemical sterilization of the root apex
    (B) root canal treatment of primary teeth
    (C) procedure performed before reinforcing an endodontically treated tooth
    (D) surgical removal of the apex of the root

81. Hemisection refers to

    (A) an irreversible pulpitis
    (B) a desensitizing solution
    (C) the removal of a root from a multirooted tooth
    (D) the removal of the root apex

82. A postextraction dressing can be used

    (A) on all surgical sites
    (B) only after third molar extractions
    (C) when blood begins to ooze from the alveolus
    (D) when there is loss of the blood clot in an extraction site

83. After an extraction, the best technique to stop bleeding is

    (A) medicating with antibiotics
    (B) applying indirect pressure
    (C) applying direct pressure
    (D) placing a drain in the extraction socket

84. Rinsing with warm salt water

    (A) causes clot formation
    (B) helps relieve pain
    (C) causes edema
    (D) decreases the number of oral microbes

85. The suture material that can be resorbed by the body is

    (A) gut
    (B) nylon
    (C) similar to floss
    (D) extra fine grade

86. Postextraction dressings are removed and changed

   (A) when the sutures are removed
   (B) every 1 to 2 days as needed
   (C) once a week
   (D) after clot formation

87. When removing sutures, you must cut

   (A) anywhere, as long as you can get the suture out
   (B) in back of the knot and pull knot through tissue
   (C) just below the knot with suture scissors
   (D) the knot off, then remove suture gently with a hemostat

88. In treatment of a dry socket, first irrigate the alveolus with

   (A) alcohol
   (B) cold water
   (C) fluoride mouthrinse
   (D) warm saline solution

89. When placing a periodontal dressing, it is necessary to

   (A) ligate with dental tape for stability
   (B) festoon the surface of the dressing for esthetics
   (C) allow sutures to be exposed
   (D) extend a large bulk of material well into the vestibule for strength

90. Instructions after periodontal surgery should include all of the following EXCEPT

   (A) no smoking
   (B) no spicy or hot foods
   (C) disclosing instructions
   (D) high protein diet

91. A periodontal dressing is analogous to

   (A) cleaning teeth
   (B) suturing
   (C) a mouth bandage
   (D) protecting the periodontium from plaque

92. Preparation of an anesthetic syringe by the assistant includes all of the following EXCEPT

   (A) engaging the stylet
   (B) placing the anesthetic in the carpule
   (C) placement of the carpule in the syringe
   (D) loosening the cap covering the needle

93. The assistant adjusts the bevel of the needle for a mandibular injection so

   (A) it is parallel to the mandible
   (B) it is perpendicular to the mandible
   (C) it is at a 45-degree angle to the mandible
   (D) it is at a 45-degree angle to the maxilla

94. Nitrous oxide is classified as a (an)

   (A) local anesthetic
   (B) analgesic
   (C) barbiturate
   (D) narcotic

95. Which of the following is a description of a patient receiving the proper level of nitrous oxide?

   (A) dilated pupils, high blood pressure
   (B) excitement, muscles relaxed
   (C) unconscious, respiration slow, blood pressure elevated
   (D) muscles relaxed, pupils normal, blood pressure lowered

96. Before administering nitrous oxide to the patient

   (A) instruct patient to breathe through mouth
   (B) give oxygen for 2 minutes
   (C) administer anesthesia
   (D) apply a rubber dam

97. Which does NOT apply to nitrous oxide sedation?

   (A) instruct patient to hold breath for 30 seconds, then inhale
   (B) instruct patient to breathe through the nose
   (C) reassure patient and project positive thoughts
   (D) never leave a room while patient is under nitrous oxide

98. What is the treatment when a patient reaches the excitement stage of nitrous oxide sedation?

   (A) no treatment necessary
   (B) give more anesthesia or wait until drug wears off
   (C) decrease nitrous flow
   (D) increase nitrous flow

99. On the nitrous oxide unit, the flowmeter

   (A) indicates the pressure of gas within the cylinder
   (B) controls the breathing bag gas reservoir flow
   (C) provides operator with a guide to the flow of volume of gas to patient
   (D) transports gas from unit to mask

100. When working with nitrous oxide, all of the following apply EXCEPT

   (A) monitor vital signs before administration
   (B) work in well-ventilated room
   (C) nosepiece must be sterilized
   (D) auxiliary may administer nitrous oxide if requested by patient

DIRECTIONS (Questions 101 through 113): For each of the items in this section, ONE or MORE of the numbered options is correct. Choose answer

A if only 1, 2, and 3 are correct
B if only 1 and 3 are correct
C if only 2 and 4 are correct
D if only 4 is correct
E if all are correct

101. Factors that determine instrument selection for restorative procedures are the

    (1) color shade of the tooth
    (2) surface of the tooth being restored
    (3) number of teeth in a patient's mouth
    (4) tooth being restored

102. The rubber cup prophylaxis is indicated before placement of the rubber dam to

    (1) polish the anterior restorations
    (2) polish the posterior restorations
    (3) remove the calculus
    (4) avoid displacement of debris under the gingiva

103. Plaque control programs should contain

    (1) oral physiotherapy instructions
    (2) nutritional counseling
    (3) behavioral modification techniques
    (4) clinical examinations

104. During coronal polishing procedures, the assistant may polish

    (1) removable appliances
    (2) fixed bridges
    (3) gold restorations
    (4) synthetic restorations

105. Using a mouth mirror during an oral examination, the dental assistant may chart

    (1) obvious lesions
    (2) existing restorations
    (3) missing teeth
    (4) periodontal pockets

106. Functions of a good recall system may include

    (1) provide reinforcement and correct any bad dental habits
    (2) a prophy and fluoride treatment
    (3) examination and evaluation by the dentist
    (4) diagnosis of x-rays by the auxiliary

107. The mouth mirror may be used to

    (1) retract the cheeks
    (2) retract the tongue
    (3) reflect light
    (4) provide indirect vision

108. Wearing gloves can aid in preventing the contraction of

    (1) epilepsy
    (2) angina
    (3) subacute bacterial endocarditis
    (4) hepatitis

109. When cementing temporary crowns

    (1) the amount of cement placed in the temporary crown depends on the type of crown
    (2) a thick mix of cement is used so the bond is stronger
    (3) the occlusion is checked after cementation and then adjusted
    (4) it is not necessary to remove excess cement interproximally because it helps maintain good contacts

110. When applying pit and fissure sealants, it is best to

    (1) use zinc phosphate cement
    (2) use protective eyewear
    (3) test occlusion and contacts
    (4) apply a rubber dam

111. Glass ionomer cements may be used for

    (1) permanent restorations
    (2) luting procedures
    (3) insulating bases
    (4) sealants

112. When teaching toothbrushing, the important emphasis should be on

    (1) brushing at least once a day
    (2) brushing three times a day
    (3) brushing before bedtime
    (4) complete removal of plaque regardless of brushing time

113. Hand cutting instruments are used in restorative dentistry to

    (1) remove deep carious lesions
    (2) refine cavity preparations
    (3) trim excess restorative material
    (4) invaginate a rubber dam

DIRECTIONS (Questions 114 through 165): Each of the questions or incomplete statements in this section is followed by four suggested answers or completions. Select the ONE lettered answer or completion that is BEST in each case. Check your answers with the correct answers that follow.

114. A supplementary finger rest is one where

   (A) the assistant assists the assistant
   (B) you use a finger of your left hand both as a retractor and as a finger rest for your right hand
   (C) the pinky is used to supplement the rest
   (D) an extra oral fulcrum is used to stabilize the instrument or handpiece

115. After topical fluoride application, the patient should be instructed not to eat, drink, rinse, or brush their teeth for

   (A) 5 minutes
   (B) 10 minutes
   (C) 30 minutes
   (D) 1 hour

116. When preparing which of the following cavity preparations would a miniature head on a handpiece be most useful?

   (A) the occlusal surface of a mandibular premolar
   (B) the buccal surface of the maxillary third molar
   (C) the incisal edge of a lower incisor
   (D) the proximal surface of an upper incisor

117. Which technique of drying a cavity preparation can be injurious to the pulp?

   (A) cotton pledgets
   (B) short blasts of air
   (C) a steady stream of air
   (D) use of 2 × 2 gauze

118. A supply company informs the office that an item that has been ordered is not available and will be shipped when it arrives. This is known as

   (A) a back order
   (B) an extra supply
   (C) deficit spending
   (D) a credit

119. Radiation exposure time for an edentulous patient should be

   (A) increased by 25%
   (B) the same as a dentulous patient
   (C) reduced by 25%
   (D) reduced by 50%

120. What part of the partial denture holds it to the abutment tooth?

   (A) the saddle area
   (B) the rigid connector
   (C) the surveyor
   (D) the clasp

121. The part of the partial denture that lies over the ridge is called the

   (A) saddle
   (B) rigid connector
   (C) surveyor
   (D) clasp

122. The function of the preliminary impression in full denture construction is to

   (A) construct wax rims
   (B) help mount final casts
   (C) construct a custom-made tray
   (D) help make adjustments after insertion

123. A facebow is used to

   (A) insert the denture in the patient's mouth
   (B) contour the wax rims
   (C) mount the upper cast on an articulator
   (D) check the bite

124. Wax bite blocks are used to

   (A) record vertical dimension
   (B) determine sore spots
   (C) construct custom-made trays
   (D) flask dentures

125. The portion of the denture that should not be polished is the

   (A) part touching the tongue
   (B) part contacting the denture-bearing mucosa
   (C) part touching the cheeks
   (D) all parts must be polished

126. The purpose of relining a denture is to

   (A) alter the occlusion
   (B) fill in the voids of the denture base for better readaptation
   (C) make a custom-made tray
   (D) take a bite registration

127. New dentures will most likely cause

   (A) sore spots
   (B) stains of the teeth
   (C) swelling of lymph nodes
   (D) occlusal trauma

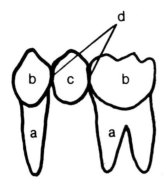

Figure 5–5.

128. An immediate denture

(A) is constructed in one visit
(B) is made of shellac
(C) replaces only the anterior teeth
(D) is inserted during the same appointment in which the remaining teeth are extracted

129. Tissue conditioning

(A) is used to help final casts
(B) takes place at the time the denture is inserted in the patient's mouth
(C) returns unhealthy tissue under a denture to a healthy state
(D) is accomplished by using wax rims

130. Shade selection is accomplished using

(A) natural light
(B) the dental light
(C) fluorescent light
(D) black light

131. A function of a fixed bridge is

(A) to help move teeth
(B) to prevent movement of teeth
(C) to make cleaning easier
(D) to improve speech

132. The teeth that support a fixed bridge are called (refer to Fig. 5–5)

(A) abutments
(B) pontics
(C) ridge laps
(D) partials

133. What type of restoration is used to reinforce an endodontically treated tooth before a crown is fabricated?

(A) an acrylic core
(B) a copper band

(C) an aluminum shell
(D) a gold post

134. Cantilever bridges

(A) are the most common bridges made
(B) are used only to replace molars
(C) always use three abutments
(D) have abutments on only one side

135. The primary function of a temporary bridge is

(A) to assist in final shade selection
(B) to help move teeth
(C) to protect teeth from thermal and contact sensitivity
(D) to improve occlusion

136. Epinephrine-impregnated cord is used to

(A) stimulate a patient who has fainted
(B) dry the prepared tooth
(C) tie stone dies together
(D) stop gingival bleeding and retract the gingiva

137. The function of the periodontium is to

(A) prevent caries
(B) support the teeth
(C) prevent vertical food impaction
(D) aid the tongue in cleansing the teeth

138. What is gingivitis?

(A) inflammation of the soft tissues surrounding the teeth
(B) inflammation of the cortical bone
(C) inflammation of the teeth
(D) inflammation around the apical foramen

139. What is periodontitis?

(A) inflammation of the soft tissue that surrounds the teeth
(B) inflammation of teeth
(C) the stage of periodontal disease involving loss of bone that supports the teeth
(D) the removal of soft tooth-accumulated material

140. Another name for Vincent's disease is

(A) acute necrotizing ulcerative gingivitis
(B) acute ear infection
(C) aphthous ulcer
(D) herpetic lesions

141. A furcation in periodontics refers to

(A) a surgical procedure
(B) mobility of anterior teeth
(C) the radicular area of multirooted teeth
(D) a dry mouth

142. A splint is an appliance that

(A) holds broken teeth together
(B) connects and stabilizes mobile teeth
(C) holds soft tissue against bone
(D) keeps sutures covered after surgery

143. Which coolant is used with the ultrasonic scaler?

(A) air
(B) water
(C) alcohol
(D) no coolant is necessary

144. Osteoplasty is the

(A) recontouring of gingival tissue
(B) recontouring of bony defects
(C) implanting of bone
(D) treatment of choice in gingivitis

145. Gingivectomy is the

(A) surgical removal of the mucogingival
    junction
(B) surgical removal of the apex of a tissue
(C) replacement of inflamed gingival tissue
(D) surgical elimination of the gingival pocket

146. Incision and drainage are used to treat a

(A) periodontal abscess
(B) granuloma
(C) cyst
(D) furcation

147. The method used to remove periodontal dressings is

(A) use beaks of cotton pliers to catch edges and
    use a teasing motion
(B) use fingernail to catch edge of dressing and
    remove
(C) with cotton pliers forcibly pull material away
    from tissue
(D) use an ultrasonic scaler

148. An abscess is

(A) a collection of serous fluid
(B) a pathway for fluid drainage
(C) a localized collection of pus
(D) always infrabony in nature

149. The armamentarium for suture removal includes

(A) periodontal probe
(B) surgical scissors

(C) surgical forceps
(D) rongeur

150. Drugs that are used for the relief of pain of low intensity are classified as

(A) hypnotics
(B) sedatives
(C) analgesics
(D) narcotics

151. The condition in which a patient lacks oxygen is called

(A) hyperventilation
(B) hypoxia
(C) anoxia
(D) syncope

152. If you had an emergency in the office involving syncope what would you be treating?

(A) headache
(B) hyperventilation
(C) cardiac arrest
(D) fainting

153. A patient having an angina attack suffers from what medical problem?

(A) diabetes
(B) heart trouble
(C) high blood pressure
(D) fever

154. Which of the following is most descriptive of someone in shock?

(A) face pale, strong pulse, breathing regular
(B) nervousness, face flushed, pulse rapid
(C) skin cool and clammy, weak pulse, breathing
    irregular
(D) nausea, rapid breathing, strong pulse

155. The average range for blood pressure is

(A) 120/80
(B) 140/100
(C) 160/80
(D) 180/60

156. The average pulse rate per minute is

(A) 60–72
(B) 93–98
(C) 50–60
(D) 72–90

157. Without premedication, subacute bacterial endocarditis is a potential danger when working on a patient with a history of

    (A) scarlet fever
    (B) heart murmur or defect
    (C) venereal disease
    (D) hepatitis

158. The Certified Dental Assistant may dispense medication to the patient

    (A) after oral surgery
    (B) by checking labels and amount of drugs
    (C) after checking for allergies the patient may have
    (D) under direct supervision of the dentist

159. The Dental Practice Act

    (A) is operated as an agency of the federal government
    (B) is under the jurisdiction of the American Dental Association
    (C) defines the practice and regulates dentistry in each state
    (D) certifies dental assistants

160. Removal of the coronal portion of the pulp is called

    (A) pulp capping
    (B) pulpotomy
    (C) apical retention
    (D) indirect pulp capping

161. What appliances are used to maintain the space of a prematurely lost second primary molar?

    (A) a space opener
    (B) a space maintainer
    (C) a space saver
    (D) it is not necessary to maintain this space

162. Full coverage of a deciduous molar usually indicates the use of

    (A) an amalgam crown
    (B) an acrylic crown
    (C) a stainless steel crown
    (D) a porcelain crown

163. A mixed dentition consists of

    (A) deciduous and permanent teeth existing simultaneously in a child's mouth
    (B) deciduous teeth in the wrong places
    (C) permanent teeth that are rotated
    (D) permanent teeth in the wrong places

164. The best way to prevent gagging during impression taking is to

    (A) use cold water when mixing the alginate
    (B) fill tray as much as possible

    (C) instruct patient to breathe through their nose and not through the mouth
    (D) take the upper arch impression first

165. Angle's classification of malocclusion is based on the

    (A) shape of the maxilla
    (B) relationship between the first molars and the orbit of the eye
    (C) relationship between the maxillary and mandibular first molars
    (D) number of teeth in the mandible

DIRECTIONS (Questions 166 through 195): Match the instruments in Column A with their primary function in Column B.

COLUMN A	COLUMN B
166. Broach	A. absorbs moisture in the root canal
167. Reamer	B. extirpates the pulpal contents
168. Luer-Lok syringe	C. carries irrigating solution to the canal
169. Paper-point	D. gains entrance and cleanses the root canal
170. Plugger	E. assists in condensing gutta percha into the canal

COLUMN A	COLUMN B
171. Matrix band	A. compresses amalgam into the cavity preparation
172. Gingival margin trimmer	B. limits the filling material to the confines of the tooth
173. Amalgam condenser	C. places amalgam into the cavity preparation
174. Cleoid-discoid carver	D. carves the restoration
175. Amalgam carrier	E. removes undermined enamel

COLUMN A	COLUMN B
176. Ultrasonic scaler	A. hand instrument used to remove supragingival calculus
177. Curette	B. measures the distance between the gingiva and the bone
178. Sickle scaler	C. removes the crevicular epithelium
179. Periodontal probe	D. used to coronal polish all surfaces of teeth
180. Rubber cup	E. its vibrating movement knocks debris off teeth

COLUMN A	COLUMN B
181. Heatless stone	A. smooths roughness in metals
182. Rag wheel	B. grossly reduces an acrylic prosthesis
183. Mandrel	C. holds unmounted stones
184. Vulcanite bur	D. polishes acrylic prosthesis with pumice
185. Rubber wheel	E. grossly reduces a metal prosthesis

COLUMN A	COLUMN B
186. Plastic instrument	A. helps seat crowns
187. Locking college pliers	B. holds medicated cotton pledgets
188. Leather mallet	C. inserts composite filling material
189. Chisel	D. carries alginate impression material
190. Rim-lock tray	E. removes unsupported enamel

COLUMN A	COLUMN B
191. Bur No. 8	A. tapered fissure bur
192. Bur No. 33	B. cross-cut fissure bur
193. Bur No. 57	C. inverted cone bur
194. Bur No. 558	D. small round bur
195. Bur No. ½	E. large round bur

DIRECTIONS: To answer questions 196 through 215, refer to the instrument tray setups in the cited illustrations.

Match the lettered illustrations in Figure 5–6 with the corresponding questions.

196. Identify the curette, periodontal probe, and syringe

   (A) B, D, and F
   (B) C, J, and N
   (C) I, K, and M
   (D) O, H, and A

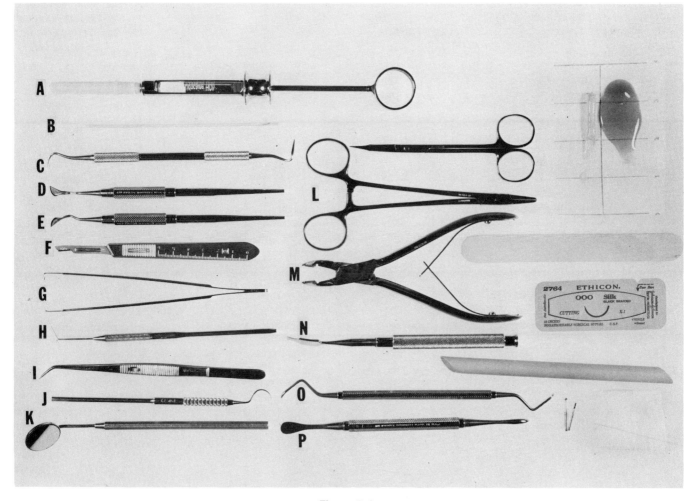

Figure 5–6.

197. Identify the interproximal knife, pocket marker, and locked college pliers

   (A) C, G, and I
   (B) E, J, and O
   (C) G, K, and M
   (D) L, M, and P

198. Identify the ronguers, scalpel, and topical anesthetic applicator

   (A) C, J, and E
   (B) I, L, and D
   (C) M, F, and B
   (D) O, K, and N

199. Identify the needle holder, periosteal elevator, and the bone chisel

   (A) C, O, and M
   (B) E, J, and K
   (C) G, D, and H
   (D) L, P, and N

Match the lettered illustrations in Figure 5–7 with the corresponding questions.

200. Identify the plastic instrument, stainless steel crowns, and spatula

   (A) B, K, and C
   (B) D, J, and G
   (C) H, E, and K
   (D) A, F, and B

201. Identify the base applicator, dappen dish, and locking pliers

   (A) B, K, and C
   (B) D, J, and G
   (C) H, E, and K
   (D) A, F, and B

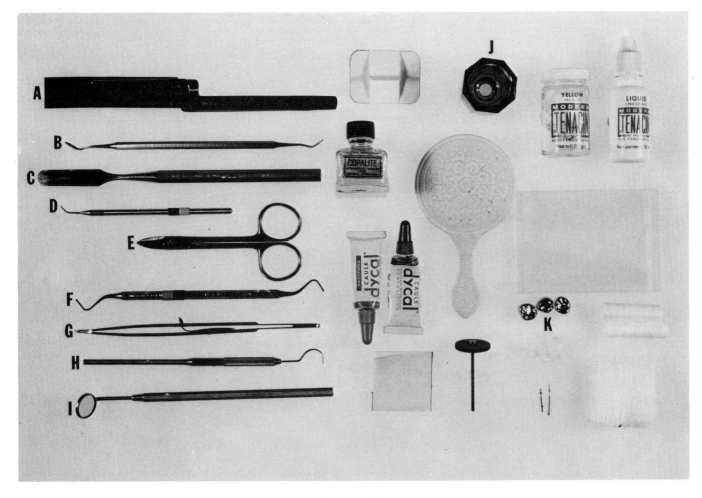

Figure 5–7.

202. Identify the explorer, spoon excavator, and crown and collar scissors

   (A) B, D, and E
   (B) D, E, and F
   (C) H, F, and E
   (D) A, F, and G

Match the lettered illustrations in Figure 5–8 with the corresponding questions.

203. Identify the anterior rubber dam clamp, high volume evacuation tip, and rubber dam frame

   (A) G, B, and F
   (B) H, E, and D
   (C) J, C, and A
   (D) K, D, and B

204. Identify the rubber dam punch, rubber dam clamp forceps, and premolar rubber dam clamp

   (A) A, F, and G
   (B) B, C, and I
   (C) C, D, and H
   (D) E, A, and J

205. Identify the rubber dam, scissors, and No. 26 molar rubber dam clamp

   (A) F, A, and K
   (B) G, H, and F
   (C) C, D, and J
   (D) D, B, and J

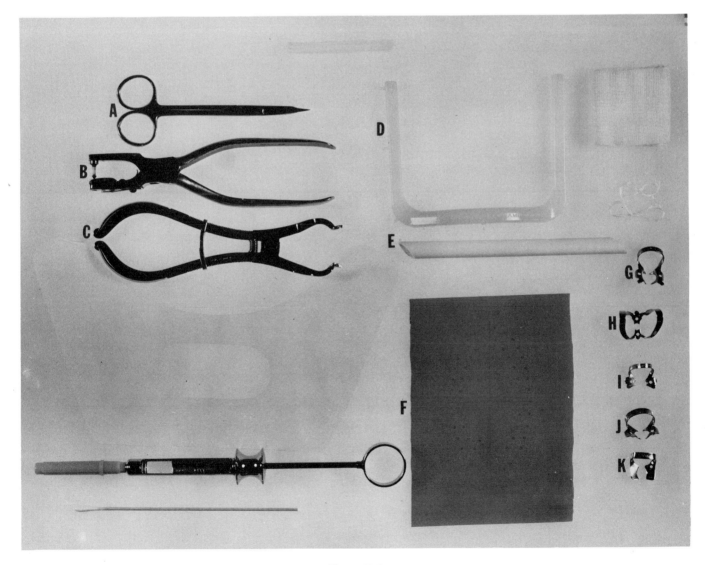

Figure 5–8.

Match the lettered illustrations in Figure 5–9 with the corresponding questions.

206. Identify the orthodontic bands, band pusher, and ligature wire

  (A) I, D, and A
  (B) H, I, and F
  (C) B, H, and D
  (D) J, E, and H

207. Identify the band removing pliers, band seater, and scaler

  (A) A, D, and I
  (B) B, A, and F
  (C) D, H, and C
  (D) E, B, and J

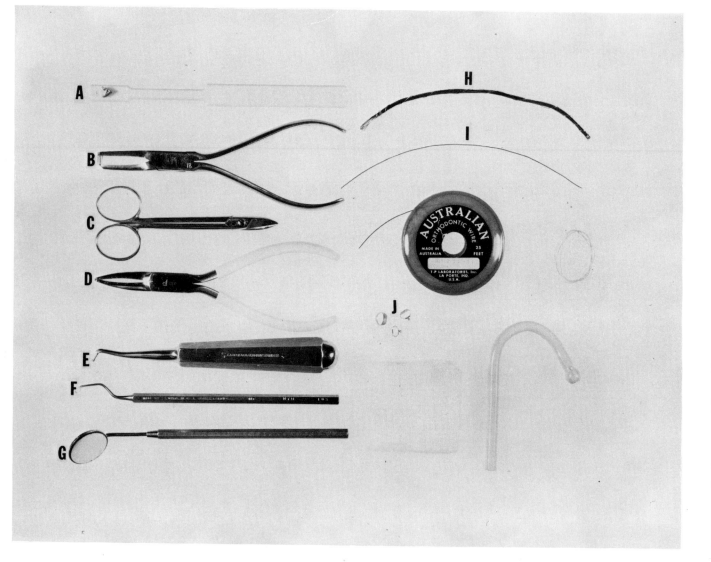

Figure 5–9.

Match the lettered illustrations in Figure 5–10 with the corresponding questions.

208. Identify the vulcanite burs, rubber impression syringe, and retraction cord

    (A) A, B, and I
    (B) D, C, and E
    (C) H, G, and B
    (D) I, A, and C

209. Identify the retraction instrument, spatula, and perforated trays

    (A) A, G, and H
    (B) C, I, and G
    (C) C, G, and H
    (D) E, C, and I

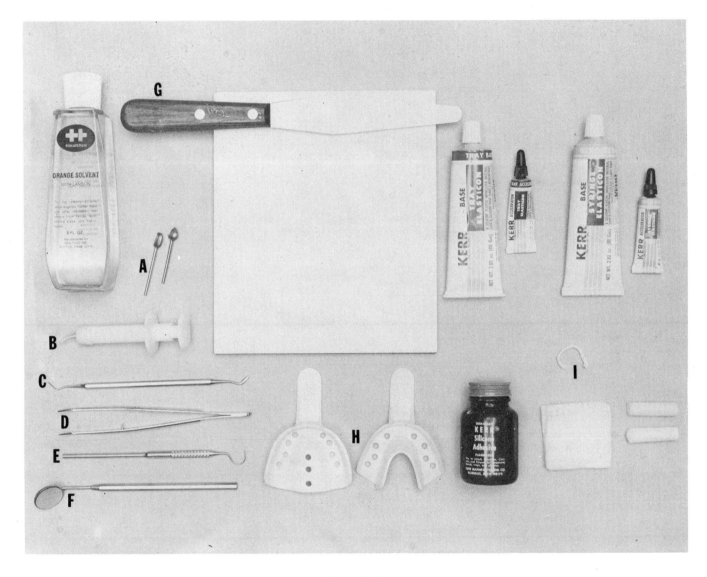

Figure 5–10.

Match the lettered illustrations in Figure 5–11 with the corresponding questions.

210. Identify the needle holder, bone file, and syringe

    (A) A, H, and L
    (B) C, E, and F
    (C) D, G, and K
    (D) I, J, and L

211. Identify the surgical curette, straight elevator, and tissue forceps

    (A) B, C, and I
    (B) K, C, and F
    (C) E, H, and J
    (D) G, I, and L

212. Identify the tissue forceps, scissors, and scalpel

    (A) J, I, and B
    (B) D, G, and L
    (C) E, H, and K
    (D) F, K, and L

213. Identify the surgical suction, mouth mirror, and periosteal elevator

    (A) C, E, and G
    (B) K, H, and E
    (C) E, G, and D
    (D) H, G, and D

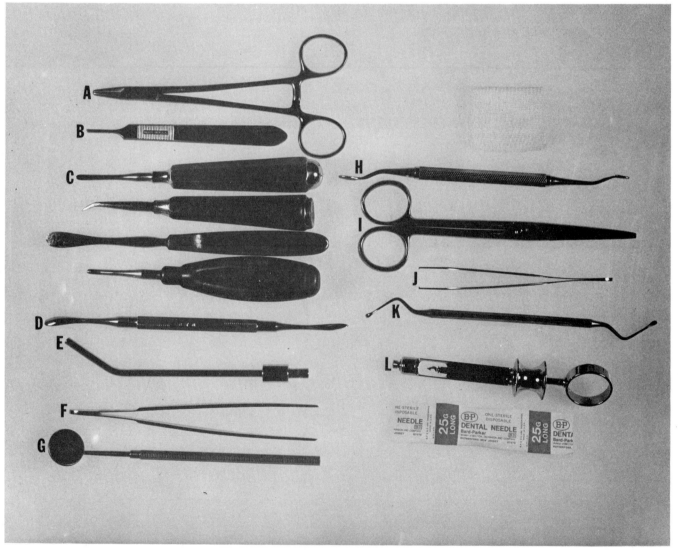

Figure 5–11.

Match the lettered illustrations in Figure 5–12 with the corresponding questions.

214. Identify the composite finishing burs, composite matrices, and straight chisel

    (A) I, M, and J
    (B) E, D, and H
    (C) C, G, and F
    (D) M, B, and H

215. Identify the composite placement instrument, enamel hoe, and No. 17 explorer

    (A) C, G, and J
    (B) F, D, and K
    (C) H, A, and I
    (D) J, B, and E

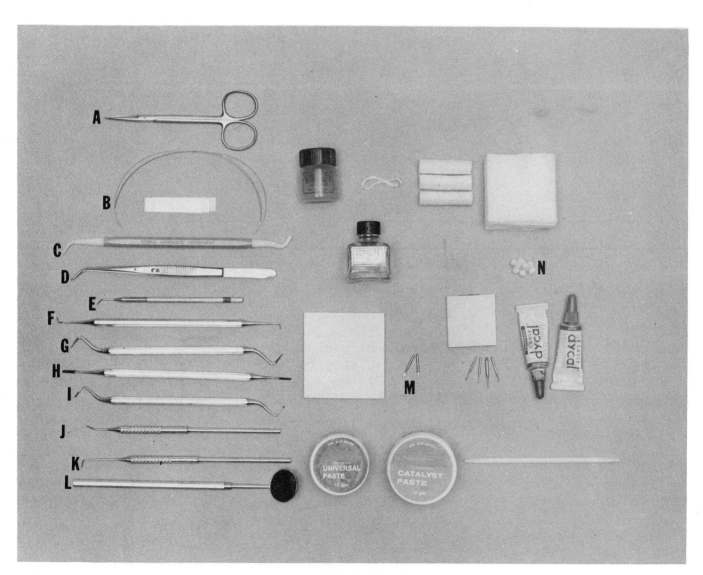

Figure 5–12.

Charting Exercises

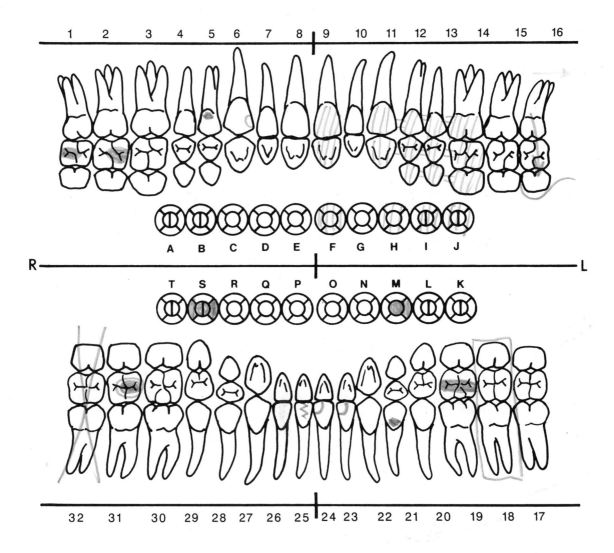

All test questions appearing on the examination related to charting use the Universal system of tooth identification. Any type of symbol or abbreviation may be used to chart items in the charting exercises. Do not use words to chart conditions. (Review pages 76 through 77 before beginning charting exercises.)

DIRECTIONS: Read each item in the charting exercise and record it on the dental chart provided. Any type of symbol or abbreviation may be used to chart conditions. Do not use words. Refer only to the dental chart you have completed when answering the charting questions for each of the charting exercises.

EXERCISE 1

Charting Items

1. The maxillary right third molar has distal occlusal decay.
2. The maxillary right second molar has a mesial occlusal amalgam restoration present.
3. The maxillary right first premolar has a Class V buccal composite restoration present.
4. The maxillary right canine has a Class III mesial composite restoration that must be replaced.
5. The maxillary left central incisor has a full crown present.
6. There is a fixed bridge between the maxillary left canine and the maxillary left first molar replacing the maxillary left first and second premolars.
7. The maxillary left third molar is vertically impacted.
8. The mandibular left second molar is missing.
9. The mandibular left first molar has a mesial occlusal distal amalgam restoration present.
10. The mandibular left first premolar has a Class V buccal gold foil restoration present and distal occlusal decay.
11. The mandibular left lateral incisor has a Class IV mesial incisal composite restoration present.
12. The mandibular left central incisor has Class IV mesial decay.
13. The mandibular right central incisor is fractured midway down the crown.
14. The mandibular right second premolar has a mesial occlusal distal amalgam restoration present.
15. The mandibular right second molar has a mesial occlusal amalgam restoration present with recurrent decay around the margins.
16. The mandibular right third molar is to be extracted.

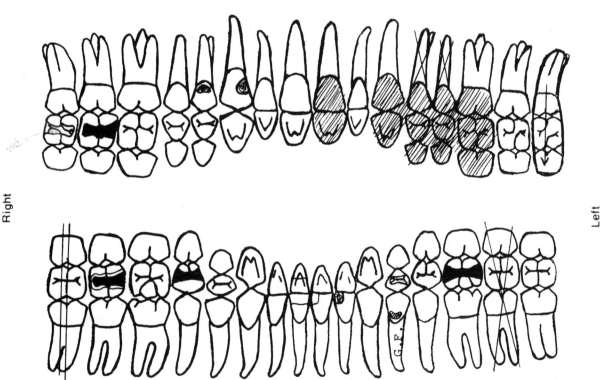

Right   Left

Figure 5–13. Sample completed chart for Exercise 1.

Charting Exercise 1

DIRECTIONS (Questions 216 through 227): Each of the questions or incomplete statements in this section is followed by four suggested answers or completions. Select the ONE lettered answer or completion that is BEST in each case. Check your answers with the correct answers that follow.

216. How many teeth are missing?

    (A) 1
    (B) 3
    (C) 5
    (D) 7

217. How many teeth need restorations?

    (A) 2
    (B) 4
    (C) 6
    (D) 8

218. How many teeth have existing restorations?

    (A) 2
    (B) 6
    (C) 10
    (D) 14

219. Which tooth is to be extracted?

    (A) maxillary left third molar
    (B) mandibular left second molar
    (C) mandibular left central incisor
    (D) mandibular right third molar

220. How many teeth are replaced with a fixed bridge?

    (A) 1
    (B) 2
    (C) 3
    (D) 4

221. What restoration exists on the mandibular left first premolar?

    (A) a composite restoration
    (B) an amalgam restoration
    (C) a gold foil restoration
    (D) a full crown

222. How many amalgam restorations are present?

    (A) 2
    (B) 4
    (C) 6
    (D) 8

223. What classification of restoration is needed on the maxillary right canine?

    (A) Class I
    (B) Class II

(C) Class III
(D) Class IV

224. How many teeth need distal occlusal restorations?

    (A) 1
    (B) 2
    (C) 3
    (D) 4

225. Which tooth is fractured?

    (A) maxillary right central incisor
    (B) maxillary left third molar
    (C) mandibular left lateral incisor
    (D) mandibular right central incisor

226. How many composite restorations exist?

    (A) 1
    (B) 2
    (C) 3
    (D) 4

227. Which tooth exhibits recurrent decay?

    (A) mandibular right second molar
    (B) maxillary right canine
    (C) mandibular left first molar
    (D) maxillary right second molar

EXERCISE 2

Charting Items

1. The maxillary right third molar is missing.
2. There is a fixed bridge between the maxillary right first premolar and the maxillary right second molar.
3. The maxillary right second premolar and first molar are missing.
4. The maxillary right lateral incisor has a Class III mesial composite restoration present.
5. The maxillary right central incisor has Class III distal decay.
6. The maxillary left canine has a porcelain jacket.
7. The maxillary left second premolar has distal occlusal decay.
8. The maxillary left second molar has a mesial occlusal distal amalgam restoration present.
9. There is a 6 mm periodontal pocket between the maxillary left second and third molars.
10. The mandibular left third molar is vertically impacted.
11. The mandibular left first molar has mesial occlusal decay and a Class III periodontal buccal furcation.
12. The mandibular left first premolar has Class V buccal decay and Class II periodontal mobility.
13. The mandibular left first premolar has Class V buccal decay.

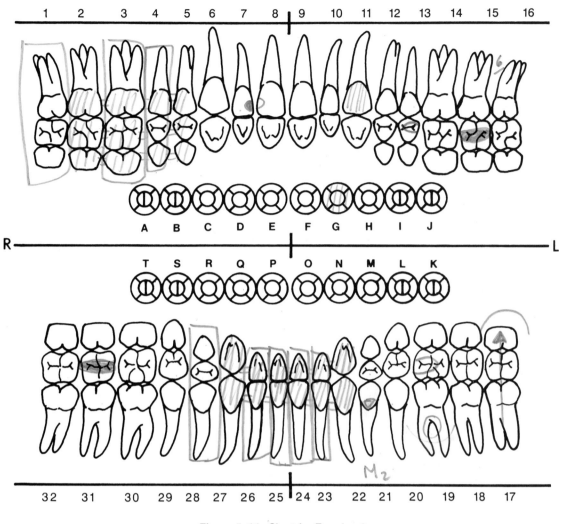

Figure 5–14. Chart for Exercise 2.

14. There is a fixed bridge between the mandibular left canine and the mandibular right canine. The mandibular left central and lateral and the mandibular right central and lateral are missing.
15. The mandibular right first premolar is not present.
16. The mandibular right second molar has a mesial occlusal distal amalgam restoration that must be replaced.

Charting Exercise 2

DIRECTIONS (Questions 228 through 239): Each of the questions or incomplete statements in this section is followed by four suggested answers or completions. Select the ONE lettered answer or completion that is BEST in each case. Check your answers with the correct answers that follow.

228. How many teeth are missing?

    (A) 2
    (B) 4
    (C) 6
    (D) 8

229. How many surfaces of teeth need restorations in the mandibular arch?

    (A) 2
    (B) 4
    (C) 6
    (D) 8

230. Which tooth is impacted?

    (A) mandibular left third molar
    (B) maxillary right third molar
    (C) maxillary left third molar
    (D) mandibular right first premolar

231. What is the classification of the cavity restoration on the maxillary right lateral incisor?

(A) Class I
(B) Class II
(C) Class III
(D) Class V

232. How many surfaces of amalgam restorations are present in the maxillary and mandibular arches?

(A) 2
(B) 4
(C) 6
(D) 8

233. Where is the periodontal pocket located?

(A) between the maxillary right second and third molars
(B) between the maxillary left second and third molars
(C) distal to the mandibular left first molar
(D) between the mandibular right canine and second premolar

234. Which teeth are abutments for a fixed bridge in the mandibular arch?

(A) mandibular right and left canines
(B) mandibular right canine and second premolar
(C) mandibular left canine and first premolar
(D) mandibular lateral incisors

235. What condition exists on the maxillary left canine?

(A) full gold crown
(B) porcelain jacket
(C) three-quarter crown
(D) gold inlay

236. Which tooth has a restoration that must be replaced?

(A) maxillary left central incisor
(B) maxillary left second molar
(C) mandibular right second molar
(D) mandibular right third molar

237. What condition exists on the mandibular left first premolar?

(A) Class II caries
(B) Class IV buccal caries
(C) Class V buccal composite
(D) Class V lingual caries

238. Where is the periodontal furcation located?

(A) maxillary right second molar buccal aspect
(B) maxillary left second molar buccal aspect
(C) maxillary left third molar buccal aspect
(D) mandibular left first molar buccal aspect

239. What periodontal condition exists on the mandibular left first premolar?

(A) Class II mobility
(B) periodontal pocket of 6 mm
(C) periodontal furcation involvement
(D) no periodontal condition exists

EXERCISE 3

Charting Items

1. The maxillary right third molar is a mesioangular impaction.
2. The maxillary right first molar needs a full crown.
3. The maxillary right second premolar has a distal occlusal amalgam restoration present.
4. The maxillary right canine has a Class III mesial composite restoration present.
5. The maxillary right central incisor has a Class V buccal composite restoration present.
6. A mesiodens tooth is present between the maxillary right and left central incisors.
7. The maxillary left central incisor has a distal incisal fracture and a periapical area.
8. The maxillary left lateral incisor has a Class III distal composite restoration that must be replaced.
9. There is a fixed bridge between the maxillary left canine and the maxillary left second premolar to replace the first premolar.
10. The maxillary left first and second molars have occlusal sealants.
11. The maxillary left third molar is missing.
12. There is a mandibular removable partial denture replacing the right first, second, and third molars and the left first, second, and third molars.
13. The mandibular left first premolar has a mesial occlusal amalgam restoration present and must be replaced.
14. The mandibular left lateral incisor has a Class IV mesial incisal composite restoration present.
15. The mandibular right canine has a Class V buccal gold foil restoration present.
16. The mandibular right second premolar has a full crown present and a 9 mm distal lingual periodontal pocket.

Charting Exercise 3

DIRECTIONS (Questions 240 through 251): Each of the questions or incomplete statements in this section is followed by four suggested answers or completions. Select the ONE lettered answer or completion that is BEST in each case. Check your answers with the correct answers that follow.

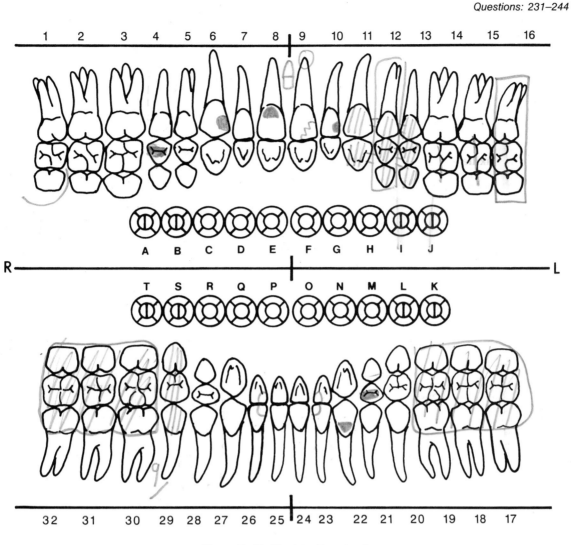

Figure 5–15. Chart for Exercise 3.

240. How many teeth are missing?

   (A) 2
   (B) 4
   (C) 6
   (D) 8

241. How many teeth need restorations?

   (A) 2
   (B) 4
   (C) 6
   (D) 8

242. How many teeth have existing restorations?

   (A) 2
   (B) 6
   (C) 10
   (D) 14

243. Which tooth is impacted?

   (A) maxillary right third molar
   (B) maxillary left third molar
   (C) mandibular right third molar
   (D) mandibular left third molar

244. What is the classification of the restoration in the lower left lateral incisor?

   (A) Class I
   (B) Class II
   (C) Class III
   (D) Class IV

245. What condition exists on the upper right second premolar?

(A) a crown is needed
(B) a distal occlusal amalgam is present
(C) a gold foil is present
(D) the tooth is missing

246. A supernumerary (mesiodens) tooth is present between the

(A) maxillary left canine and left second premolar
(B) maxillary central incisors
(C) mandibular central incisors
(D) maxillary right lateral incisor and right central incisor

247. How many restorations must be replaced?

(A) 2
(B) 4
(C) 6
(D) 8

248. Which tooth has a periapical area?

(A) maxillary right canine
(B) maxillary left central incisor
(C) mandibular left canine
(D) mandibular right second premolar

249. Which tooth is fractured?

(A) maxillary left central incisor
(B) maxillary right canine
(C) mandibular left canine
(D) mandibular right second premolar

250. What condition exists on the maxillary left first molar?

(A) a full crown is indicated
(B) occlusal caries is present
(C) a sealant restoration is present
(D) no clinical condition exists

251. Where is the periodontal pocket located?

(A) between the maxillary right and left central incisors
(B) distal to the maxillary right second molar
(C) between the mandibular left first and second molars
(D) distal of the mandibular right second premolar

EXERCISE 4

Charting Items

1. The maxillary right second primary molar has a mesial occlusal amalgam restoration present.

2. The maxillary right first primary molar has a distal occlusal amalgam restoration that must be replaced.
3. The maxillary right canine has Class V buccal decay.
4. The maxillary right central incisor has an incisal fracture.
5. The maxillary left central incisor has mesial and distal decay.
6. The maxillary left lateral incisor has mesial decay.
7. The maxillary left first primary molar needs a pulpotomy and full stainless steel crown.
8. The maxillary left second primary molar is to be extracted.
9. The mandibular left second primary molar is missing.
10. The mandibular left first primary molar has a stainless steel crown present.
11. The mandibular left lateral incisor has mesial decay.
12. The mandibular left central incisor has distal decay.
13. The mandibular right central incisor is missing.
14. The mandibular right first primary molar has a stainless steel crown present.
15. The mandibular right second primary molar has a mesial occlusal distal amalgam restoration present.

Charting Exercise 4

DIRECTIONS (Questions 252 through 258): Each of the questions or incomplete statements in this section is followed by four suggested answers or completions. Select the ONE lettered answer or completion that is BEST in each case. Check your answers with the correct answers that follow.

252. Which tooth is to be extracted?

(A) maxillary right first primary molar
(B) maxillary left first primary molar
(C) maxillary left second primary molar
(D) mandibular left second primary molar

253. How many surfaces of teeth need restorations in the mandibular arch?

(A) 2
(B) 3
(C) 4
(D) 5

254. What condition exists on the maxillary right canine?

(A) Class V buccal amalgam restoration
(B) Class V buccal caries
(C) Class I caries
(D) Class V buccal composite restoration

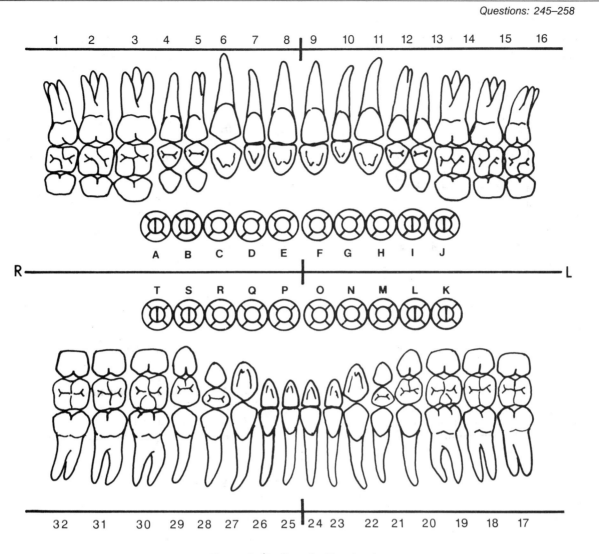

Figure 5–16. Chart for Exercise 4.

255. Which tooth needs a stainless steel crown?

(A) mandibular left first primary molar
(B) maxillary left second primary molar
(C) maxillary left first primary molar
(D) mandibular right first primary molar

256. How many surfaces of amalgam restorations are present?

(A) 4
(B) 5
(C) 6
(D) 7

257. Which tooth is fractured?

(A) maxillary left central incisor
(B) maxillary right central incisor
(C) mandibular left central incisor
(D) mandibular right central incisor

258. What is the classification of the restoration on the upper right first molar?

(A) Class II
(B) Class III
(C) Class V
(D) full crown coverage

EXERCISE 5

Charting Items

1. The maxillary right second primary molar is partially erupted.
2. The maxillary right first primary molar has occlusal decay.
3. The maxillary right lateral incisor has Class V buccal decay.

4. The maxillary right central incisor is missing (exfoliated).

5. The maxillary left central incisor is missing (exfoliated).

6. The maxillary left canine has a Class III mesial composite restoration present.

7. The maxillary left first primary molar is missing.

8. The maxillary left second primary molar has a stainless steel crown present.

9. The mandibular left second primary molar has a band with a soldered fixed loop space maintainer that extends to the mandibular left canine.

10. The mandibular left first primary molar is missing.

11. The mandibular left canine has a Class III distal amalgam restoration present.

12. The mandibular right canine has Class V buccal decay.

13. The mandibular right first primary molar has a mesial occlusal amalgam restoration present.

14. The mandibular right second primary molar has an occlusal amalgam restoration that has recurrent decay.

Charting Exercise 5

DIRECTIONS (Questions 259 through 265): Each of the questions or incomplete statements in this section is followed by four suggested answers or completions. Select the ONE lettered answer or completion that is BEST in each case. Check your answers with the correct answers that follow.

259. How many teeth are missing?

   (A) 2
   (B) 3
   (C) 4
   (D) 5

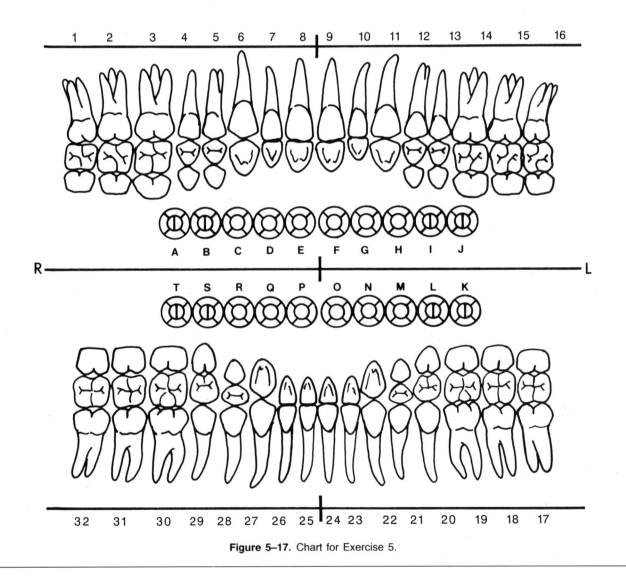

Figure 5–17. Chart for Exercise 5.

260. A Class III composite exists on which tooth?

   (A) mandibular left canine
   (B) maxillary left canine
   (C) mandibular right canine
   (D) maxillary right canine

261. Which tooth has a restoration that must be replaced?

   (A) mandibular right first primary molar
   (B) mandibular right second primary molar
   (C) maxillary right first primary molar
   (D) maxillary right second primary molar

262. What condition exists on the maxillary right second primary molar?

   (A) the molar is partially erupted
   (B) the molar has a stainless steel crown
   (C) the tooth has exfoliated
   (D) the molar has recurrent decay

263. How many teeth need restorations?

   (A) 2
   (B) 3
   (C) 4
   (D) 5

264. What tooth space is being retained by a soldered fixed loop space maintainer?

   (A) mandibular left first molar
   (B) maxillary left first molar
   (C) mandibular left second molar
   (D) maxillary left second molar

265. What is the classification of the cavity restoration on the mandibular right first primary molar?

   (A) Class I
   (B) Class II
   (C) Class III
   (D) Class V

Answers and Explanations

1. **(A)** A complete medical history is required before rendering any type of dental treatment on a patient. Potential life-threatening situations can be avoided by being alert to medical complications identified from a medical health questionnaire. The medical history provides information regarding premedication requirements, heart conditions, infectious diseases, and other related illnesses that are critical for the dental auxiliary to acknowledge before seating the patient for dental treatment.

2. **(B)** Color coding trays allows easy identification of the procedure the tray is prepared for (eg, blue tray for amalgam restoration, white tray for prophylaxis).

3. **(A)** Hand instruments are placed on the prepared tray in their order of use and on the side of the tray closest to the patient. After a hand instrument is used, it is replaced in its original position.

4. **(C)** The assistant, when working with a right-handed operator, holds the suction tip in the right hand with a thumb to nose grasp. For finer tactile sense, the assistant may hold the suction tip in a grasp in which all the fingertips are on the tip.

5. **(D)** The assistant's eye level is 4 to 6 inches above the dentist's eye level. This permits the assistant to have maximum visibility of the operating field and not interfere with the dentist's visibility.

6. **(A)** When working on the lower right molars, the operator is in the 9 o'clock position, and the assistant retracts the tongue as the operator retracts the right cheek. The operator working on the lower left quadrant retracts the tongue while the assistant retracts the left cheek.

7. **(D)** Protective barriers are necessary when sterilizing instruments. Heavy-duty utility gloves should be worn when handling soiled armamentarium and scrubbing instruments before sterilization. A face mask and safety glasses also may be used.

8. **(C)** The best position of the instrument tray is over the assistant's lap.

9. **(B)** When working in the anterior area of the mouth, the suction tip is placed on the opposite side of the tooth being prepared and parallel to the labial or lingual surface of the tooth being prepared. The lumen should bisect the incisal edge of the tooth being prepared.

10. **(A)** As indicated in the manufacturer's directions on maintenance, the high-speed handpiece should be cleaned and lubricated daily for optimum use and long mechanical life.

11. **(B)** Indirect vision refers to seeing by looking into a mirror. Often, dental work must be accomplished in this manner because of the shape and location of structures in the oral cavity. Direct vision refers to seeing without the use of a mirror.

12. **(C)** The purpose of aspiration is to find out if the lumen of the needle is in a blood vessel. If blood is aspirated, the needle is moved to another location before the local anesthetic is deposited.

13. **(A)** The reading that is recorded first when taking blood pressure is the systolic measurement. Systolic blood pressure is the pressure exerted on the walls of arteries when the heart contracts. In healthy young adults, the average blood pressure is 120/80. The measurement is recorded as a fraction, with 120 representing the systolic measurement and the number 80 representing the diastolic measurement.

14. **(B)** The patient's clinical record must include an updated medical health questionnaire. The medical health questionnaire should be reviewed and updated periodically as indicated by office policy. The date and signature of the patient also are required. Potential medical emergencies can be avoided by reviewing the medical history of each patient before

treatment. Legal requirements for the health professional necessitate accurate clinical record keeping, including updated medical health questionnaires on every patient. The signature of the reviewing clinician also is required on the form.

15. **(A)** When transferring an instrument, the assistant holds it between the thumb and forefinger, parallel to the instrument being used, close to the operating field, and opposite the working end, which is pointed toward the surface at which it will be used.

16. **(D)** The fulcrum digit used in the modified pen grasp is the fourth finger, or ring finger. A fulcrum serves as the pivotal point or support for stabilizing a particular finger rest.

17. **(C)** Class I caries is classified according to G.V. Black as cavities that occur on the occlusal surfaces of premolars and molars. Pits or fissures on the lingual surfaces of incisors near the cingulum also are classified as Class I caries.

18. **(B)** Contraindications to topical anesthetic agents include a patient history of allergy to the topical medication, and such agents should not be used.

19. **(C)** The matrix band is removed slowly and carefully teased off the tooth in an occlusal direction. As the matrix band becomes free, the marginal ridge of the amalgam restoration must be held in place with an instrument to avoid accidental fracture of the restoration during matrix band removal procedures.

20. **(A)** The color of the nitrous oxide cylinder tank is always blue. The color blue identifies the cylinder as containing nitrous oxide gas. Nitrous oxide gas is nonflammable and is used as an inhalation agent.

21. **(C)** If a patient jumps out of the chair after being treated in a supine position, he or she will not have an opportunity to regain circulatory equilibrium. This can cause fainting due to lack of blood to the brain.

22. **(D)** Materials should be mixed just before use and be brought as close to the area of operation as possible. This will minimize the motion necessary for the operator to obtain these materials.

23. **(B)** Class II cavity preparations include the occlusal and one or two proximal surfaces of premolars and molars.

24. **(B)** When placing a rubber dam, a blunt type of instrument may be used to invert the dam around the teeth being prepared. Inversion of the dam places the free edge of the dam into the gingival sulcus and thereby prevents leakage.

25. **(C)** The rubber dam napkin is used to avoid irritation around the patient's mouth by absorbing fluids and avoiding direct contact of the rubber dam with the patient's face.

26. **(D)** A lubricant can be placed around the holes punched in the rubber dam to facilitate the placement of the rubber dam between the teeth. A lubricant also can be used at the corners of the patient's mouth to help avoid irritation.

27. **(D)** Class IV cavity preparations involve the proximal surface and the incisal angle of incisors and canines.

28. **(C)** Debridement of the cavity preparation refers to cleaning and drying the preparation. This is accomplished by washing the preparation with water or hydrogen peroxide, followed by drying the preparation with intermittent blasts of air.

29. **(D)** A fulcrum is the stationary point of a lever. Examples of fulcrums in dentistry are the condyle of the mandible and the finger rests on a tooth during instrumentation.

30. **(A)** The rubber dam is removed after condensation of a Class II amalgam preparation in order to check the patient's occlusion.

31. **(B)** Burnishers are not used to evaluate amalgam restorations. They are used to adapt restorative materials, such as amalgam and gold foil, to the margins of the cavity preparation.

32. **(C)** When applying a rubber dam, the anchor tooth (tooth that is clamped) selected is one or two teeth distal to the tooth being prepared.

33. **(A)** Before removing the rubber dam clamp, the interseptal rubber dam material is cut carefully by stretching the rubber dam material toward the operator and cutting away from the gingiva with crown and collar scissors.

34. **(D)** The following pieces of equipment should be disinfected after treatment of each patient: light handles, chair controls, countertops, and chair headrest. Handpieces, curettes, and filmholders must be sterilized.

35. (B) The purpose of palpating the neck of a patient is to feel for enlarged lymph nodes, which may indicate a localized dental infection in the oral cavity or face and neck area. The lymph nodes are palpated either bidigitally or bimanually during an extraoral examination and are located on either side of the neck and under the chin. As part of the body's immune system, the lymph nodes become filled with lymphocytes to fight the foreign bodies causing the infection. The increased number of lymphocytes in one localized area results in tender, swollen nodes.

36. (A) Dental plaque is a soft white deposit that collects around the gingival margins of teeth. The bacteria in plaque are directly responsible for dental caries and gingival disease. Calculus is classified as a hard deposit, and leukoplakia refers to whitish lesions of the oral mucosa.

37. (A) Coronal polishing procedures require the use of a bristle brush attached to the dental handpiece to effectively remove soft deposits from the pits and fissured grooves of the occlusal surfaces. The rubber polishing cup may be used on all other surfaces of the teeth.

38. (D) Steam sterilization (autoclave) is the best method of sterilization because it provides the largest margin of safety by effectively destroying the hepatitis B virus. All autoclaves and chemiclaves must be biologically monitored on a periodic basis to ensure continued effective sterilization of instruments and destruction of infectious pathogens. All health care workers who are exposed frequently to blood or other body fluids should be immunized with the hepatitis B vaccine as an additional safety measure from occupational exposure to bloodborne pathogens. Appropriate disposal methods for infectious waste also must be enforced.

39. (D) To prevent a mouth mirror from fogging, gently rub the face of the mouth mirror against the buccal mucosa to coat it with a thin transparent film of saliva.

40. (C) A cavity varnish (liner) is applied to all surfaces, including the walls and floor of a cavity preparation. The thin liquid varnish is composed of a resin base suspended in an organic solvent.

41. (D) Calcium hydroxide is used because it stimulates the formation of secondary dentin. When used as a liner in a cavity preparation, calcium hydroxide does not aid in reducing marginal leakage around the restoration because the application site is limited to the deepest portion of the cavity preparation only. The lining material does not seal dentinal tubules or provide sufficient thermal insulation.

42. (B) To prevent gagging or excess flow of alginate impression material down the back of the throat, the patient should be seated in an upright position with the head tilted slightly forward.

43. (B) The appropriate trays for obtaining alginate impressions are perforated Rim-lock (autoclavable) trays or perforated plastic (disposable) trays. Water-cooled trays are used for final hydrocolloid impressions, and styrofoam disposable trays are used for fluoride treatments. Custom-made dental compound trays are best suited for edentulous impressions with a zinc-oxide eugenol impression paste material.

44. (C) Composite resin materials must be mixed using a folding motion with a plastic type of spatula only. Metal mixing spatulas tend to discolor the resin material and are contraindicated. Placement procedures for composite resins also require the use of plastic application instruments.

45. (A) Criteria for a properly placed wedge (either wooden or plastic) requires that the wedge ensure stability of the matrix band and separate the adjacent teeth slightly.

46. (C) The matrix band best suited for molars with deep gingival preparations is the metal molar band with wide gingival extensions.

47. (A) A Tofflemire matrix properly prepared for the mandibular right quadrant also can be used in the maxillary left quadrant. If prepared for the mandibular left quadrant, the Tofflemire matrix may be adapted also to the maxillary right quadrant.

48. (B) An intraoral fulcrum placed as close to the working site as possible is best for proper stability and control of the dental handpiece or dental instruments.

49. (D) Fogged x-ray films have an overall graying image on the processed film. This is due to the use of outdated films, stray radiation, or exposure to light in the darkroom.

50. (B) All dental personnel working with dental x-ray equipment should wear a radiation detection badge to estimate the radiation absorbed by the wearer. The film badge is worn during x-ray exposure procedures and removed at either weekly, biweekly, or monthly intervals for evaluation.

51. (C) A topical anesthetic is used before administration of a local anesthetic injection for temporary surface numbness of the oral tissues. The oral tissue is dried with a 2×2 gauze before applying the topical anesthetic agent.

52. **(B)** A temporary filling is best packed (filled) with a condenser type of instrument. The appropriate condenser should be selected to adapt to the size of the cavity preparation.

53. **(D)** The best instruments for removing excess cement from teeth are a scaler and an explorer. Dental floss is effective for removing residual cement debris from interproximal surfaces. A knot may be formed in the dental floss before running the floss interproximally for removal of embedded deposits.

54. **(A)** When removing excess cement from teeth, maintain a fulcrum as close as possible to the working site. The ring finger serves as the fulcrum for the established finger rest. Soft tissues are not stable enough to support a fulcrum.

55. **(A)** When placing a temporary filling, it is not important to carve detailed anatomy, since the filling material is not permanent and will need to be replaced in a short period of time. Occlusion should be functional and checked before dismissing the patient. Margins must be sealed and a proper contact maintained.

56. **(B)** The primary use of a matrix band is to provide the missing wall in a proximal surface cavity.

57. **(C)** A properly placed Tofflemire matrix band should be placed at least 1 mm above the occlusal ridge to ensure proper contour and occlusion of the final restoration. The matrix band also extends 1 mm beyond the gingival margin of the preparation to ensure an appropriate seal at the base of the preparation without impinging on the actual cavity preparation, which may lead to a final restoration with inadequate or open gingival margins.

58. **(A)** Greenstick compound may be heated slightly and used to stabilize the matrix band and wedge. A burnisher type of instrument is used for adapting and contouring the greenstick compound.

59. **(D)** The beavertail burnisher is not a handcutting instrument. The primary function of a burnishing instrument is to smooth out a metal surface while it is still malleable. The spoon excavator is used to remove soft carious dentin from a cavity preparation, and the hoe and gingival margin trimmer are used to bevel and redefine a cavity preparation.

60. **(D)** When assembling a Tofflemire matrix retainer, the diagonal slot always will face toward the gingival tissue.

61. **(C)** Wet agents cause less frictional heat than do dry agents. A suitable wet agent for flour of pumice may include water, glycerin, or mouthwash.

62. **(D)** Light pressure is used during coronal polishing procedures to avoid any unnecessary frictional heat, which may cause injury to the dental pulp.

63. **(A)** Extrinsic stains of the teeth are removed during coronal polishing procedures. Blackline stain is an extrinsic stain that often occurs around the cervical surfaces of maxillary and mandibular molars.

64. **(B)** Tin oxide is a white powder polishing agent for metallic restorations. Water is added to the powder to reduce frictional heat to the teeth during polishing procedures.

65. **(C)** A safety precaution that may be used during application of a rubber dam clamp is to loop a strand of dental floss around the bow of the clamp, then secure the floss by tightening. This safety measure will assist in quickly retrieving the clamp should it become dislodged during the application phase of rubber dam placement.

66. **(B)** Inverting the rubber dam material around the neck of each tooth provides for a tighter seal and prevents the leakage of saliva from coming through the rubber dam. A blunt instrument may be used to invert the rubber dam material.

67. **(B)** The rubber dam clamp is placed around the neck of the tooth approximately 1 mm above the gingival margin and just below the height of contour of the tooth. The jaws of the clamp should come in contact with the tooth and fit securely so as not to rock back and forth.

68. **(A)** When seating a rubber dam clamp, the lingual jaws are placed first, then the buccal jaws are adapted. A properly placed clamp should be stable and not impinge on soft gingival tissues.

69. **(D)** Acidulated phosphate fluoride gel is the most common form of fluoride used with the rigid tray system. The gel is dispensed into the trays, and the patient is instructed to close and bite once the tray has been properly seated to allow the gel to penetrate and saturate all occlusal tooth surfaces. Sodium fluoride and stannous fluoride frequently are in a liquid form or rinse.

70. **(C)** Flour of pumice is gray in color and comes from volcanic stone. Pumice is used as an abrasive agent for polishing tenacious stains of the teeth. Pumice is available in various grades. Fine flour of pumice is used for polishing teeth, and coarser grades of pumice are used for laboratory procedures only and are contraindicated for oral use. All dry powdered abrasives must be mixed with a liquid lubricant, such as water or glycerin, to reduce frictional heat during polishing procedures.

71. **(B)** Before applying a vitalometer to the teeth, it is necessary to dry the teeth with a 2 × 2 gauze or cotton roll. The vitalometer should contact the enamel surface only and is not recommended on metallic restorations. The vitalometer is used to determine (test) the vitality or life of a tooth. Small electrical impulses are conducted by adjusting the vitalometer monitor dial. A low reading (1–2) indicates pupal vitality, and a high reading (9–10) indicates degeneration of the pulp, or pulpal death.

72. **(A)** A very low reading (1–2) on the vitalometer indicates pulpal hyperemia. Hyperemia indicates an increase in the amount of blood in the vessels of the pulp cavity. This may be due to an inflammatory process or an irritation to the pulp.

73. **(C)** A high reading (10) on an electric pulp tester (vitalometer) indicates that the tooth is nonvital.

74. **(D)** Before placing a x-ray film in the patient's mouth, it is not necessary to chart the existing restorations of the patient. A visual oral inspection of the soft tissues is recommended to assist the auxiliary in appropriate film size selection and film placement principles. Always place a lead apron on the patient before exposure and remove any appliances from the patient's mouth.

75. **(B)** Obtaining a measurement (or length) of the root canal will avoid the possibility of irritating periapical tissues by overextending instruments beyond the apex of the root. Measurement is obtained by placing a reamer in the canal and taking a radiograph.

76. **(C)** An important principle of root canal instrumentation is the sequential use of instruments. The operator begins instrumentation with the instrument with the smallest diameter and gradually enlarges the canal using instruments with progressively larger diameters.

77. **(A)** Three endodontic instruments are used in the root canals: files are used to enlarge and shape the canal, broaches are used to remove pulpal tissue from the canal, and reamers are used to check the path and length of the canal.

78. **(B)** The rubber dam is used in root canal therapy to maintain asepsis and protect the patient from swallowing instruments.

79. **(C)** The material commonly used to fill root canals is gutta percha.

80. **(D)** An apicoectomy is the surgical removal of the apex of the root. The procedure consists of flapping the gingival tissue over the designated area and removing bone to gain access to the root apex. The operator then cuts the root apex off and curettes the periapical infection. The flap is then sutured closed over the designated area.

81. **(C)** Hemisection is performed when the periodontal condition of one root threatens the survival of the tooth. Hemisection requires that root canal therapy be performed before surgical removal of a root.

82. **(D)** A dry socket (alveolar osteitis) is a breakdown of a blood clot in an extraction socket. It may be caused by infection, poor blood supply to the area, excessive trauma during extraction or improper postoperative care. Treatment of a dry socket consists of irrigation of the socket and packing it with gauze and an anodyne.

83. **(C)** Application of direct pressure is the best technique to stop bleeding after extractions. Direct pressure is applied by having the patient bite on a gauze compress, which is placed directly over the extraction site for 30 to 45 minutes. This process leads to formation of a blood clot in the extraction site, which is the first step in healing.

84. **(D)** Rinsing with warm salt water decreases the number of microorganisms in the mouth and thereby promotes healing and helps prevent infection.

85. **(A)** A suture material that is resorbed by the body is gut. Other suture materials are silk, cotton, nylon, and wire. Sutures are used to approximate closely the edges of a wound.

86. **(B)** Postextraction dressings are removed and changed every 1 to 2 days as needed or until healing occurs. A postextraction dressing is used to soothe a painful condition known as alveolar osteitis, or dry socket, that may occur after the extraction of a tooth. The tooth socket is cleansed, irrigated, dried, and then packed with a medicated surgical gauze or Gelfoam. This procedure is repeated as often as necessary.

87. **(C)** When removing sutures, never pull the knot through the tissues. Single interrupted sutures are removed with sterile suture scissors and a pair of cotton pliers. The area is first cleansed gently with a Q-Tip dipped in peroxide to remove surface plaque and debris that has collected over the suture material. Grasp the suture with cotton pliers just below the knot and snip suture with scissors. Gently pull through tissue. Continuous sutures require several small cuts before removal. The patient is allowed to rinse with warm water, and appropriate postoperative hygiene instructions must be given before dismissing the patient.

88. **(D)** In treatment of a dry socket, the alveolus may be irrigated with a warm saline solution or hydrogen peroxide and warm water.

89. **(B)** When placing a periodontal dressing, it is necessary to festoon the material around the neck of each tooth. The dressing material should not be excessively bulky or extend into the vestibule areas of the oral cavity. For esthetic purposes, the dressing material should closely follow the natural contours of the dentition and not overextend onto the labial, buccal, or lingual surfaces of the teeth.

90. **(C)** Following periodontal surgery, the patient is instructed to omit hot, spicy, or sticky foods. All alcohol and tobacco products should be avoided, since they interfere with healing. Foods that have high nutritional value and are rich in protein are recommended to promote healing. Oral hygiene instructions include the use of a soft toothbrush dipped in water to clean off surface debris from the dressing. Disclosing agents are contraindicated during this postoperative healing time period.

91. **(C)** A periodontal dressing is analogous to a mouth bandage. The dressing makes the patient more comfortable by protecting the surgical area from trauma, mouth fluids, and other irritants. A periodontal dressing may be lightly brushed with a moist toothbrush to remove plaque accumulation and other soft deposits.

92. **(B)** The assistant prepares the syringe by placing the carpule in the syringe, placing the needle on the syringe, engaging the stylet in the rubber plunger of the carpule, loosening the needle cover, and testing the syringe to be sure the anesthetic comes out. The auxiliary does not place the anesthetic solution in the carpule.

93. **(A)** After the assistant has passed the syringe to the operator, the bevel of the needle should be parallel to the mandible when the anesthetic is injected.

94. **(B)** The term relative analgesia or analgesia is used to classify nitrous oxide, an inhalation sedation drug. Nitrous oxide is effective in reducing anxiety during dental treatment. The inhalation agent is easy to administer and allows for rapid recovery. Indications for use of nitrous oxide sedation may include to control gagging, to raise pain threshold, to reduce fear and anxiety concerning dental treatment, to stabilize blood pressure in patients with a history of hypertension, and to control excess salivary flow.

95. **(D)** A patient receiving the proper level of nitrous oxide will be conscious and relaxed and have normal pupils. The administration of nitrous oxide tends to lower the blood pressure slightly.

96. **(B)** During the induction phase of nitrous oxide administration, the patient is given approximately 5 to 8 liters of oxygen for 1 to 2 minutes. The patient is instructed to breathe deeply once the nosepiece is in place. Nitrous oxide is administered at the rate of 1 liter per minute while the oxygen flow is decreased by 1 liter intervals in the same manner. Vital signs must be monitored before the induction phase.

97. **(A)** Instructing the patient to hold his or her breath for 30 seconds, then inhale deeply does not apply to the correct procedure for the induction phase of nitrous oxide sedation.

98. **(C)** If the patient exhibits signs and symptoms of the excitement stage of nitrous oxide sedation, the nitrous flow must be decreased immediately. The objective of nitrous oxide sedation is to achieve a baseline level of sedation where dental treatment may be administered in a relaxed setting with as little discomfort to the patient as possible. Preexcitement or excitement signs and symptoms exhibited by the patient may include giddiness, laughter, tingling sensations in hands and feet, and difficulty in communication.

99. **(C)** The flowmeter controls the volume of gas administered to the patient. The flow of each gas—oxygen and nitrous oxygen—is indicated in liters per minute when regulated by the control dials. By observing the positions of the floats in the flowmeter columns of each cylinder gauge, it is possible for the operator to determine the appropriate volume of gas necessary for effective sedation and dental treatment.

100. **(D)** The dental auxiliary may not administer nitrous oxide to a patient if requested to do so by the patient. Under the doctor's direct supervision and orders, the dental auxiliary may assist in the administration of nitrous oxide sedation. The doctor must be present at the patient's chairside during the procedure of nitrous oxide administration. The State Dental Practice Act should be consulted for further definition of the individual responsibilities and acceptable duties of the doctor and dental auxiliary regarding the administration of nitrous oxide.

101. **(C)** Factors that determine instrument selection for restorative procedures are the tooth and the surface being restored and the type of restoration being placed.

102. **(D)** The rubber cup prophylaxis is indicated before placement of the rubber dam to avoid displacement of debris under the gingiva. By removing the plaque and other soft deposits from the teeth, application of the rubber dam is completed in a plaque-free environment. The dental floss used to seat the interseptal rubber dam material does not, therefore, force any soft debris into the gingival sulcus.

103. **(A)** Plaque control programs should contain oral physiotherapy instructions, nutritional counseling to decrease the intake of sugars and carbohydrates, and behavior modification techniques to motivate patients into practicing good daily oral hygiene habits. A clinical examination is performed by the doctor before implementing a plaque control program and is not a part of the patient's plaque control appointment.

104. **(E)** During coronal polishing procedures, the assistant may polish fixed bridges, gold restorations, and synthetic restorations. Removable appliances also may be polished outside the mouth to remove soft deposits and stains. When polishing removable appliances, care must be taken not to polish any surface of the appliance that comes in direct contact with the soft tissues. Avoid excess heat or friction when polishing any acrylic surfaces on the appliance. It is best to hold the removable appliance over a sink filled with water or a towel-lined tray to buffer an accidental slip of the appliance or breakage.

105. **(A)** The dental auxiliary may examine the oral cavity with a mouth mirror to chart existing restorations, missing teeth, and obvious lesions. Periodontal pockets must be measured first with a periodontal probe before charting. This procedure is performed by a doctor or a dental hygienist only.

106. **(A)** Functions of a good recall system may include a prophy and fluoride treatment, evaluation and examination by the dentist, and positive reinforcement of good oral hygiene habits and correction of any bad dental habits. The auxiliary cannot diagnose x-rays.

107. **(E)** The mouth mirror may be used to retract the buccal mucosa and tongue and to reflect or illuminate light in the oral cavity. The mouth mirror is used for indirect vision while working on the lingual surfaces of the maxillary anterior teeth and in other areas where direct vision is not possible.

108. **(D)** Protective barriers include gloves, masks, and protective eyewear. The barriers assist in controlling cross-contamination and preventing contraction of hepatitis. Subacute bacterial endocarditis is a microbial infection of the heart valves that occurs in patients with a history of valvular defects or a weakened endocardium due to congenital heart defects. The early onset of rheumatic fever often leads to permanent heart valvular damage, which may in turn lead to subacute bacterial endocarditis (SBE) if prophylactic antibiotic coverage is not administered before dental treatment. Wearing protective barriers does not prevent the contraction of SBE, angina, or epilepsy, since these illnesses are not contracted in this manner.

109. **(B)** When cementing temporary crowns, the consistency and amount of cement placed in the temporary crown depend on the type of crown to be seated. After cementation, the occlusion is checked and adjusted.

110. **(C)** During the application of pit and fissure sealants, which are polymerized by an ultraviolet light, it is necessary to use protective shaded eyewear. In order to keep the teeth as dry as possible before sealant application, a rubber dam may be applied.

111. **(A)** Glass ionomer cements are used for permanent restorations, luting procedures, and insulating bases. The powder is made from aluminosilicate glass, and the liquid is polyacrylic acid and water base. The cement exhibits physical properties of high compressive strength and adhesion to reduce marginal leakage. Secondary decay is also controlled by the ionomer cements, which incorporate fluoride in the powder composition, which is slowly leached into the enamel surface after placement.

112. **(D)** When teaching toothbrushing, the important emphasis should be on the complete and thorough removal of dental plaque regardless of brushing time.

113. **(A)** Handcutting instruments used in restorative dentistry are the spoon excavator to remove carious lesions, the hoe, the hatchet, and the chisel to refine the cavity preparation, the knife and file to remove excess restorative material, and the cleoid-discoid to carve restorative material.

114. **(B)** The supplementary finger rest used in the lower anterior area of the mouth requires the use of the operator's left hand to serve as a retractor and a finger rest for the right hand. The left-handed operator reverses the procedure, with the right hand positioned to retract the lower lip and serve as a finger rest for the left hand.

115. **(C)** After a topical fluoride application, the patient is instructed not to eat, rinse, or brush teeth for approximately 30 minutes. This allows for further penetration of the fluoride ion into the enamel.

116. **(B)** When preparing a cavity preparation on the buccal surface of the maxillary third molar, there is usually little room to operate, and a miniature head on a handpiece is useful. The anatomic restrictions in this area include the cheek and the ramus of the mandible.

117. **(C)** A steady stream of warm air may desiccate the dentin and be injurious to the pulp. The correct way to dry a cavity preparation is to use cotton pledgets or short blasts of air or both.

118. **(A)** A back-ordered item is a supply that currently is unavailable and will be shipped when it is available.

119. **(C)** Radiation exposure time for an edentulous patient should be reduced by 25%.

120. **(D)** The clasp of the partial denture contacts the abutment teeth. It functions to stabilize and retain the denture.

121. **(A)** The saddle of the partial denture contacts the edentulous ridge. Replacement teeth are placed on the saddle area.

122. **(C)** The function of the preliminary impression is to obtain a model on which a custom-made tray is fabricated. The custom-made tray is used to make a second and more accurate impression of the denture-bearing surface.

123. **(C)** A facebow is used to mount the upper cast on an articulator. This mounting should transfer the relationship of the maxilla to the temporomandibular joint accurately to the articulator.

124. **(A)** Wax bite blocks are used to record vertical dimension, centric relation, and facial contour and to set up denture teeth.

125. **(B)** The portion of the denture that should not be polished is the part contacting the denture-bearing mucosa. If adjustments are made on the tissue side of the denture, they can be smoothed with a small rubber wheel.

126. **(B)** A denture is relined to improve the readaptation of the denture base to the underlying tissue. The procedure is made necessary by the resorption of bone in the denture-supporting area.

127. **(A)** Sore spots are common after dentures are inserted. This should be explained to patients, and they should be told to return to the office for denture adjustments when this occurs. After inserting new dentures, often a series of visits is necessary to alleviate sore spots and make the patient comfortable.

128. **(D)** An immediate denture is inserted into the patient's mouth during the same appointment in which the remaining teeth, usually anterior, are extracted. Some advantages are improved healing at the extraction sites, greater patient comfort, shorter adaptation period, improved function, and improved appearance.

129. **(C)** Tissue conditioning is used to return unhealthy tissue, caused by an ill-fitting denture, to a healthy condition. This procedure must be accomplished before final impressions are made to construct a new denture. The treatment entails placing a soft material in the patient's present denture that will permit the unhealthy tissue to recover.

130. **(A)** Shade selection is accomplished in natural light with the aid of a shade guide. The shade of the acrylic or porcelain will depend on several factors, some of which are the shade of adjacent teeth, the shade of the patient's face, and the individual teeth involved (central incisors might be lighter than canines).

131. **(B)** Fixed bridges function to prevent movement of the remaining teeth, restore function of the missing teeth, and create an esthetic appearance.

132. **(A)** Teeth that support a fixed bridge are called abutments. Other parts of a fixed bridge are retainers (Fig. 5–4b), which are restorations, crowns, or inlays that are permanently cemented on abutments (Fig. 5–4a), pontics (Fig. 5–4c), which are the replacements for the missing teeth and are connected to the retainers, and connectors (Fig. 5–4d), which attach the pontics and retainers.

133. **(D)** A gold post is used to reinforce an endodontically treated tooth before a crown preparation is made. Endodontically treated teeth are more brittle than are nonendodontic treated teeth. To prevent further fractures of these teeth, they should be reinforced before a crown is fabricated for them.

134. **(D)** Cantilever bridges are fixed bridges with abutments on only one side. These bridges are used for esthetics and to eliminate the need for a removable bridge.

135. **(C)** Temporary bridges are used for esthetics, mastication, decreased thermal sensitivity, stabilizing teeth, as a model for the permanent bridge, and for decreased contact sensitivity.

136. **(D)** Epinephrine-impregnated cord is used to stop gingival bleeding and to retract the gingiva before taking an impression with an elastic impression material. Epinephrine is a vasoconstrictor that stops the bleeding, and the physical presence of the cord causes the gingival retraction.

137. **(B)** The function of the periodontium is to support the teeth. Periodontal disease is the destruction of this supporting mechanism, which can lead to the loss of a tooth.

138. **(A)** Gingivitis is inflammation of the gingival tissues surrounding the teeth. The etiology is usually poor oral hygiene, which allows plaque to remain on the teeth. If treated in its early stages by removal of the irritants, the disease process is reversible.

139. **(C)** Periodontitis is a stage in periodontal disease wherein there is a destruction of bone supporting the teeth. This condition is often the extension of untreated gingival inflammation (gingivitis). If periodontitis is not treated, it will progress until teeth are lost due to lack of supporting bone. The formation of periodontal pockets also occurs with periodontal disease. A pocket is a pathologic condition that cannot be cleansed by the patient. If not eliminated, pockets usually progress and cause further destruction of the supporting apparatus of the teeth.

140. **(A)** Another name for Vincent's disease is acute necrotizing ulcerative gingivitis (or trench mouth). It is caused by poor oral hygiene, physical stress, mental stress, and smoking. The gingival tissue is red and puffy. It bleeds easily, lacks interdental papillae, is painful, and has a fetid odor.

141. **(C)** A furcation refers to the radicular area of multirooted teeth. Furcations in teeth with two roots are called bifurcations. Furcations in teeth with three roots are called trifurcations.

142. **(B)** A splint is an appliance that connects and stabilizes mobile teeth. Splints are made of various materials, including cast gold, wire, and amalgam.

143. **(B)** A coolant is needed to dissipate the heat produced around the tip of the ultrasonic scaler as a result of its rapid back-and-forth motion.

144. **(B)** Osteoplasty is the recontouring of bony defects. The procedure is performed to obtain an anatomic condition that can be maintained in health by the patient.

145. **(D)** Gingivectomy is the surgical elimination of a gingival pocket so the patient can completely eliminate the plaque surrounding his or her teeth.

146. **(A)** Incision and drainage are used to treat a periodontal abscess. A periodontal abscess, part of the body's defense mechanism, forms when a foreign body, food, calculus, or other particle becomes lodged in a periodontal pocket.

147. **(A)** The beaks of the cotton pliers are used to gently remove a periodontal dressing. Suture removal scissors may be used to trim suture material that may become enmeshed in the periodontal dressing material.

148. **(C)** An abscess is a localized collection of pus. The specific name of the abscess is derived from its location. It can be periapical, periodontal, pericoronal, or subperiosteal.

149. **(B)** The armamentarium for suture removal includes surgical scissors and cotton pliers. The perio probe is used to measure periodontal pocket depths, and the surgical forceps and rongeurs are used during surgical procedures for tooth or bone removal.

150. **(C)** Analgesics are drugs that may be used for the relief of pain of low intensity. Analgesic drugs as a rule are also antipyretics.

151. **(B)** The condition in which a patient lacks oxygen is called hypoxia. Hypoxia is reduced oxygen within the circulatory system.

152. **(D)** Fainting also is known as syncope. Syncope is a temporary loss of consciousness due to an insufficient supply of blood to the brain. Treatment of syncope includes placing the patient in a position where the feet are elevated higher than the head to cause the flow of blood toward the head instead of the stomach. Spirits of ammonia may be used by passing the vial just under the patient's nostrils. The ammonia vapors are strong and allow for the quick inhalation of additional oxygen. Vital signs, including pulse and blood pressure, must be monitored.

153. **(B)** An angina attack signals a heart problem. Angina pectoris is a painful condition of the heart caused by a lack of blood to the heart muscles. Patients with a history of angina may take special medications, such as nitroglycerin, which is administered sublingually.

154. **(C)** Symptoms of shock include cold clammy skin, weak pulse, and irregular breathing. Low blood pressure is also a sign of shock.

155. **(A)** An average range for blood pressure if 120 for systolic pressure and 80 for diastolic pressure. The reading when monitored is recorded as a fraction: 120/80. Vital signs should be monitored routinely before dental treatment and recorded in the patient's dental record.

156. **(A)** An average range for a pulse rate is 60 to 80 beats per minute for an adult. The radial artery on the thumb side of the wrist is used most frequently to monitor the pulse reading.

157. **(B)** Subacute bacterial endocarditis (SBE) is a microbial infection of the endocardium or heart valves. Bacteremia in the bloodstream may be caused by any routine dental procedure in which bleeding occurs. The bacterial microorganisms initiate an inflammatory reaction around the heart and heart valves, leading to dysfunction of the heart and serious illness or death, depending on the severity of the infection and heart damage. Patient's at high risk for SBE have a history of a congenital heart defect (heart murmur) or other related heart conditions, such as a prosthetic heart valve. Rheumatic fever also weakens the heart, causing irreversible damage and leaving the patient at high risk for SBE. Prophylactic premedication with an antibiotic is required before beginning any type of dental treatment in order to prevent SBE. The patient's medical history must be reviewed and the physician consulted if necessary for the proper premedication regimen.

158. **(D)** The Certified Dental Assistant may dispense medication to the patient under the direct supervision of the dentist only. All medications dispensed to the patient must be documented in the patient dental record, including date, name of drug, and amount dispensed. If an office drug log is kept, the dispensed medication must be recorded and initialed by two staff members.

159. **(C)** Each state is governed by a State Dental Practice Act, which defines the duties, responsibilities, and restrictions of the dental auxiliary and dentist. The State Dental Practice Act serves as a regulatory body, which monitors the practice of dentistry in the state. The Dental Board of Examiners for each individual state is appointed to serve, interpret, and enforce the regulations of the State Dental Practice Act.

160. **(B)** The removal of the coronal portion of the pulp is called pulpotomy. In pedodontics, there are several types of pulpal therapies possible: direct pulp capping, in which a small exposure of a vital pulp is medicated with calcium hydroxide, indirect pulp capping, in which dentin affected by the carious process is medicated with calcium hydroxide or zinc oxide-eugenol, and pulpectomy, which is complete removal of a necrotic pulp and filling of the root canals with an inert material.

161. **(B)** If a second primary molar is lost prematurely, a space maintainer is placed in the mouth to maintain the room necessary for the normal eruption of the permanent second premolar. The use of either a removable or a fixed space maintainer is dictated by the situation.

162. **(C)** A stainless steel crown usually is indicated for full coverage of a deciduous molar. This restoration is less expensive and easier to construct than a cast gold restoration. It protects the deciduous molar, enabling it to function and permitting normal eruption of the succedaneous tooth.

163. **(A)** A mixed dentition exists when there are deciduous and permanent teeth existing simultaneously in a child's mouth. This condition begins when the first permanent molars erupt, at age 6, and lasts until the second primary molars are exfoliated, at about age 12.

164. **(C)** The best way to prevent gagging during impression taking is to seat the patient in an upright position with the head tilted slightly forward. Ask the patient to breathe normally through the nose. Do not overfill the tray with impression material to prevent an excess flow down into the oropharynx area. Talk to the patient in a reassuring positive manner during the procedure to further relax the patient with a high gag reflex. It is best to take the lower impression first and the upper arch last. Cold water will retard the set and prolong the procedure. A fast set impression mix is recommended to reduce chair time for the patient.

165. **(C)** Angle's classification of malocclusion is based on the relationship between the maxillary and mandibular first molars. When the teeth are in normal occlusion (Class I neutroclusion), the mesiobuccal cusp of the maxillary molar fits in the buccal groove of the mandibular first molar. Deviations of occlusion classification include: the mandibular molars are one cusp distal to their normal position (Class II distoclusion) and the mandibular molars are one cusp mesial to their position (Class III mesioclusion).

166. **(B)**

167. **(D)**

168. **(C)**

169. **(A)**

170. **(E)**

171. **(B)**

172. (E)

173. (A)

174. (D)

175. (C)

176. (E)

177. (C)

178. (A)

179. (B)

180. (D)

181. (E)

182. (D)

183. (C)

184. (B)

185. (A)

186. (C)

187. (B)

188. (A)

189. (E)

190. (D)

191. (E)

192. (C)

193. (A)

194. (B)

195. (D)

196. (D)

197. (A)

198. (C)

199. (D)

200. (A)

201. (B)

202. (C)

203. (B)

204. (B)

205. (A)

206. (D)

207. (B)

208. (A)

209. (C)

210. (A)

211. (B)

212. (A)

213. (C)

214. (D)

215. (A)

216. (B)

217. (C)

218. (C)

219. (D)

220. (B)

221. (C)

222. (B)

223. (C)

224. (B)

225. (D)

226. (C)

227. (A)

228. (D)

229. (C)

230. (A)

231. (C)

232. (C)

233. (B)

234. (A)

235. (B)

236. (C)

237. (B)

238. (D)

239. (A)

240. (D)

241. (B)

242. (C)

243. (A)

244. (D)

245. (B)

246. (B)

247. (A)

248. (B)

249. (A)

250. (C)

251. (D)

252. (C)

253. (A)

254. (B)

255. (C)

256. (D)

257. (B)

258. (A)

259. (C)

260. (B)

261. (B)

262. (A)

263. (C)

264. (A)

265. (B)

BIBLIOGRAPHY

Carter LM, Yaman P, Ladley BA, eds. *Dental Instruments.* St. Louis: CV Mosby Co, 1981.

Chasteen, JE. *Essentials of Clinical Dentistry Assisting,* 4th ed. St. Louis: CV Mosby Co, 1989.

Chasteen, JE. *Four Handed Dentistry in Clinical Practice.* St. Louis: CV Mosby Co, 1978.

Davis K. *Training Manual for Oral and Maxillofacial Surgery Assistants,* 2nd ed. Bellflower, Calif: Bellflower Training Manual Publishing Co., 1988.

Hooley J, Whitacre R. *Medications Used in Oral Surgery,* 3rd ed. Seattle: Stoma Press, Inc, 1983.

Ladley BA, Wilson SA. *Review of Dental Assisting.* St. Louis: CV Mosby Co, 1980.

Linkow L. *Theories and Techniques of Oral Implantology.* St. Louis: CV Mosby Co, 1970, Vols 1, 2.

Miller BF, Keane CB. *Encyclopedia and Dictionary of Medicine, Nursing, and Allied Health,* 4th ed. Philadelphia: WB Saunders Co, 1987.

Richardson RE, Barton RE. *The Dental Assistant,* 5th ed. New York: McGraw-Hill Inc, 1978.

Robinson GE, et al. *Four Handed Dentistry Manual,* 4th ed. Birmingham: University of Alabama School of Dentistry, 1978.

Spohn EE, Halouski WA, Berry TC. *Operative Dentistry Procedures for Dental Auxiliaries.* St. Louis: CV Mosby Co, 1981.

Torres H, Ehrlich A. *Modern Dental Assisting,* 4th ed. Philadelphia: WB Saunders Co, 1990.

Wolfson E. *Four Handed Dentistry for Dentists and Assistants.* St. Louis: CV Mosby Co, 1974.

Zwemer TJ. *Boucher's Clinical Dental Terminology.* St. Louis: CV Mosby Co, 1982.

Oral and Maxillofacial Surgery

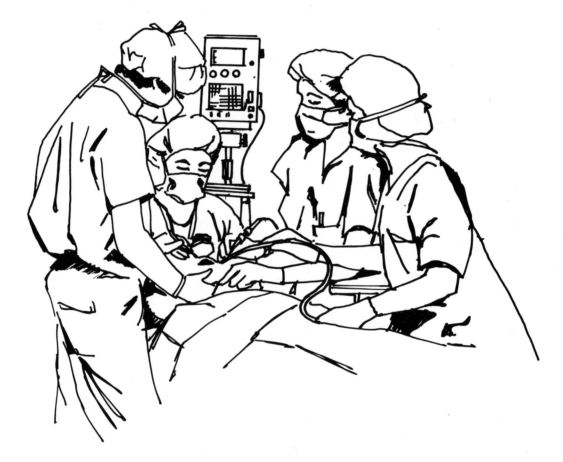

To assist you in preparing for the Specialty Examination in Oral and Maxillofacial Surgery, it is recommended that you review Chapter 1, General Anatomy, Chapter 2, Dental Anatomy, Chapter 4, Biomedical Sciences, Chapter 5, Chairside Assisting, Chapter 6, Dental Radiology, and Chapter 8, Medical Emergencies.

Questions

DIRECTIONS (Questions 1 through 10): Each of the questions or incomplete statements in this section is followed by four suggested answers or completions. Select the ONE lettered answer or completion that is BEST in each case. Check your answers with the correct answers that follow.

1. An impaction is

(A) a succedaneous tooth
(B) a tooth that will not erupt fully
(C) any tooth that is ankylosed
(D) a supernumerary tooth

2. The basic components of a surgical elevator are

(A) handle, shank, and tip
(B) handle, hinge, and beak
(C) handle, shank, and beak
(D) handle, shank, and point

3. Rongeurs forceps are designed for

(A) gross bone removal
(B) splitting teeth in bone
(C) cutting and contouring bone
(D) removing root tips

4. An instrument that holds a tissue flap away from the operating field is called a

(A) pick
(B) retractor
(C) elevator
(D) hemostat

5. A biopsy is

(A) any lesion in the oral cavity
(B) the surgical removal of an abscessed tooth
(C) the removal of tissue for diagnostic purposes
(D) the radical removal of a cancerous lesion

6. Surgical burs are specifically designed with

(A) prepackaged sterile pouches
(B) extra long shanks
(C) long cutting blades
(D) pretreated metal alloys

7. The basic components of an extraction forcep are

(A) handle, shank, and tips
(B) handle, hinge, and beaks
(C) handle, shank, and beak
(D) handle, shank, and point

8. General anesthetics are administered

(A) for nerve blocks
(B) routinely in most dental offices
(C) to render the patient unconscious
(D) without any risks

9. Before assisting in surgery, the auxiliary should perform a thorough surgical scrub for approximately

(A) 1 minute
(B) 3 minutes
(C) 5 minutes
(D) 10 minutes

10. Instrument transfer of surgical forceps is done using a

(A) two-handed palm grasp
(B) one-handed modified pen grasp
(C) two-handed pen grasp
(D) stable fulcrum

DIRECTIONS (Questions 11 through 15): Match each item in Column A with the appropriate explanation in Column B.

COLUMN A

11. Local anesthesia
12. General anesthesia
13. Nitrous oxide
14. Intravenous sedation
15. Narcotic analgesic

COLUMN B

A. weakest of the inhalation anesthetic agents
B. primarily intravenous barbiturates as a group
C. vasoconstrictors allow profound analgesia, remove pain but not pressure sensation
D. induces loss of sensation and consciousness
E. conscious but extremely drowsy, reduces state of awareness and anxiety

DIRECTIONS (Questions 16 through 39): Each of the questions or incomplete statements in this section is followed by four suggested answers or completions. Select the ONE lettered answer or completion that is BEST in each case. Check your answers with the correct answers that follow.

16. Monitoring a patient during general anesthesia or intravenous sedation is the primary responsibility of the

    (A) surgeon
    (B) Certified Dental Assistant
    (C) anesthetic team
    (D) monitoring surgical assistant

17. The three body systems that are monitored on a patient during general anesthesia or intravenous sedation are the

    (A) cardiovascular, lymphatic, and peripheral systems
    (B) cardiovascular, central venous, and muscular systems
    (C) cardiovascular, central nervous, and respiratory systems
    (D) digestive, respiratory, and lymphatic systems

18. The pulse is monitored by palpating the

    (A) radial or carotid veins
    (B) radial or temporal arteries
    (C) radial or carotid arteries
    (D) carotid or temporal veins

19. When palpating the pulse, you should be aware of the

    (A) location, placement, and strength of the pulse
    (B) rate, rhythm, and strength of the pulse
    (C) respiration rate per minute
    (D) patient's body temperature

20. The characteristics of a laryngospasm are

    (A) snoring, gurgling, and high-pitched crowing
    (B) snoring, gasping, and high-pitched crowing
    (C) gasping, sneezing, and high-pitched crowing
    (D) gurgling, wheezing, and high-pitched crowing

21. The electrocardiogram is a graphic tracing of the electrical activity of the

    (A) brain
    (B) pulse
    (C) central nervous system
    (D) heart

22. After surgery, the patient is instructed not to drink liquids using a straw because it may cause

    (A) premature healing
    (B) a dry socket

    (C) bleeding to occur
    (D) an initial infection

23. Intravenous barbiturates are classified as

    (A) analgesics
    (B) anesthetics
    (C) sedative-hypnotics
    (D) unconscious producing hypnotics

24. The greatest potential danger of a narcotic analgesic is depression of the

    (A) central nervous system
    (B) respiratory system
    (C) cardiovascular system
    (D) peripheral system

25. Common complications that may occur during the postoperative recovery period are

    (A) respiratory obstruction, bodily injury, and hemorrhage
    (B) abdominal pain, vomiting, and giddiness
    (C) gastroenteritis and elevated blood pressure
    (D) vomiting and postoperative pain

26. The most common complication associated with implants is the lack of

    (A) good oral hygiene
    (B) osseointegration
    (C) gingival support
    (D) esthetics

27. Which of the following metals used for implants possesses favorable biomechanical and biocompatible properties?

    (A) titanium
    (B) surgical silver
    (C) stainless steel
    (D) carbonium

28. Dental implants are classified in the following three categories

    (A) endosteal, periosteal, and transosteal implants
    (B) subperiosteal, transosteal, and subendosteal implants
    (C) endosteal, subperiosteal, and transosteal implants
    (D) subperiosteal, endosteal, and subtransosteal implants

29. The most common general anesthetic agents used in oral and maxillofacial surgery are

    (A) Anectine and Brevital
    (B) Brevital and Pentothal
    (C) Valium and Brevital
    (D) atropine sulfate and Brevital

30. A narcotic antagonist drug is

    (A) Vistaril
    (B) Ketamine
    (C) Fentanyl
    (D) Narcan

31. The treatment of fractures is

    (A) the placement of a drain
    (B) immediate mobilization
    (C) immobilization
    (D) bony transplants

32. The Caldwell-Luc procedure is performed to remove a

    (A) full bony impacted tooth
    (B) partial bony impacted tooth
    (C) displaced mesiodens
    (D) displaced tooth in the maxillary sinus

33. A hand instrument used for gross bone removal and to split teeth is called a

    (A) periosteal elevator
    (B) surgical chisel
    (C) surgical bur
    (D) rongeurs

34. An instrument used to effectively remove debris and diseased tissue from a tooth socket is

    (A) surgical curette
    (B) scalpel
    (C) elevator
    (D) curved hemostat

35. An elevator instrument is designed to luxate and remove

    (A) impacted wisdom teeth
    (B) deciduous teeth

    (C) root tip fragments only
    (D) roots, teeth, and root tip fragments

36. A particular elevator used to loosen the gingival tissue surrounding the tooth before an extraction is the

    (A) angular elevator
    (B) periosteal elevator
    (C) cross-bar elevator
    (D) east-west elevator

37. A drain is placed in a surgical site to

    (A) hold bone fractures together
    (B) treat gingival grafts
    (C) treat dry sockets
    (D) create a pathway for fluid to leave the body

38. Before dismissing a patient immediately after surgery, the dental auxiliary must check the patient for all of the following EXCEPT

    (A) swelling
    (B) excessive bleeding
    (C) dizziness
    (D) postoperative instruction have been read and reviewed

39. Nitrous oxide is used primarily in oral surgery as

    (A) a local anesthetic
    (B) an inhalation sedation agent
    (C) a sedative agent to bring the patient to an unconscious state
    (D) an inhalation agent to assist the patient with respiratory problems

ORAL AND MAXILLOFACIAL SURGERY ASSISTING INSTRUMENT IDENTIFICATION

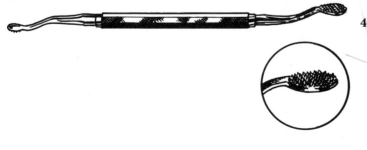

40. Identify the instrument shown

    (A) bone file
    (B) chisel
    (C) tissue retractor
    (D) surgical curette

41. The instrument shown is designed primarily to

   (A) stabilize implant abutments
   (B) clamp blood vessels and arteries
   (C) hold a suture needle
   (D) extract deciduous teeth

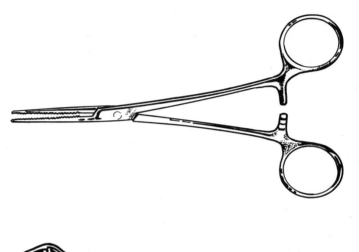

42. The surgical tips of the forcep shown is used to extract which teeth?

   (A) the mandibular third molars
   (B) the maxillary molars
   (C) the maxillary anteriors
   (D) the mandibular anteriors

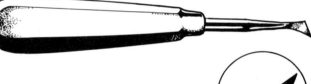

43. Identify the instrument shown

   (A) rongeur
   (B) periosteal elevator
   (C) crossbar elevator
   (D) Cryer elevator

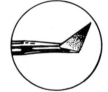

44. The instruments shown are designed primarily for

   (A) surgical biopsies requiring bone removal
   (B) soft tissue retraction
   (C) elevation of periodontally involved teeth
   (D) taking intraoral photographs

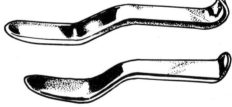

45. Identify the No. 12 surgical blade

   (A)
   (B)
   (C)
   (D) the No. 12 surgical blade is not shown

A.

B.

C.

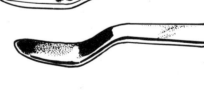

46. The instrument shown is designed primarily to

(A) remove a suture
(B) place periodontal dressings
(C) remove necrotic tissues
(D) place postextraction dressings

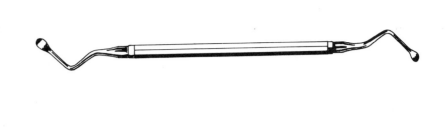

47. The primary function of the forceps shown is

(A) to remove palatal tori
(B) to cut alveolar bone
(C) to remove maxillary anterior teeth
(D) to remove mandibular anterior teeth

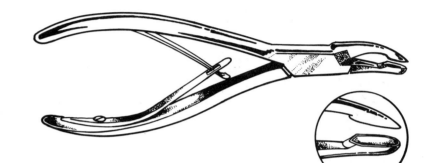

48. The No. 23 cowhorn surgical forcep is used to remove mandibular molars. Identify the No. 23 cowhorn surgical forcep.

(A)
(B)
(C)
(D) No. 23 forcep is not shown

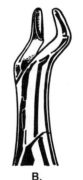
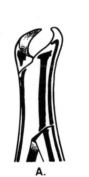
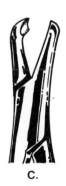

A.   B.   C.

49. The forcep shown is designed to extract

(A) maxillary anterior teeth
(B) mandibular first primary molars
(C) mandibular primary second molars
(D) mandibular first molars

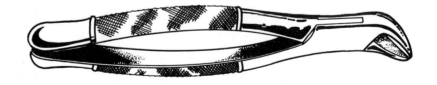

50. Identify the No. 15 surgical blade

    (A)
    (B)
    (C)
    (D) No. 15 surgical blade is not shown

A.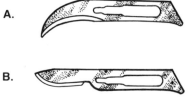

B.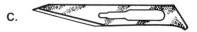

C.

51. The instrument shown is designed primarily to

    (A) loosen the tooth from the bony socket
    (B) remove cysts
    (C) recontour bone
    (D) separate fused roots

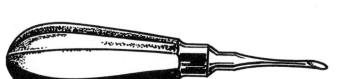

52. The surgical mallet and chisel are used specifically during surgical procedures for

    (A) dental implants
    (B) resetting fractured
        mandibles
    (C) bone removal and
        recontouring
    (D) removal of posterior teeth

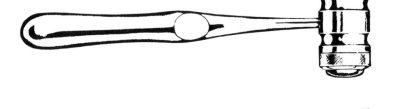

53. Identify the instrument shown

    (A) surgical curette
    (B) periosteal elevator
    (C) straight elevator
    (D) bone file

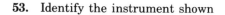

Answers and Explanations

1. **(B)** An impaction is a tooth that will not erupt fully. Most impacted teeth are third molars. These teeth are removed surgically because of pain, to avoid damage to adjacent teeth, or to prevent future complications.

2. **(A)** The basic components of a surgical elevator are the handle, shank, and tip (blade).

3. **(C)** Rongeurs forceps are designed for cutting and contouring bone during a surgical procedure. Rongeurs are shaped as a side or end cutting instrument with spring action handles.

4. **(B)** An instrument that holds a tissue flap away from the operating field is called a retractor. Proper retraction offers the operator better access and visibility to the surgical site while protecting the flap and surrounding tissue from unnecessary trauma.

5. **(C)** A biopsy is a surgical procedure that removes tissue for diagnostic purposes. There are several types of biopsies: *excisional*, in which the entire lesion is removed, *incisional*, in which a wedge-shaped piece of a large lesion is removed, *aspiration biopsy*, in which a piece of lesion is removed with a large-lumen needle, and *exfoliative cytology*, in which cells of a lesion are scraped off.

6. **(B)** Surgical burs are designed with extra long shanks to enable the surgeon to keep the handpiece head in visual field during operational procedures.

7. **(B)** The basic components of an extraction forcep are the handle, hinge, and beaks, which may vary in design. The extraction forcep is used to remove teeth.

8. **(C)** General anesthetics render patients unconscious by their effect on the central nervous system. These anesthetics can be administered by inhalation or by intravenous injection. The administration of general anesthetics requires special equipment and training and has a risk that limits its use in the general dental office.

9. **(D)** Before assisting in surgery, the auxiliary should perform a thorough surgical scrub for approximately 10 minutes. Hands, wrists, and arms approximately 2 inches above the elbow must be cleansed with a surgical scrub soap or solution.

10. **(A)** Instrument transfer of surgical forceps is done using a two-handed palm grasp.

11. **(C)**

12. **(D)**

13. **(A)**

14. **(E)**

15. **(B)**

16. **(A)** Although monitoring of a patient during surgery is done by the anesthetic team, the surgeon takes full responsibility for all surgical procedures, including patient monitoring and related complications if they should occur.

17. **(C)** The body systems monitored during general anesthesia or intravenous sedation are the respiratory system, cardiovascular system, and central nervous system.

18. **(C)** The pulse is monitored by palpating the radial or carotid arteries with the fingertips.

19. **(B)** When palpating the pulse you should be aware of the rate, rhythm, and strength of the pulse. The normal rate for an adult is 60 to 100 beats per minute. The rhythm should be constant and regular, with the strength ranging anywhere from very strong to very weak.

20. **(A)** The characteristics of a laryngospasm are snoring, gurgling, and high-pitched crowing sounds. These sounds indicate that the patient has a partially obstructed airway and immediate emergency treatment must be administered.

21. **(D)** The electrocardiogram is a graphic tracing of the electrical activity of the heart. The electrocardiogram machine produces the graphic tracing and is used during extensive surgical procedures.

22. **(C)** After surgery, the patient is instructed not to spit or drink through a straw because this action causes suction and negative pressure in the mouth, resulting in possible bleeding. Postoperative instructions must always be reviewed thoroughly with the patient before beginning surgical procedures.

23. **(C)** Intravenous barbiturates are classified as sedative-hypnotics. These drugs produce a conscious but sleeplike state.

24. **(B)** The greatest potential danger of a narcotic analgesic is depression of the respiratory system.

25. **(A)** Common complications that can be anticipated and prevented during the postoperative recovery period are respiratory obstruction, bodily injury, and hemorrhage. Patients must be monitored closely after surgery to prevent serious postoperative complications.

26. **(B)** The most common complication associated with implant surgery is the lack of osseointegration, a direct structural and functional connection between living bone and the surface of a dental implant.

27. **(A)** Titanium is a metal that is used for dental implants. Titanium exhibits favorable biomechanical and biocompatible properties.

28. **(C)** Dental implants are classified in the following three categories: endosteal, subperiosteal, and transosteal implants. Endosteal implants (endosseous) are surgically placed within the bone, and transosteal (transosseous) implants are placed through the bone. The subperiosteal dental implant is placed over the bone.

29. **(B)** The most common anesthetic agents used in oral and maxillofacial surgery are Brevital and Pentothal. Both drugs are ultrashort-acting intravenous barbiturates that produce general anesthesia with greater dosages than for sedation.

30. **(D)** Narcan (naxolone) is one of three narcotic antagonists that may be given to reverse the action of a narcotic-based drug.

31. **(C)** The treatment of fractures is the approximation of the parts (reduction) followed by immobilization (fixation) until the bone heals. Reduction can be accomplished by closed reduction, manipulation of the fracture without exposing the bone, or by open reduction, in which the fractured ends of the bones are exposed. Immobilization of the mandible or maxilla is accomplished by wiring the upper and lower teeth together.

32. **(D)** The Caldwell-Luc procedure is performed to remove a displaced tooth in the maxillary sinus.

33. **(B)** Surgical chisels are used in conjunction with a surgical hand mallet to remove bone and split teeth. Some surgical chisels may be driven by a special handpiece.

34. **(A)** The surgical curette is generally used to remove debris, granulomas, and enucleation of small cysts and diseased tissue. The surgical curette also may be used to debride bony tooth sockets after an extraction.

35. **(D)** Elevators are designed in various shapes, sizes, and working angles, and their function is to luxate and remove teeth. The elevator is effective also in the removal of roots and root fragments during surgical procedures.

36. **(B)** The periosteal elevator is used to reflect the mucoperiosteum and the gingival tissue from around the neck of the tooth before extraction.

37. **(D)** A drain is a piece of material, usually rubber or gauze, that creates a pathway whereby fluid can leave the body.

38. **(A)** Before dismissing a patient immediately after surgery, the dental auxiliary must check the patient to see that he or she is not feeling dizzy or experiencing unusual or excessive bleeding. Postoperative instructions must be explained to the patient thoroughly before the surgical procedure begins, and a written copy of the postoperative instructions is given to the patient. If indicated, appropriate arrangements regarding transportation must be made before dismissing the patient if the patient is unable to drive due to medications administered during the surgical procedure. Swelling is a common symptom after any type of surgical procedure and should not present a serious concern.

39. **(B)** Nitrous oxide is used primarily in oral surgery as an inhalation sedation agent.

40. **(A)**

41. **(C)**

42. **(B)**

43. **(D)**

44. **(B)**

45. **(A)**

46. **(C)**

47. **(B)**

48. **(A)**

49. **(D)**

50. **(B)**

51. **(A)**

52. **(C)**

53. **(B)**

Orthodontics

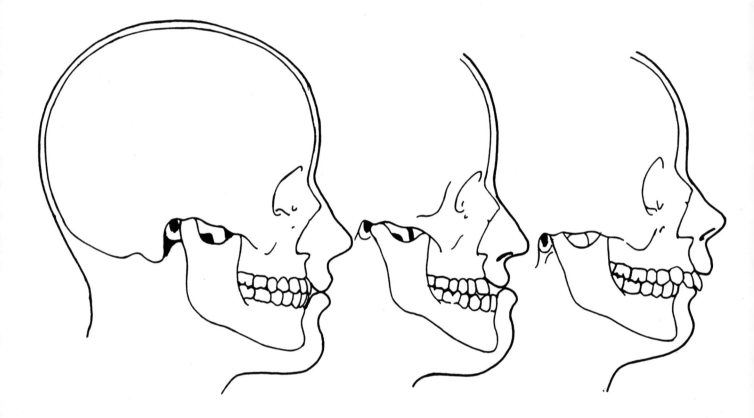

To assist you in preparing for the Specialty Examination in Orthodontics, it is recommended that you review Chapter 3, Preventive Dentistry, Chapter 4, Biomedical Sciences, Chapter 5, Chairside Assisting, Chapter 6, Dental Radiology, Chapter 7, Dental Materials, Chapter 8, Medical Emergencies, and Chapter 10, Dental Practice Management.

Questions

DIRECTIONS (Questions 1 through 44): Each of the questions or incomplete statements in this section is followed by four suggested answers or completions. Select the ONE lettered answer or completion that is BEST in each case. Check your answers with the correct answers that follow.

1. Orthodontics is the dental specialty that deals with

   (A) the diseases and abnormal conditions of the hard and soft tissues of the oral cavity
   (B) the treatment of pulpal and periapical diseases of the teeth
   (C) the growth and development of the jaws and face
   (D) the prevention and education of dental health problems on a community level

2. The condition in which the mandible is located ahead of the maxilla is called

   (A) prognathism
   (B) micrognathism
   (C) retrusion
   (D) centric relation

3. On which surface(s) is the archwire located?

   (A) incisal surfaces only
   (B) labial surfaces only
   (C) lingual surfaces only
   (D) labial or lingual surface

4. Removal of bands may be accomplished with

   (A) band seater
   (B) explorer
   (C) bird beak pliers
   (D) anterior band slitting pliers

5. A headgear appliance is worn

   (A) during active play and while sleeping
   (B) as the orthodontist prescribes
   (C) a minimum of 8 hours a day, 5 days a week
   (D) 24 hours a day except while eating

6. A positioner is worn

   (A) in place of a fixed appliance
   (B) for gross tooth movement
   (C) to separate the teeth before banding
   (D) after the removal of fixed appliances

7. In placing TP springs, an important consideration is

   (A) to place them from the lingual surface
   (B) to place them from the buccal surface
   (C) the placement should be above the contact area
   (D) to place them below the contour of the tooth and above the interdental papilla

8. The instrument of choice in ligating an archwire is

   (A) How plier
   (B) separating plier
   (C) ligature-typing pliers
   (D) utility pliers

9. Direct bracket bonding is advantageous because the procedure

   (A) does not add to arch length
   (B) permits movement of teeth that will not accept bands
   (C) is much more esthetic than traditional cemented brackets
   (D) allows the dentist less clinical chair time

10. The attachment either welded or soldered to the bands that secure the archwire is the

    (A) bracket
    (B) separator
    (C) retainer
    (D) coil spring

11. Brass separators are removed by

    (A) brass separating pliers
    (B) cutting opposite the pigtail with ligature cutters
    (C) surgical scissors
    (D) sickle scaler

12. What instrument is used to place elastic separators?

   (A) mosquito hemostat
   (B) sickle-type scaler
   (C) elastic separating pliers
   (D) ligature pliers

13. The patient should be instructed to clean his or her retainer

   (A) with an electric toothbrush
   (B) using hot water
   (C) with an immersion agent
   (D) after each meal

14. Cephalometry is

   (A) taking measurements of the skull
   (B) compression of the skull
   (C) the study of the soft tissues of the head
   (D) a technique of maintaining orthodontic movement

15. Cephalometric tracings are made over

   (A) silk screens
   (B) extraoral radiographs
   (C) articulating paper
   (D) special acetate paper

16. The cephalometric headplate taken most often is the

   (A) frontal headplate
   (B) posteroanterior
   (C) lateral skull headplate
   (D) cephalostats

17. An open bite refers to a condition wherein

   (A) there are no posterior teeth
   (B) there are spaces between teeth in the same arch
   (C) the anterior teeth do not contact
   (D) the teeth contact only during mastication

18. Overjet is the

   (A) horizontal distance between maxillary and mandibular teeth
   (B) coronal length of maxillary anterior teeth
   (C) vertical overlap of maxillary and mandibular anterior teeth
   (D) labioversion of the mandibular teeth

19. A type of measuring device commonly used to take intraoral measurements is a (an)

   (A) protractor
   (B) flexible millimeter ruler
   (C) Boone gauge
   (D) inch ruler

20. When seating and sizing bands using a band pusher type of instrument, it is necessary to maintain control by

   (A) using extraoral finger rests
   (B) holding the instrument with both hands
   (C) establishing a stable fulcrum before applying pressure
   (D) using the patient's chin as support

21. Class III malocclusion is

   (A) abnormal crowding of teeth with a normal jaw relationship
   (B) a protruded position of the mandible in relation to the maxilla
   (C) retruded position of mandible in relation to maxilla
   (D) based on relationship between maxillary and mandibular second molars

22. Vertical overbite refers to the

   (A) horizontal distance between the posterior teeth
   (B) coronal length of maxillary anterior teeth
   (C) vertical overlap of the incisal edges of maxillary and mandibular anterior teeth
   (D) labioversion of mandibular teeth

23. Class II malocclusion is

   (A) based on the relationship between maxillary and mandibular first bicuspid
   (B) a protruded position of the mandible in relation to the maxilla
   (C) also known as neutroclusion
   (D) retruded position of the mandible in relation to the maxilla

24. The head-stabilizing device used in cephalometrics is called a

   (A) cephalostat
   (B) angle board
   (C) cassette
   (D) articulator

25. During cementation of bands, the cement is placed

   (A) on the brackets
   (B) on the tooth
   (C) on the outer surface of the band
   (D) on all surfaces within the band

26. The attachment of anterior plastic brackets directly to teeth can be accomplished by

   (A) zinc phosphate cementation
   (B) soldering
   (C) acid etch bonding
   (D) spot welding

27. Cervical anchorage (headgear) is an

    (A) appliance that exerts distal forces on maxillary teeth
    (B) intraoral appliance that constricts the mandible
    (C) intraoral appliance that moves teeth anteriorly
    (D) appliance that enlarges the palate

28. After active orthodontic treatment is finished, what appliance is used to stabilize the teeth?

    (A) thin rubber bands
    (B) a retainer
    (C) a night guard
    (D) molar bands

29. When determining the length of a preformed archwire, you measure the distance from

    (A) central to central
    (B) first premolar to first premolar
    (C) first molar to first molar
    (D) tuberosity to tuberosity

30. In the removal of an archwire

    (A) ligature ties, then the archwire, are removed one side at a time from the buccal tube
    (B) the separators and ligature ties are removed first
    (C) the archwire is removed, then the bands are removed
    (D) the anterior portion of the archwire is removed before the posterior archwire is removed

31. The most common type of removable retainer is

    (A) headgear appliance
    (B) Hawley retainer
    (C) positioner
    (D) space maintainer

32. What is used to tie the archwire onto orthodontic brackets?

    (A) separating wire
    (B) buccal tubes
    (C) ligature wire
    (D) finger springs

33. When removing separators, care must be taken to

    (A) prevent the space from closing too quickly
    (B) avoid injuring the interdental papillae
    (C) avoid creating too much interdental space
    (D) avoid stripping the gingival sulcus

34. A useful instrument for removing elastic separators is

    (A) a gold knife
    (B) a sharp explorer
    (C) crown and collar scissors
    (D) a sickle scaler

35. TP springs are a type of

    (A) separator
    (B) matrix holder
    (C) removable appliance
    (D) mouth prop

36. An elastic separator is placed by

    (A) snapping through the contacts
    (B) gently threading through the contact with floss threaders
    (C) first removing the archwire
    (D) stretching and pushing through the contacts

37. When placing an archwire, one should

    (A) position wire into brackets, then guide the wire carefully into the buccal tubes
    (B) use a three-pronged plier
    (C) insert wire into one side of the buccal tubes, then guide it into the brackets
    (D) use the How pliers

38. The importance of the ligature wire is that it

    (A) provides tension for moving teeth
    (B) holds archwire in place
    (C) holds brackets on bands
    (D) holds headgear in place

39. When ligating with a tie wire, the tie wire should be

    (A) straight
    (B) bent at a 45-degree angle
    (C) bent at a 90-degree angle
    (D) applied with a separating plier

40. Select the instrument used to check for loose bands

    (A) band remover
    (B) bird beak pliers
    (C) How pliers
    (D) pin and ligature pliers

41. After cutting brass wire separators, the pigtails are cut to

    (A) 3–5 mm
    (B) 1–2 mm
    (C) 2–3 mm
    (D) length of archwire

42. What instrument is used to cut ligature ties in the removal of an archwire?

    (A) pin and ligature cutters
    (B) mosquito forceps
    (C) explorer
    (D) band removing pliers

43. When placing headgear

    (A) always ligate to molar tubes
    (B) insert one side of facebow first, then the other
    (C) pull facebow upward till it snaps into place
    (D) make sure inner bow is resting on top of lower lip

44. The type of appliance that has cemented bands and lingual or labial archwires is referred to as

    (A) a fixed appliance
    (B) a removable appliance
    (C) Hawley appliance
    (D) Crozat appliance

DIRECTIONS (Questions 45 through 59): For each of the items in this section, ONE or MORE of the numbered options is correct. Choose answer

    A if only 1, 2, and 3 are correct
    B if only 1 and 3 are correct
    C if only 2 and 4 are correct
    D if only 4 is correct
    E if all are correct

45. If an orthodontic elastic separator has been swallowed or has disappeared, the assistant should

    (1) look for the elastic separator in the oral cavity
    (2) call a physician
    (3) inform the dentist if not located in the oral cavity
    (4) do nothing—losing elastic is not important

46. To check for loose bands

    (1) use band remover pliers to see if cementation is complete
    (2) look at the bands to see if one is higher or lower than the rest
    (3) ask the patient if he or she has any loose bands
    (4) use the How pliers in an occlusal and gingival direction to see if the band moves

47. Which of the following are used to determine if an alginate impression tray is the correct size for the maxillary arch?

    (1) tray must extend slightly mesial to the last molar
    (2) tray extends to cover maxillary tuberosity
    (3) tray must extend slightly to the floor of mouth
    (4) tray should fit well up into the periphery

48. When inspecting and evaluating an alginate impression, the assistant must check for the following

    (1) surface detail
    (2) proper extension over retromolar area and peripheral roll
    (3) deficiencies in the peripheral impression
    (4) the final impression must have a granular surface

49. The brass separating wire should NOT interfere with

    (1) occlusion
    (2) gingival tissue
    (3) chewing
    (4) speech

50. Which of the following are correct procedures for mixing zinc phosphate cement for band seating?

    (1) spatulate over large area of slab
    (2) mix to putty consistency
    (3) use cool slab
    (4) incorporate large increments of powder into mix

51. The information needed for the diagnosis and treatment planning of an orthodontic case includes

    (1) complete medical history
    (2) radiographs and tracings
    (3) study models
    (4) photographs

52. An important function of the dental assistant in an orthodontic practice is

    (1) to keep instruments well sharpened
    (2) to administer fluoride treatments
    (3) to chart existing restorations
    (4) to motivate and reinforce oral hygiene home care

53. A finished Hawley retainer may have

    (1) acrylic palate
    (2) labial wire
    (3) arrow clasps
    (4) split palate

54. Before cementation

    (1) brackets are waxed
    (2) bands are arranged in cementation order
    (3) teeth are isolated and dried
    (4) teeth are coronal polished

55. Orthodontic bands with metallic bracket attachments are designed to be

(1) placed on occlusal surfaces of the teeth
(2) cemented on teeth to hold the cervical neck collar
(3) held in place by elastic and finger springs
(4) cemented on teeth as a means of anchoring archwires

56. In reference to an orthodontic study cast model

(1) trimmed models must be polished and labeled
(2) a model trimmer is used to establish right angles
(3) white orthodontic plaster is used
(4) wax bite is used to occlude models while trimming heel

57. If an archwire does not go in

(1) check for a crushed bracket
(2) molar band tube is blocked
(3) check width/diameter of archwire
(4) check tongue

58. In the placement and removal of elastic ligatures, which of the following instruments may be used?

(1) locking hemostat
(2) pigtail explorer
(3) scaler
(4) ligature-tying pliers

59. After removal of the orthodontic bands, all excess cement should be removed because

(1) gingival irritation may occur
(2) teeth will not occlude properly
(3) teeth may appear discolored
(4) cement is irritating to interproximal surfaces of teeth

ORTHODONTIC INSTRUMENT IDENTIFICATION

60. Identify the instrument shown

(A) rubber dam clamp forceps
(B) ligature-tying pliers
(C) separating pliers
(D) mosquito hemostat

61. Name the orthodontic instrument shown

(A) elastic separator
(B) brass wire separator
(C) coil spring
(D) TP spring

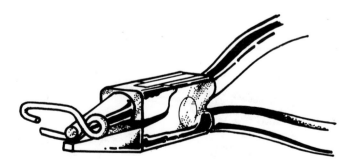

62. The orthodontic pliers shown are designed primarily for

(A) removal of orthodontic bands
(B) attachment of ortho brackets
(C) removal of headgear
(D) cementation of ortho bands

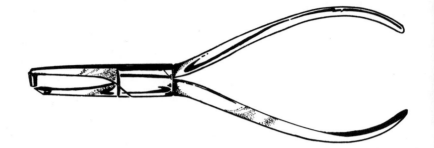

DIRECTIONS: Refer to the following figure to answer Questions 63 through 67.

63. Locate the orthodontic bracket

(A) 1
(B) 2
(C) 3
(D) not shown

64. Locate the orthodontic archwire

(A) 1
(B) 2
(C) 3
(D) 4

65. Locate the orthodontic tie wire

(A) 1
(B) 2
(C) 3
(D) 4

66. Locate the headgear tube

(A) 1
(B) 2
(C) 3
(D) not shown

67. Locate the orthodontic band

(A) 1
(B) 2
(C) 3
(D) not shown

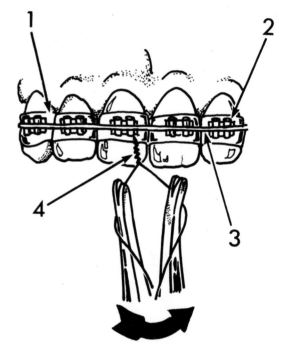

68. Figure shown indicates placement of a (an)

(A) positioner
(B) elastic separator
(C) elastic rubber band
(D) separating wire

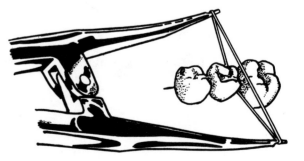

69. In reference to the two figures shown all of the following are true EXCEPT

(A) the high-pull headgear does not require a face bow

(B) headgear appliances must not be worn during contact sports

(C) the cervical neck band design is attached to the outer face bow by hooks

(D) the number of hours the headgear is to be worn is determined by the doctor

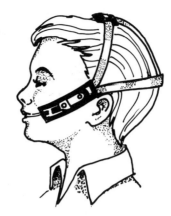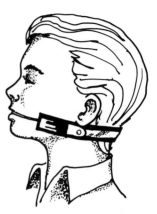

70. The primary function of the cervical face bow shown is to

(A) stabilize an extraoral radiograph

(B) serve as an anchor for the mandibular archwire

(C) apply direct force to the maxillary molars and restrain maxillary anterior growth

(D) apply direct force to the lower lip and mandibular arch

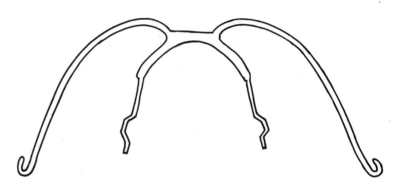

Answers and Explanations

1. **(C)** Orthodontics is the dental specialty that deals with the growth and development of the jaws and face. Treatment includes correction of occlusion and facial contour.

2. **(A)** Prognathism is the condition in which the mandible is located ahead of the maxilla. The correction of this bony defect is a combination of surgery and orthodontic treatment. The mandible is cut bilaterally and moved posteriorly to a position of desired occlusion. The mandible is then stabilized for approximately 6 weeks.

3. **(D)** The archwire can be located on either the labial or lingual surface. When activated, an archwire applies force to slowly move teeth.

4. **(D)** Removal of bands may be accomplished with anterior band slitting pliers or posterior band removing pliers, or both.

5. **(B)** A headgear appliance is to be worn as the orthodontist prescribes. Most headgear appliances are worn 24 hours a day except while eating. The headgear appliance is accompanied by a wired face bow. The headgear appliance may encircle the neck or the head or both. The patient must be cautioned not to engage in contact sports while using orthodontic headgear.

6. **(D)** A positioner is worn after orthodontic treatment has been completed. The primary function of the orthodontic positioner is to allow the alveolar bone to become stronger around the teeth before the patient wears an orthodontic retainer. The patient is instructed to wear the appliance for long periods of time and to exercise the jaws by chewing up and down vigorously.

7. **(A)** Steel spring separators, such as TP springs, should be inserted from the lingual surface and below the contact point of the tooth.

8. **(C)** The instrument of choice in ligating an archwire is the ligature-tying plier. The hemostat occasionally is used to tighten or twist the archwire.

9. **(D)** Direct bracket bonding is advantageous because the procedure allows the dentist less clinical chair time.

10. **(A)** Brackets are either welded or soldered to the orthodontic bands. Anterior band brackets differ from molar brackets (buccal tubes) on orthodontic bands.

11. **(B)** Brass separators are removed by cutting with a ligature cutter or wire cutter. Avoid trauma to soft gingival tissues when removing brass separators.

12. **(C)** Elastic separating pliers are used to place elastic separators.

13. **(D)** The patient should be instructed to clean the retainer after every meal. Toothpaste and cold water or a mild soap and cold water may be used to brush off soft deposits.

14. **(A)** Cephalometry is the part of orthodontic diagnosis that studies the measurement of the skull to determine skeletal patterns. The measurements are taken from tracings of extraoral radiographs (lateral plates and posteroanterior plates).

15. **(B)** Cephalometric tracings are made over extraoral radiographs on special acetate paper or orthodontic tracing paper. Landmarks of the skull are transferred onto the orthodontic tracing paper with a white tracing pencil.

16. **(C)** The cephalometric headplate taken most often is the lateral skull headplate.

17. **(C)** An open bite refers to an orthodontic problem wherein the anterior teeth do not contact each other.

The etiology may be a habit, such as thumbsucking or tongue thrusting. The treatment may include discontinuance of the habit and orthodontic intervention.

18. **(A)** Overjet, also known as horizontal overbite, is the horizontal distance between the incisal edges of the maxillary and mandibular anterior teeth when they are in occlusion.

19. **(B)** A type of measuring device commonly used to take intraoral measurements is the flexible millimeter ruler. The protractor is used to make cephalometric tracings. The Boone gauge is used to measure the height of orthodontic bands.

20. **(C)** When seating and sizing bands using a band pusher type of instrument, it is necessary to maintain control by establishing a stable fulcrum before applying pressure. A stable fulcrum prevents accidental slippage and laceration of the soft tissues. An intraoral fulcrum close to the working site should always be maintained.

21. **(B)** Class III malocclusion, or mesioclusion, indicates that the mesiobuccal cusp of the maxillary first molar occludes in the interdental space between the distal cusp of the mandibular first permanent molar and the mesial cusp of the mandibular second permanent molar, giving the appearance of a protruded mandible in relation to the maxilla.

22. **(C)** Vertical overbite refers to the vertical overlap of the incisal edges of the maxillary and mandibular anterior teeth when the teeth are in occlusion.

23. **(D)** Class II malocclusion is also known as distoclusion. Class II malocclusion indicates that the mesialbuccal cusp of the maxillary first molar is mesial to the buccal groove of the mandibular first molar, giving the appearance of a retruded mandible in relation to the maxilla.

24. **(A)** The stabilizing head device used for cephalometric radiography is called a cephalostat or cephalometer.

25. **(D)** During cementation of orthodontic bands, the cement is mixed to a creamy consistency and placed on all surfaces within the band. At least two bands are filled with cement simultaneously during the cementation procedure.

26. **(C)** Acid etch bonding currently is being used to attach clear plastic brackets directly to anterior teeth. This technique is more esthetically pleasing to many patients than the metal bands and brackets.

27. **(A)** Cervical anchorage is an appliance that attaches intraorally to the maxillary molars and protrudes extraorally to attach to an elastic band that fits around the patient's neck. This appliance provides distal forces to move the molars.

28. **(B)** After orthodontic treatment is finished, a retainer is used to stabilize the teeth in the correct position.

29. **(C)** When determining the length of a preformed archwire, you measure the distance from first molar to first molar.

30. **(A)** In the removal of an archwire, the ligatures, then the archwire, are removed one side at a time from the buccal tube.

31. **(B)** The Hawley retainer is the most common type of orthodontic removable appliance. The Hawley retainer is made of clear acrylic and contouring wire and is worn after removal of orthodontic bands to maintain teeth in their new position. The Hawley retainer also is used for minor orthodontic corrections of the teeth.

32. **(C)** Ligature wire is used to tie the archwire into brackets. Rubber bands also can be used to hold the archwire in the brackets and tubes.

33. **(B)** When removing separators, care must be taken to avoid injuring the interdental papillae.

34. **(D)** A useful instrument for removing elastic separators is the sickle scaler. The sickle scaler is used to gently lift the elastic separator away from between the contact area of the teeth. The elastic separator should be removed in an occlusal direction. A stable fulcrum point is necessary to prevent injury to the soft tissues. The number of elastic separators removed must correspond to the number of separators originally placed.

35. **(A)** TP springs are a type of orthodontic separator. Orthodontic separators are placed between the teeth before orthodontic banding procedures to allow for adequate separation of the teeth when the bands are ready to be cemented. Separators may be made of elastic or wire.

36. **(D)** An elastic separator is placed with the elastic separating pliers by stretching and pushing through the contacts of the teeth in a buccolingual motion. Correct placement should be checked with a mouth mirror and explorer.

37. **(C)** When placing an archwire, one should insert the archwire into one side of the buccal tubes, then guide it into the brackets. The same procedure is repeated on the other side.

38. **(B)** The ligature tie wire is a fine gauge wire used to tie the main preformed archwire onto the brackets of the cemented orthodontic bands. Ligature wire holds the archwire securely in place.

39. **(B)** Ligature tie wires are applied with ligature tying pliers. A tie wire loop is bent at a 45 degree angle and carefully inserted over and around the fixed bracket of the orthodontic band. The wire is guided behind the bracket and over the archwire, ligated to 4 mm, then cut with ligature cutters to a 2 mm pigtail. The ends are tucked under to avoid irritation to the soft tissues.

40. **(C)** The How pliers are used to check for loose orthodontic bands.

41. **(C)** After cutting brass wire separators, the pigtails are cut approximately 2 to 3 mm long. The free end of the pigtail is then tucked in a gingival direction with a condenser type of instrument.

42. **(A)** Pin and ligature cutters (pliers) are used to cut ligature ties for the removal of an archwire. The cut should be made as close to the pigtail as possible. After snipping the wire, use a hemostat to pull free. Instruct the patient to keep eyes closed during procedure to avoid accidental injury to the eye. Protective eyewear should be worn by the auxiliary.

43. **(B)** When placing headgear, insert one side of the inner face bow first, then the other side. Once the inner face bow is in place, apply straps over the hooks for placement of outer bow of headgear appliance.

44. **(A)** A fixed appliance has cemented bands and a lingual or labial archwire. The Hawley and Crozat appliances are designed to be removable.

45. **(B)** If an orthodontic elastic separator has been swallowed or has disappeared, the assistant should look for the elastic separator by examining the oral cavity and inform the dentist of the missing separator.

46. **(D)** To check for loose bands, examine the mouth carefully to see if bands are properly aligned and use the How plier in an occlusal/gingival direction to see if the orthodontic band moves.

47. **(C)** If an alginate impression tray is the correct size for the maxillary arch, the tray should extend to cover the maxillary tuberosity and fit well up into the periphery to obtain the proper study cast model.

48. **(A)** When inspecting and evaluating an alginate impression, the assistant must check for surface detail, proper extension over retromolar area and periphery borders, and any type of surface deficiencies or impression discrepancies.

49. **(E)** Brass separators should be placed carefully in the mouth so as not to interefere with occlusion, gingival tissues, chewing, and speech.

50. **(B)** When mixing zinc phosphate cement for band seating, use a cool glass slab approximately 70°F and spatulate cement over a large area of the slab to dissipate heat. Mix enough cement to a creamy consistency for multiple band seating.

51. **(E)** To diagnose and plan treatment for an orthodontic case, it is necessary to have a complete medical history, extraoral radiographs, cephalometric tracings, study models, and photographs showing facial profiles.

52. **(D)** An important function of the dental assistant in an orthodontic practice is to motivate and reinforce home oral hygiene care and plaque control. Patient education in proper nutrition and maintenance and care of orthodontic appliances is also a responsibility of the orthodontic dental assistant.

53. **(A)** A finished Hawley retainer may have an acrylic palate, labial archwire, and arrow clasps. The Crozat appliance (or jackscrew) has a split palate design to widen a narrow palate.

54. **(E)** Before cementation of bands, brackets must be waxed, teeth must be thoroughly polished and dried, and the orthodontic bands must be arranged in the order of cementation.

55. **(D)** Orthodontic bands with metallic bracket attachments are designed to be cemented on the teeth and serve as a support for anchoring and stabilizing the orthodontic archwires.

56. **(E)** In reference to an orthodontic study cast model, the impressions should be poured in white orthodontic plaster of Paris. Models are trimmed on a model trimmer and are occluded together while trimming the heels of the maxillary and mandibular cast. A wax bite is used to prevent accidental fracture of the teeth during this trimming procedure. Orthodontic study models must be polished and labeled properly, including patient's full name, age, and date.

57. **(A)** If an archwire does not go in properly, check for a crushed bracket, possible blocked molar tube, and inadequate length of archwire.

58. (B) Elastic ligatures are placed over the bracket wings once the archwire has been secured. Hemostats may be used for application. Removal of the elastic ligatures is done with a sickle scaler. Ligature-tying pliers are used for anchoring ligature tie wires only.

59. (E) Teeth should be thoroughly scaled and polished after removal of cemented orthodontic bands. Excess residual cement will cause gingival irritation and be visibly unesthetic, causing possible discoloration of the teeth. Occlusion and contacts also are affected by residual cement deposits. Appropriate oral hygiene instructions should be given to the patient immediately after orthodontic treatment.

60. (B)

61. (D)

62. (A)

63. (B)

64. (C)

65. (D)

66. (D)

67. (A)

68. (B)

69. (A)

70. (C)

CHAPTER 6

Dental Radiology

INTRODUCTION

Through the diligent work of leaders in the scientific field and through advanced technology, x-ray films have become an important and sophisticated diagnostic tool in dentistry. Knowledge and an understanding of x-ray production are critical for the proper exposure of radiographs and the practice of radiation safety. Dental auxiliaries and dentists must be aware of the potential radiation hazards in order to protect themselves and their patients. This chapter presents an overview of the principles of x-ray production, x-ray film processing techniques, methods of evaluation in identifying exposure errors, and occupational radiation safety.

BASIC PRINCIPLES OF RADIOLOGY

Knowledge and understanding of basic principles of x-ray production are essential for the proper exposure of radiographs. X-rays belong to a group of radiations called *electromagnetic radiations*. Electromagnetic radiations or waves occur in different wavelengths and in both natural and manufactured forms. X-rays are manufactured and have short wavelengths. The short wavelength gives off high energy, which allows x-rays to travel through solid objects and penetrate dense tissues, including bone. Key characteristic properties of x-rays include the following.

1. X-rays have no mass (weight) and are not perceptible to any of the senses.
2. X-rays travel in straight lines and cannot be seen in the visible light spectrum.
3. Like light, x-rays are capable of producing images on photographic film.
4. X-rays can ionize atoms or molecules.
5. X-rays are capable of causing biologic changes in the person exposed to radiation.
6. X-rays in high concentrated doses are used on human tissue to destroy areas of neoplastic cells (tumors) in the treatment of cancer.

The dental x-ray machine houses an x-ray tube where electrical energy is converted into beams of energy (x-rays), which can penetrate solid substances. There are three basic components in an x-ray tube that are necessary for the production of x-rays.

1. A cathode and tungsten filament to supply the electrons
2. A high voltage to accelerate or speed up the electrons
3. An anode, or target (focal spot), on which the electrons are focused and where they interact to generate x-rays

X-rays are produced when electrons strike the target. This produces a beam of x-rays that the operator directs toward the patient to record an image on the film (Fig. 6–1).

Primary radiation refers to the main beam of x-ray energy emitted from the x-ray tubehead. The primary radiation records an image on the x-ray film.

Secondary radiation occurs when primary radiation collides with matter. Scattered radiation is a form of secondary radiation and denotes x-ray beams that have traveled or been deflected in all different directions. Scatter radiation is difficult to confine and may be scattered throughout the dental operatory.

All x-rays generated are not equal. Some have high energy, and others do not. Lower-energy rays, those with longer wavelengths, are not useful because they have a lower penetration power and represent a radiation hazard. An aluminum disk 2 mm to 2.5 mm thick filters out the less penetrating rays before they leave the x-ray machine while letting the more penetrating rays through.

Since the film to be illuminated is approximately $1\frac{1}{4} \times 1\frac{5}{8}$ inches, the spread or divergency of the x-ray beam must be controlled. Otherwise, areas peripheral to the targeted area would be exposed and would increase patient exposure. This process, called *collimation,* is accomplished by a lead diaphragm located within the x-ray tube, which limits the size of the x-ray beam.

Three parameters are controlled by the operator of an x-ray unit.

1. Quality (penetrating power) of the x-ray beam, expressed as kilovoltage (kVp)
2. Quantity (number) of x-rays produced, expressed as milliamperage (mA)

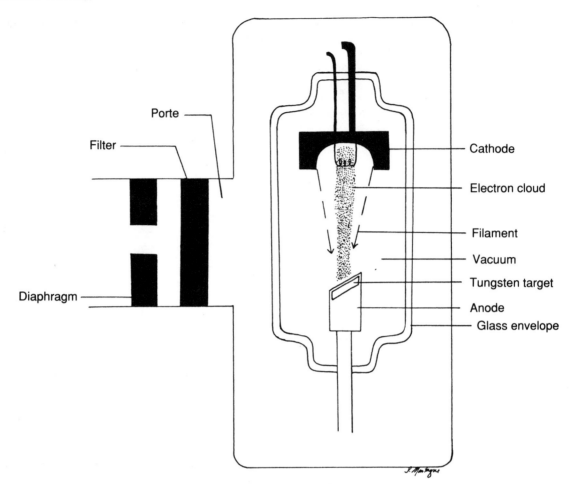

Figure 6–1. Diagram of x-ray head.

3. Length of time the x-rays are produced, expressed as exposure time

The exposure time usually is the only parameter that is varied within a dental office. Suitable penetrating power for dental x-rays ranges from 50 kVp to 100 kVp and 5 mA to 15 mA.

RADIATION EFFECTS AND SAFETY

Radiation can be a useful tool for diagnosis and treatment planning in dentistry. Dental assistants must be aware of potential hazards associated with radiation in order to protect themselves and their patients.

Harmful effects of radiation become manifest in tissues as a direct or indirect result of exposure to x-rays. The degree to which radiation effects occur depends mainly on the total amount of x-ray exposure, the rate of exposure, and the type and number of cells irradiated. Cell sensitivity to radiation exposure varies with cell types and, in general, is directly proportional to their reproductive capacity. The cells most sensitive to radiation are young growing cells, reproductive cells, and blood-forming cells. Young growing cells are found in the pregnant dental patient, and such a patient should not have radiographs taken except in emergency situations.

The National Council on Radiation Protection has established specific radiation limits for operators of radiation equipment. The maximum permissible dose (MPD) for occupational exposure is 5 rem per year or 0.1 rem per week. The dental auxiliary is responsible for assuring safe use of radiation in the dental office. Radiation safety includes three main elements.

1. Limitation of the radiation exposure
2. Limitation of the size of the primary radiation beam
3. Minimizing exposure to secondary or scatter radiation

Protective measures for radiation safety also involve both time and distance factors. The time factor represents the total history of radiation exposure. The operator must consider the patient's past history of radiation exposure, the number of films needed to obtain diagnostic information, the kVp, and the exposure time and film speed.

Distance factors affect the intensity of the x-ray beam. The *inverse square law* states that the intensity of the primary beam decreases in proportion to the square of the distance from the source. The dental auxiliary must understand this law in order to reduce his or her exposure to scatter or secondary radiation.

Radiation can produce both short-term and long-term effects. The term *latent period* is used to describe the time lapse from x-ray exposure until there is observable damage. *Short-term effects*, or acute effects of radiation, result from very high doses of radiation, as from a nuclear accident. Dental radiographs are not capable of such acute effects. Long-term or chronic effects occur years after exposure. Such long-term or chronic effects have been seen in operators who have held x-ray film in the patient's mouth during x-ray exposures. A dermatitis and subsequent development of cancerous lesions of the fingers is a result of this procedure. Other long-term effects of radiation exposure may include

1. Reddening of the skin
2. Hair loss
3. Split fingernails
4. Blindness
5. Sterility

Additional specific radiation protection measures for the patient and operator are as follows.

Radiation exposure to the *patient* is minimized by the following procedures.

1. Follow federal regulations and guidelines when purchasing x-ray units.
2. Periodically check x-ray machines for leakage.
3. Check machines to ensure that filters and collimators are placed properly.
4. Drape patients with leaded lap aprons and lead thyrocervical collars.
5. Use fast-speed film.
6. Employ lead-shielded, open-ended cones, which reduce scattered radiation.
7. Avoid retakes.

Radiation exposure to the *operator* is minimized by the following steps.

1. Stand at least 6 feet away or behind a lead shield, or both.
2. Do not hold the film for a patient during an exposure.

No working area should be in the direct line of the x-ray machine. As a further precaution, all personnel should wear film badges that periodically monitor dosages. Workers who follow radiation safety measures should receive no unnecessary exposure to radiation.

RADIOGRAPHIC EXPOSURES

The dental auxiliary needs to understand that x-rays penetrate objects differently. This knowledge is used to adjust exposure factors to produce a high-quality radiograph. A high quality radiograph has good density. *Density* is described as the degree of blackness on the radiograph. Exposure factors affect the image on a radiograph.

The number of x-rays that hit the film determines the degree of blackening, or density, of the radiograph. Areas and structures that are denser, such as bone and metallic restorations, absorb more x-rays. Therefore, few x-rays reach the film, making the film appear *radiopaque* (white) in these areas. Structures and areas that are less dense, such as pulp chambers and sinus cavities, appear *radiolucent* (black) on radiographs.

The range of shades from white to black, including all shades of gray, is called *contrast.* The contrast of the radiograph is controlled by kilovoltage adjustment. Increasing the kilovoltage darkens the radiograph and decreases contrast. The density is increased slightly. Decreasing the contrast lightens the radiograph and produces more shades of gray and, therefore, the radiograph is more diagnostic.

Changes in milliamperage affect the amount of radiation produced. Increasing the milliamperage darkens the radiograph and increases the density. The contrast is slightly increased and produces fewer shades of gray. Density of radiographs is best controlled by adjusting the milliamperage.

Changes in exposure time affect density. Increasing the exposure time increases the density and darkens the radiograph. Conversely, decreasing the exposure time decreases density and lightens the radiograph. Milliamperage and exposure time work together to determine the amount of radiation produced.

It is important to minimize the degree of distortion in radiographs. Minimum distortion can be accomplished by meeting three criteria.

1. Only the most parallel rays strike the object and, subsequently, the film.
2. A minimum distance is maintained between the object and the film.
3. The object and the film are parallel to each other.

However, these criteria present problems. A lengthy focal–film distance (FFD) is necessary for the most parallel rays to reach the object.

The inverse-square law, which relates energy and distance, demonstrates that large FFDs require very high levels of energy. Therefore, an increased FFD necessitates increased exposure, resulting in increased radiation to the patient. The most commonly used FFDs in dentistry are 8, 12, and 16 inches.

Maintenance of a minimum distance between the object and the film (object–film distance) and parallelism between the object and the film are two criteria that compromise each other. The anatomy of intraoral structures prevents the film from being parallel to the object and, hence, being as close as possible to the object (Fig. 6–2).

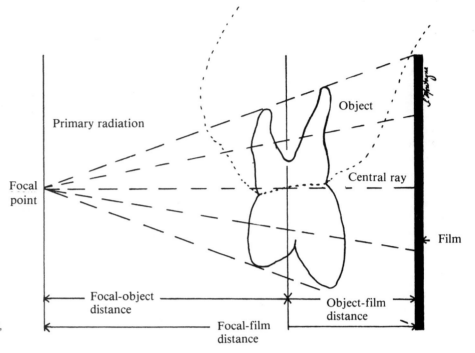

Figure 6–2. Relationship among focal point, object, and film.

THE FILM PACKET

The film packet must be moisture and light resistant, flexible, and easy to open in the darkroom. The packet contains a waterproof outer covering, black paper, the film, and a piece of lead foil that absorbs any unused radiation. The foil backing also serves to reduce background scatter and thereby prevents film fogging.

The film itself is composed of a silver halide emulsion, covered by gelatin on a cellulose acetate film. The size of the silver halide crystals determines the film speed, or sensitivity. This film speed affects the amount of radiation and the length of time (milliamperes) required to produce an image on the film. Faster films have larger crystals and give poorer definition or detail on a film. Slower films, which have smaller crystals, give more detail and require more milliamperes.

Film speed is designated by the American National Standards Institute (ANSI) by letter groups A–F, with speed increasing incrementally with the alphabet. Fast films D–E are used most often in the dental office, combining fast film speed with an acceptable level of detail.

Dental films should always be stored in a lead-lined container or compartment. Films that are outdated or affected by undesired radiation or light become fogged, compromising their diagnostic value.

Quality assurance measures can be implemented to avoid problems with x-ray film quality by periodic test film runs on selected film packets.

TYPES OF INTRAORAL RADIOGRAPHS

Periapical radiographs provide information used to diagnose pathologic conditions of alveolar bone and teeth, including tumors, cysts, developmental abnormalities, and presence of infection. Diagnostic periapical radiographs show the entire tooth or teeth from the incisal/occlusal edge to the apex (Fig. 6–3).

Bite-wing radiographs provide information useful in detecting the presence of interproximal caries and periodontal disease. Dimensional accuracy, clarity, image density, and contrast must be of excellent quality (Fig. 6–4).

Occlusal radiographs are used frequently to survey larger areas of the jaw (Table 6–1). The following is a list of indications for use (Figs. 6–5, 6–6).

1. Locate supernumerary teeth, impacted teeth, retained roots, foreign bodies, salivary gland calcifications, and other pathoses
2. Determine extent and shape of cystic neoplastic and infectious lesions
3. Locate and determine type and extent of jaw fractures in tooth-bearing areas
4. Provide a means of radiographic examination for a patient who is unable to open the mouth wide enough for periapical radiographs
5. Record changes in size and shape of dental arches
6. Minimize the number of radiographs made during a pedodontic survey

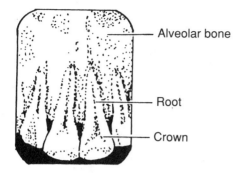

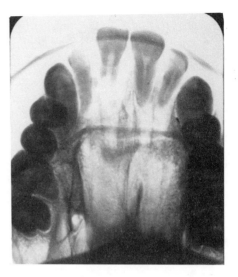

Figure 6–3. Periapical film.

Figure 6–5. Maxillary occlusal radiograph. (Courtesy of Cerritos College Dental Assisting Department.)

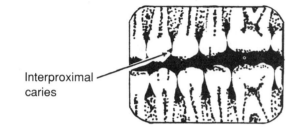

Interproximal caries

Figure 6–4. Bite-wing film.

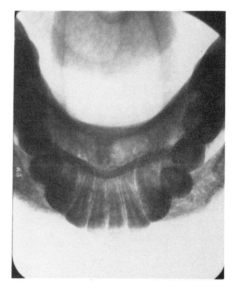

Figure 6–6. Mandibular occlusal radiograph. (Courtesy of Cerritos College Dental Assisting Department.)

TABLE 6–1. FEATURES OF OCCLUSAL FILMS

Arch	Film Packet Placement	Direction of Central Ray
Maxillary	On occlusal surfaces of maxillary teeth; patient bites down on film packet	Perpendicular to film packet; cone is 2–4 inches away from face; occlusal plane parallel to floor
Mandibular	On occlusal surfaces of mandibular teeth; patient bites down on film packet	Beneath mandible; perpendicular to film packet; cone is 2–4 inches away from face; inferior border of mandible aligned perpendicular to floor

EXTRAORAL FILMS

Extraoral films are radiographs taken with the film outside the patient's mouth. The size of these films varies from 5 × 7 inches to 8 × 10 inches to 5 × 12 inches. These films are held in cassettes that perform the same function as the film packet. Most cassettes are metal, but lightweight plastic cassettes are used when taking a panoramic radiograph. Intensifying screens in the cassettes are used to intensify the radiation and, therefore, decrease the exposure time. Table 6–2 describes features of extraoral films (Figs. 6–7, 6–8, 6–9).

TABLE 6–2. EXTRAORAL FILMS

Type of Film	Area Visualized
Lateral skull	Whole skull pathologic survey
Anterior-posterior	Anterior-posterior plane of skull fracture survey
Water's view	Sinuses
Lateral oblique of mandible	One side of mandible, usually for third molar impaction
Temporomandibular joint (TMJ)	TMJ in various positions
Cephalometric (usually a lateral skull plate)	Identifies anthropometric landmarks essential to orthodontic diagnosis

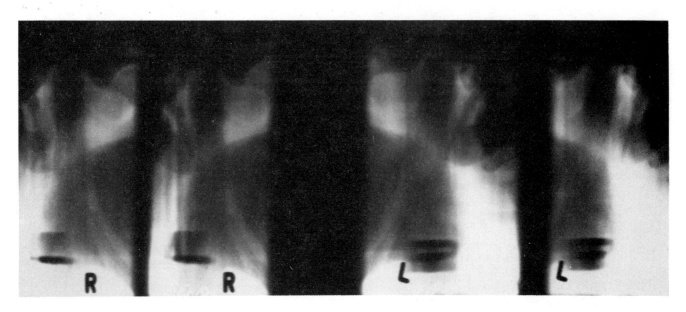

Figure 6–7. Extraoral film of temporomandibular joint. (Courtesy of Veterans Administration Medical Center, West Los Angeles.)

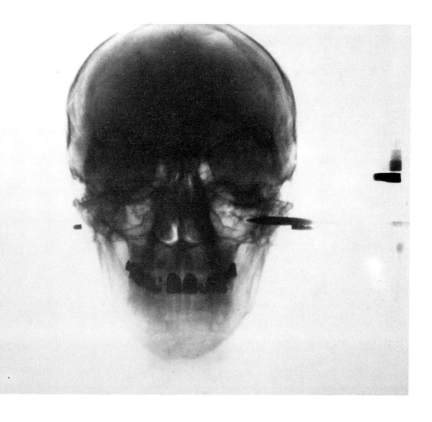

Figure 6–8. Cephalometric film, PA view. (Courtesy of Veterans Administration Medical Center, West Los Angeles.)

PANORAMIC RADIOGRAPHY

Innovations in radiography have led to the ability to take a film of the complete upper and lower jaw simultaneously. This procedure is accomplished by using a panoramic x-ray unit. In essence, the patient's head is fixed and the x-ray tube and film focus and rotate around the patient's head. As a result, a continuous picture is produced on a single film. Such a film is excellent for evaluation of facial trauma (fractures), cysts, and tumors. It is

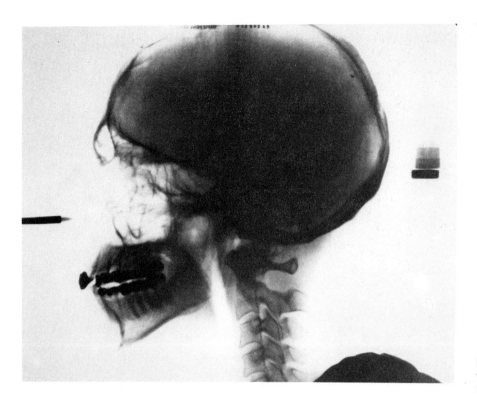

Figure 6–9. Cephalometric film, lateral view. (Courtesy of Veterans Administration Medical Center, West Los Angeles.)

also a very useful film to assess maxillary and mandibular dentition development and to evaluate the jawbones of the edentulous patient.

Some types of machines produce a film displaying a continuous image of the patient's jaws. In these types of units, the x-ray source rotates around the patient's face in a continuous elliptical arch (Fig. 6–10). Other machines are designed so that the x-ray source rotates halfway across the patient's face and stops while the patient's chair moves laterally to a second center of rotation, then continues to expose the other half of the patient's face. Because of the interruption in the exposure, a clear unexposed strip is created vertically down the center of the film (Fig. 6–11).

A panoramic radiograph of diagnostic quality includes the following features.

1. The condyles, inferior border of the mandible, maxilla including zygomatic arches, sinuses, and lower portions of both orbits should be present on the film.
2. The occlusal plane should show a slight upward curve.
3. The teeth are the same size bilaterally without excessive overlap of interproximal contacts.
4. The anterior teeth are of normal size and are not distorted.
5. The condyles are approximately equal distance from the top of the film.
6. The contrast and density allow visualization of the soft tissue structures, such as the tongue, earlobes, and dental pulp tissue.

Advantages and disadvantages of panoramic radiography include the following.

Advantages

1. Areas not seen on a routine full mouth series are shown.
2. Both upper and lower teeth are shown on one film.
3. Less patient cooperation is required.
4. Gagging is eliminated.
5. Less time is required.
6. The patient is exposed to minimum amounts of radiation.

Disadvantages

1. The radiograph is not as diagnostic as individual films for caries or bone height.
2. Images of teeth are enlarged or distorted.
3. There is overlapping of contacts in premolars and molars.
4. Anterior teeth are difficult to see when they have pronounced inclinations.
5. Decreased sharpness and generalized haziness occur.

Positioning Errors

Common positioning errors in panoramic radiography include improper chin tilt, noncentered patients, and tilting of the head to one side. Each error allows structures to appear distorted or to be projected off the film.

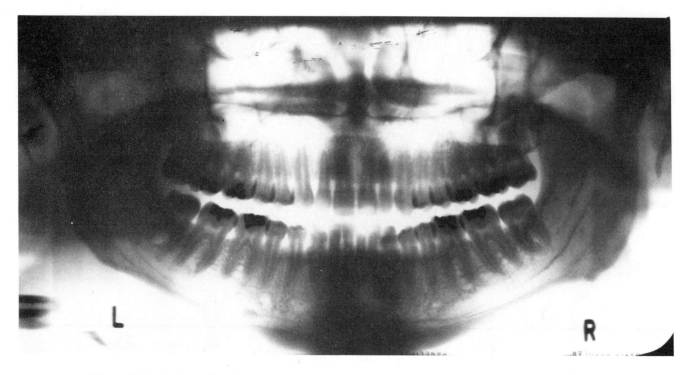

Figure 6–10. Panelipse film of adult dentition. (Courtesy of Veterans Administration Dental Service, West Los Angeles.)

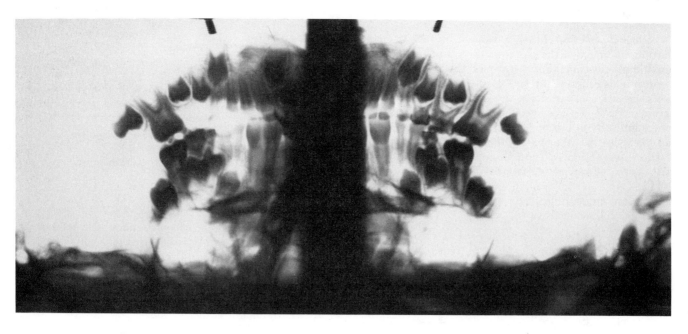

Figure 6–11. Panorex film of mixed dentition. (Courtesy of Cerritos College Dental Assisting Department.)

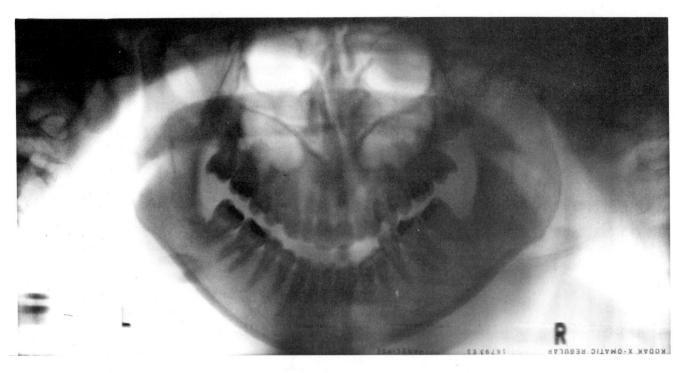

Figure 6–12. Chin tilted downward. (Courtesy of Veterans Administration Dental Service, West Los Angeles.)

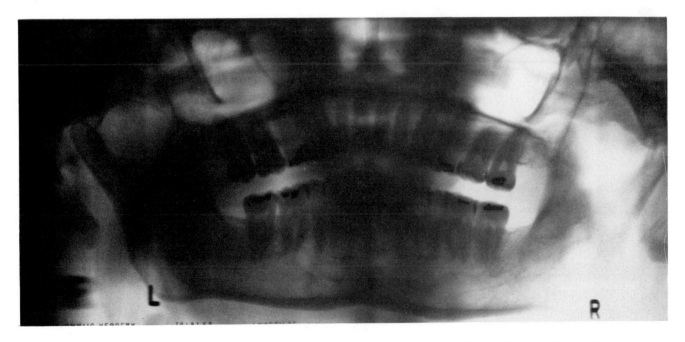

Figure 6–13. Chin tilted upward. (Courtesy of Veterans Administration Dental Service, West Los Angeles.)

Chin tilted too far downward (Fig. 6–12)

1. Mandibular symphysis is projected off the film.
2. Occlusal plane may exhibit an exaggerated curve.
3. Condyles may not be present on the film.
4. Anteriors may be distorted.
5. Excessive overlap of interproximal contacts exists.

Chin tilted too far upward (Fig. 6–13)

1. There is reverse occlusal plane curve.
2. Mandibular structures may appear narrower than normal, whereas maxilla structures appear widened, the palate appears thickened, and the film lacks bilateral image symmetry.

Head turned slightly

1. Images of structures on the side farther from the film appear wider and may be out of focus.
2. Superior portion of the condyle heads may be projected off the film.

TECHNIQUES OF INTRAORAL RADIOGRAPHY

Two techniques are used to take a series of radiographic films: paralleling and bisecting the angle.

The *paralleling technique* is based on the principle that the object (tooth) and the film are parallel to each other, and the central ray is directed perpendicular to both (Fig. 6–14). Increased object–film distance results in loss of image detail, which is compensated for by using a long cone.

Advantages and disadvantages to the paralleling technique are as follows.

Advantages

1. The image formed on the film will have dimensional accuracy.
2. Owing to minimum distortion, periodontal bone height can be diagnosed accurately.
3. On maxillary molar projection, there is little or no root superimposition.

Disadvantages

1. Intraoral film-holding devices must be used. These devices can be difficult to work with and uncomfortable for the patient.
2. Some patients have anatomic features, such as low palatal vaults, that prevent proper placement of film.
3. The use of a long cone necessitates an increase in exposure time.

In the *bisecting the angle technique,* an imaginary line is identified that bisects the angle formed by the long axis of the tooth and the film. The central ray is directed perpendicularly to the imaginary line. This technique uses a short cone (Fig. 6–15).

Advantages and disadvantages to the bisecting the angle technique are as follows.

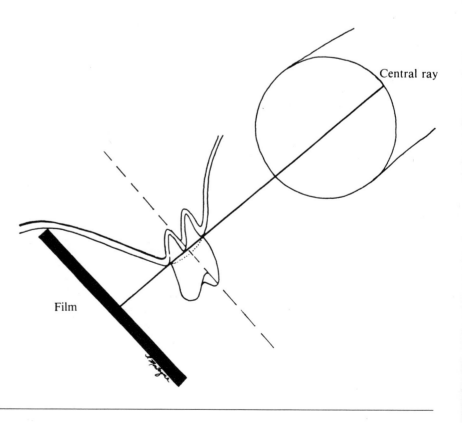

Figure 6–14. Central ray, tooth, and film packet in parallel angle technique.

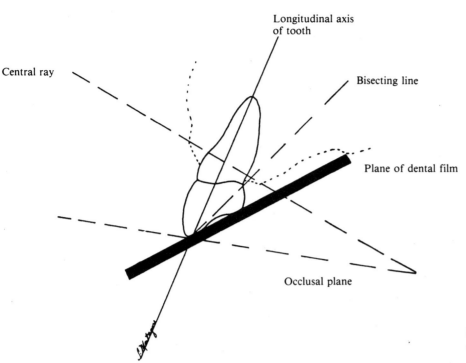

Longitudinal axis
of tooth

Central ray

Bisecting line

Plane of dental film

Occlusal plane

Figure 6–15. Bisecting the angle technique of intraoral radiography.

Advantages

1. Decreased exposure time.
2. Less cumbersome film holder.
3. Anatomic features usually do not interfere with film placement.

Disadvantages

1. The image projected on the film is dimensionally distorted in varying degrees.
2. True alveolar bone height can be misinterpreted.
3. The use of a short cone results in divergent rays. Therefore, the image is not an optimum reproduction of the object.

STANDARD FULL SERIES RADIOGRAPH SURVEYS

A full mouth series of radiographs for an adult with a full complement of teeth usually is composed of at least 14 to 16 periapical films and 4 bite-wing films (Fig. 6–16). Periapical films show the entire tooth and the supporting alveolar bone. They are used to diagnose bone and root pathologic conditions and to provide information on tooth formation and eruption.

Bite-wing films show upper and lower teeth in occlusion. The full roots of the teeth are not visible on the film. Bite-wing films are useful in identifying recurrent decay, proximal decay, the proximal gingival marginal fit of restorations, and periodontal bone loss.

The following projections constitute a typical full series for a patient with a complete dentition.

Maxillary periapicals

- Right and left central and lateral incisors
- Right and left canines
- Right and left premolars
- Right and left molars

Mandibular periapicals

- Right and left central and lateral incisors
- Right and left canines
- Right and left premolars
- Right and left molars

Bite-wings

- Right and left premolars
- Right and left molars

A suggested sequence is as follows.

1. Maxillary right projections
2. Maxillary left projections
3. Bite-wings (left, then right)
4. Mandibular right projections
5. Mandibular left projections

The pedodontic full mouth survey differs from the adult full mouth survey in the number of radiographs and the size of film packets used. The number of radiographs and the film size depend on the age of the child and the stage of dental development (Fig. 6–17).

The edentulous full mouth survey usually consists of 14 periapical films. Bite-wing films are not taken. Other modifications when taking an edentulous series include increase the vertical angulation, decrease the exposure time, and replace the occlusal plane with the crest of the

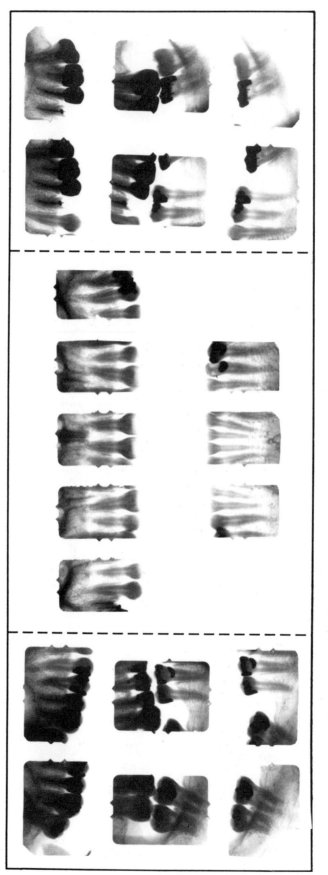

Figure 6–16. Adult full mouth survey. (Courtesy of Veterans Administration Dental Service, West Los Angeles.)

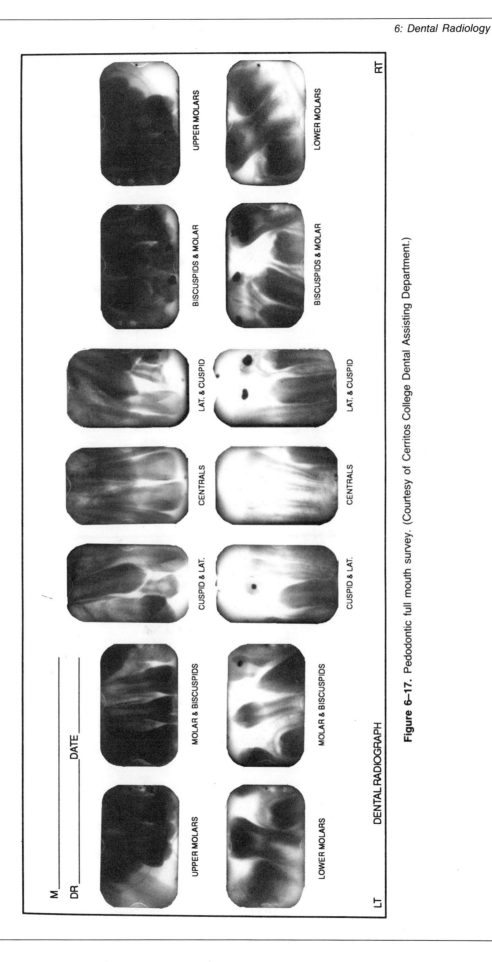

Figure 6–17. Pedodontic full mouth survey. (Courtesy of Cerritos College Dental Assisting Department.)

edentulous ridge. The edentulous survey is important in diagnosing pathologic conditions, such as cysts and abscesses, and locating retained root tips and impacted teeth.

RULES FOR EXPOSING RADIOGRAPHS

Regardless of whether the paralleling technique or bisecting the angle technique is used, certain procedures and rules must be followed.

1. Seat the patient with head positioned so that the occlusal plane of the jaw being radiographed is parallel to the floor and the midsagittal plane is perpendicular to the floor.
2. Remove any eyeglasses or removable prosthetic appliances.
3. Drape the patient with a leaded lap apron that extends from the neck past the genital area and thyrocervical collar.
4. Turn the knob to the desired exposure time before placing the film in the patient's mouth. (A chart listing the desired exposure times for each area to be radiographed should be posted near the machine.)
5. After an exposure is made, remove the film from the patient's mouth. Dry the film and place it in a lead-lined container or disposable cup.
6. Never place films, either exposed or unexposed, within an operatory where exposures are made.
7. Follow a definite order when taking a full series. Do not shift from area to area.
8. Use appropriate infection control techniques and protective barriers when exposing radiographs.

Common Errors in Exposure of a Full Mouth Series of Radiographs

Table 6–3 lists errors commonly made in the exposure of a full mouth series, as well as the reasons for these errors.

THE DEVELOPMENT PROCESS

A latent image exists on the film after it is exposed in the patient's mouth. The energized silver halide crystals must be processed through chemical reactions so that the latent image becomes a visible image. This developing process occurs in the darkroom. The darkroom is a separate room used specifically for processing exposed radiographs. The following components and requirements are essential.

1. No light leaks (films out of their holders are light sensitive)
2. Safelight (usually a 10-watt or 15-watt bulb with a red filter placed about 3 to 4 feet from the working surface)
3. Developing tank with three compartments
   a. Developer (usually on the right)
   b. Wash
   c. Fixer
4. Timing device
5. Thermometer (in developing solution)
6. Rack on which to place films
7. Clean working surface
8. Sink (for cleaning tanks)
9. View box
10. Storage space

Before developing films, all solutions should be stirred to ensure that the solutions are homogeneous and that the temperatures are equalized. Failure to maintain accu-

TABLE 6–3. ERRORS IN EXPOSURE OF FULL MOUTH SERIES OF RADIOGRAPHS

Common Error	Reasons
Elongation (most common error)	Too little vertical angulation; occlusal plane not parallel to floor; film not against tissue; poor film placement
Foreshortening	Too much vertical angulation; poor chair position
Cone cutting (clear film, curved line)	Beam not aimed at center of film
Film reversal or herringbone effect	Film placed in mouth backward
Film placement	Film not placed far enough in patient's mouth
Sagittal plane orientation (occlusal surfaces appear because patient has leaned over; elongation and distortion)	Plane not perpendicular to floor
Overlapping	Incorrect horizontal angulation (central ray not perpendicular to center of film)
Crescent-shaped marks (black lines)	Overbent films; cracked emulsion
Light films (underexposed) (image not dense enough)	Incorrect milliamperes (too low) or time (too short); cone not approximating patient's face; incorrect focal film distance (FFD)
Dark films (overexposed) (image too dense)	Incorrect milliamperes (too low) or time (too long)
Double exposure	Film used twice
Fogged films	Exposure to radiation other than primary beam
Artifacts	Failure to remove prosthetic appliances, earrings, or eyeglasses
Clear films	Unexposed
Blurred image	Caution patient to avoid movement; adjust tube head and extension arm to prevent drifting
Poor contrast	Incorrect, kVp—too high; to correct, decrease kVp

rate records or to process films correctly will result in unnecessary radiation to the patient because radiographs will have to be retaken.

Film Processing

Under the safelight conditions, each film should be carefully unwrapped and placed on the film rack. The development process for films is then accomplished in five steps.

1. *Developing.* The developing solution is a basic solution of Elon or metal hydroquinone that reduces the energized silver halide crystals to silver. The silver is precipitated on the film base and appears black (radiolucent). Since this precipitation process is dependent on the concentration and temperature of the development fluid, the radiograph is very sensitive to both the length of time in the developer and the temperature of the solution. The optimum time–temperature relationship is 4½ minutes at 68°F.
2. *Washing.* The developed film is then washed for approximately 20 to 30 seconds in running water. Washing stops the developing stage and removes any remaining developing solution that might contaminate the fixer.
3. *Fixing.* The fixing solution is an acidic solution that contains sodium thiosulfate and sodium sulfite, which removes the unexposed (or unenergized) silver halide crystals from the emulsion and preserves the picture. There is potassium aluminum in the solution for the purpose of shrinking and hardening the film. Radiographs must be placed in the fixer for a minimum of 10 minutes, since inadequate fixation will cause the films to turn brown. Films may be removed from the fixer for inspection 1 minute after exposure but should be replaced for 10 minutes to complete fixation.
4. *Washing.* Films must be placed in running water for at least 20 minutes. This final wash ensures removal of the fixing solution from the emulsion.
5. *Drying.* Films must be dried in a dust-free, clean area either by air drying or machine drying.

Table 6–4 lists common errors made in the darkroom.

Automatic Processing

In recent years, automatic processing equipment has become available that permits films to be carried on a series of rollers from solution to solution. The appropriate time–temperature relationship is set, and dry films emerge in approximately 5 minutes. These machines save time, but they require periodic cleaning, and solutions must be changed regularly.

STEPS FOR MOUNTING RADIOGRAPHS

1. Separate the films into three piles.
   a. Anterior periapicals. The teeth are shown on the film vertically (up and down).

TABLE 6–4. COMMON ERRORS IN THE DARKROOM

Error	Causes
Record keeping	Racks not labeled
Fogged film	White light leak; faulty safelight
Underdeveloped film	Incorrect time (short) and temperature (cold); expended solutions (weak solutions)
Overdeveloped film	Incorrect time (long) and temperature (hot)
Developer cutoff (top of film is clear straight line)	Solutions too low
Clear films (emulsion washed away)	Films left in wash (running rinse water) for more than 24 hours
Stained film	Sloppy or dirty working surface
Scratched film	Racks hit; fingernails too long
Brown films	Films have not had adequate fixation
Torn emulsion	Films touching or overlapping while drying
Static marks (multiple black linear streaks)	Static electricity caused by friction when opening film packet
Lost films	Films not placed carefully in rack

   b. Posterior periapicals. The teeth are shown on the film horizontally (across).
   c. Bite-wings. The crowns of both the upper and lower teeth are shown on the film (the roots are not visible).
2. View the anterior films with the dot facing outward (labial mounting). Separate the maxillary films from the mandibular films. They can be identified by referring to anatomic landmarks (Tables 6–5 and 6–6).
3. Mount the anterior periapical films. The incisal edges of the maxillary anteriors are to be facing downward. The incisal edges of the mandibular anteriors are to be facing upward. (This is the same position as the teeth in the mount.)
4. View the posterior films with the dot facing outward. Separate the mandibular films from the maxillary films.
5. Mount the posterior periapicals. The occlusal surfaces of the maxillary teeth are to be facing downward. The occlusal surfaces of the mandibular teeth are to be facing upward.
6. View the bite-wing films with the dot facing outward.
7. Mount the bite-wings. The bite-wings should match with the crowns of the periapical films directly above.
8. Check the mounted radiographs to be sure
   a. All dots are facing same direction.

TABLE 6–5. RADIOLUCENT ANATOMIC LANDMARKS

Area	Landmarks
Mandibular molar	1. Mandibular canal (inferior alveolar canal)
	2. Mandibular foramen
Mandibular premolar	1. Mental foramen
	2. Mandibular canal
Mandibular cuspid	1. Mental foramen (position varies)
Mandibular incisor	1. Lingual foramen
Maxillary premolar	1. Anterior portion of maxillary sinus
Maxillary cuspid	1. Nasal fossae
	2. Maxillary sinus
Maxillary incisor	1. Incisive foramen and portion of incisive canal
	2. Median palatine suture
	3. Nasal fossae
	4. Outline of nasal shadow

TABLE 6–6. RADIOPAQUE ANATOMIC LANDMARKS

Area	Landmarks
Mandibular molar	1. Anterior border of ramus
	2. External oblique line
	3. Mylohyoid line—internal oblique
	4. Impacted third molar
Mandibular premolar	1. Inferior border of mandible
	2. Mylohyoid line or ridge
	3. Mandibular tori
Mandibular cuspid	1. Mental process
	2. Inferior border of mandible
Mandibular incisor	1. Genial spine or tubercle
	2. Mental prominence
	3. Inferior border of mandible
	4. Mental symphysis
Maxillary molar	1. Coronoid process
	2. Pterygoid hamulus
	3. Zygomatic arch
	4. Maxillary tuberosity
	5. Outline of maxillary sinus
Maxillary premolar	1. U-shaped zygomatic process
	2. Floor of nasal cavity
	3. Outline of maxillary sinus
Maxillary cuspid	1. Inverted Y-formation of maxillary sinus
Maxillary incisor	1. Median nasal septum
	2. Outline of soft tissue of nose

b. All incisal and occlusal surfaces are facing in the proper direction.
c. Radiographs on right side of mount are matching (restorations, missing teeth, impactions, and so on).
d. Radiographs on left side of mount are matching.

Landmarks to Facilitate Mounting

Anatomic landmarks are those normal structures and areas that appear in a routine series of radiographs. However, these structures will not appear with the same clarity for all patients. The terms *radiolucent* and *radiopaque* refer to the penetration ability of x-rays. The term radiolucent describes the dark areas that appear on the radiograph. Tissues such as oral mucosa, pulp, and gingiva provide little or no resistance, and, therefore, x-rays can easily penetrate these thin or less dense objects. This is in contrast to the very light areas on the film. Structures that are very thick or dense, such as amalgam restorations, enamel, and bone, absorb most x-rays and do not permit them to reach the film. These structures are termed radiopaque and appear white. Tables 6–5 and 6–6 list radiopaque and radiolucent anatomic landmarks that can be identified on a series of radiographs.

Additional Guidelines to Facilitate Mounting

1. The slight curve upward from the cuspid area toward the molar area, formed by the occlusal (biting) surfaces of the teeth
2. The upward curve of bone at the end of the mandibular arch
3. The appearance of the area behind the maxillary molar (shadows formed) as compared with the appearance of the area behind the mandibular molars (definite shape of the mandible)
4. The root difference between maxillary and mandibular teeth
5. Root tips that usually curve toward the distal
6. The differing bone densities in the mandibular and maxillary arches
7. The differences in size of anterior teeth (mandibular anterior teeth are smaller than the maxillary anterior teeth)
8. The darkened area (maxillary sinus is radiolucent) usually visible above and between the roots of the maxillary premolars and molar areas
9. The white lines (floor and walls of the cavities and sinuses) visible on the maxillary arch
10. Maxillary first premolars usually have two roots, whereas mandibular premolars have one root
11. Mandibular first and second molars usually have two divergent curved roots with bone clearly visible between them. This is particularly true of the first molar. Maxillary molars have three roots, two buccal and one palatal. The large palatal root obscures the intraradicular bone.

INFECTION CONTROL AND RADIOGRAPHS

Although exposing, processing, and mounting dental radiographs are not considered a primary source for disease transmission, proper infection control procedures should always be followed. The barriers for the tube head and exposure control switch are more easily protected than trying to disinfect them using chemicals. Of course, protective attire (ie, gloves, mask, and protective eyewear) must be worn during patient contact.

After exposing intraoral radiographs, the exposed film should be placed in a paper cup for processing. Once in the darkroom, carefully unwrap the film packets, spill the untouched film on an uncontaminated flat surface, and dispose of the wrappings in a waste receptacle as you proceed. When all of the films have been unwrapped, remove and discard gloves in the waste receptacle and deposit the film in the automatic processor or place on film racks. If the automatic film processor has a daylight loader, the constant contamination of the fabric light shield must be recognized. When gloved, contaminated hands are inserted through the elastic light shield, the fabric is repeatedly soiled, and there is no practical way to disinfect this material. The following procedure is suggested.

1. Place the exposed film in a paper cup and remove soiled gloves.
2. Use clean gloved hands to place cup inside the daylight loader and close lid.
3. Clean gloved hands pass through the light shield to unwrap the film.
4. Drop the film onto the uncontaminated surface inside the loader.
5. Place the soiled film wrapping in the cup.
6. Remove soiled gloves and place them in the paper cup.
7. Place film into the chute for developing.

Questions

DIRECTIONS (Questions 1 through 121): Each of the questions or incomplete statements in this section is followed by four suggested answers or completions. Select the ONE lettered answer or completion that is BEST in each case. Check your answers with the correct answers at the end of the chapter.

1. A dental assistant may expose radiographs

   (A) if the dentist gives permission
   (B) if he or she is a certified dental assistant
   (C) if it is permissible in the state in which he or she is employed
   (D) if he or she is supervised by the dentist or hygienist

2. The most sensitive cells to ionizing radiation are

   (A) bone cells
   (B) muscle cells
   (C) nerve cells
   (D) reproductive cells

3. The best type of x-ray to penetrate body tissue is

   (A) low frequencies
   (B) hard rays, short wavelength
   (C) long wavelength
   (D) soft rays, long wavelength

4. X-rays are made up of

   (A) electrons
   (B) protons
   (C) photons
   (D) neutrons

5. The cathode is a filament composed of

   (A) tungsten
   (B) silver
   (C) copper
   (D) aluminum

6. Milliamperage controls

   (A) the speed with which electrons move from cathode to anode
   (B) cooling of the anode
   (C) heating of the anode
   (D) heating of the cathode

7. Collimation of the primary beam

   (A) decreases the exposure time
   (B) restricts the shape and size of the beam
   (C) makes the primary beam more difficult to connect
   (D) dictates the contrast of the final radiograph

8. The lead diaphragm determines the size and shape of the

   (A) electron cloud
   (B) film used
   (C) x-ray beam
   (D) filament

9. The portion of the target that is struck by electrons is called the

   (A) focal spot
   (B) photon point
   (C) principal point
   (D) end point

10. Proper collimation for the film size and target–film distance will

    (A) increase the wavelength
    (B) decrease the wavelength
    (C) increase the kVp
    (D) decrease the radiation received by the patient

11. To increase the penetrating quality of an x-ray beam, the auxiliary must

    (A) increase kVp
    (B) decrease kVp
    (C) increase mA
    (D) increase FFD

12. The x-ray at the center of the primary beam is called

    (A) photon ray
    (B) central ray

(C) secondary ray
(D) restricted beam

13. The housing of the x-ray tube is

(A) copper
(B) plastic
(C) tungsten
(D) glass

14. Filtration of the x-ray beam protects the patient by

(A) eliminating all radiation from the x-ray head
(B) eliminating weak wavelength x-rays from the x-ray beam
(C) eliminating short wavelength x-rays from the x-ray beam
(D) decreasing exposure time

15. The size of the collimated beam for intraoral radiology measured at the patient's skin is

(A) 1.5–1.75 inches
(B) 2.0 2.25 inches
(C) 2.75–3.0 inches
(D) 3.25–3.5 inches

16. Scatter radiation is a type of

(A) secondary radiation
(B) primary radiation
(C) stray radiation
(D) filtered radiation

17. The quality, or penetrating power, of secondary radiation is

(A) more than that of primary radiation
(B) less than that of primary radiation
(C) the same as that of primary radiation
(D) unrelated to that of primary radiation

18. The first sign of x-ray dermatitis is

(A) alopecia
(B) erythema
(C) dry skin
(D) pain

19. The time period between the effects of cumulative radiation and visible tissue damage is the

(A) short-term period
(B) acute effect period
(C) latent period
(D) long-term period

20. The amount of radiation a person receives

(A) begins anew each day
(B) is cumulative only on the skin
(C) is cumulative in the entire body
(D) is not harmful in small doses

21. Maximum protection of the patient requires that the x-ray beam pass through a

(A) shielded open-ended cone
(B) plastic closed-ended cone
(C) shielded closed-ended cone
(D) lead apron

22. A technique used to measure the operator's exposure to radiation is

(A) to check the color of the operator's fingernails
(B) for the operator to wear a radiation film badge
(C) to multiply the number of films the operator has exposed by 0.1 rem
(D) to count the number of full mouth x-ray series taken

23. Accumulated radiation dosage for those who work with radiation may not exceed

(A) 0.1 rem/week
(B) 1 rem/week
(C) 10 rems/week
(D) 100 rems/week

24. The operator must avoid all of the following EXCEPT

(A) stray radiation
(B) secondary radiation
(C) the primary beam
(D) natural sunlight

25. To avoid exposure to secondary radiation, the operator should stand

(A) at least 6 feet from the x-ray head
(B) 2 feet to the right of the primary beam
(C) any distance in back of the x-ray head
(D) 4 feet in front of the patient

26. The most effective way to reduce gonadal exposure from x-rays is to

(A) increase the kVp
(B) use a leaded lap apron
(C) increase vertical angulation
(D) use ultraspeed film

27. After each use, the leaded lap apron must be

(A) stored in the darkroom
(B) folded neatly and stored in the operatory
(C) draped over a support rod unfolded
(D) discarded for appropriate infection control

28. Which characteristic of x-rays makes them both beneficial and hazardous?

    (A) they cause tissue regeneration
    (B) they dehydrate tissue
    (C) they destroy tissue
    (D) they can penetrate metallic restorations

29. The best technique for reducing the radiation exposure to both patient and operator is the use of

    (A) an automatic timer
    (B) fast film
    (C) thinner films
    (D) a thicker cellulose acetate base

30. Film speed is determined by the

    (A) amount of silver bromide salt
    (B) thickness of cellulose acetate base
    (C) size of the silver bromide crystal
    (D) side of the film exposed

31. The radiographic film is covered with an emulsion of

    (A) silver bromide salts
    (B) cellulose
    (C) silver acetate
    (D) potassium bromide

32. The raised button on the radiograph aids in

    (A) determining film speed
    (B) processing
    (C) drying
    (D) mounting

33. The purpose of the lead foil in dental film is to

    (A) provide stiffness to the film
    (B) reduce film fogging
    (C) absorb the primary beam
    (D) prevent scattered radiation to the patient

34. The detection of interproximal caries is seen best with a (an)

    (A) occlusal film
    (B) panorex film
    (C) bite-wing film
    (D) lateral head plate

35. Which extraoral film is used to visualize the sinus?

    (A) Water's film
    (B) lateral skull film
    (C) occlusal film
    (D) posterior-anterior film

36. X-ray films should be kept by the dentist along with other records for

    (A) 1 year
    (B) 2 years
    (C) 5 years
    (D) indefinitely

37. If a patient expresses concern about the hazards of radiation, the patient can be assured that

    (A) only those films necessary for proper diagnosis will be exposed
    (B) automatic film processors will be used
    (C) the auxiliary is wearing a safety monitor
    (D) the walls of the operatory are lead lined

38. The periapical film reveals

    (A) the entire jaw
    (B) upper and lower teeth in the same film
    (C) interproximal caries
    (D) the entire tooth, including the apex

39. Interproximal film may show all of the following EXCEPT

    (A) incipient caries
    (B) root tip fractures
    (C) crest of alveolar bone
    (D) recurrent decay under existing restorations

40. Which of these is not a factor when considering what size film to use?

    (A) patient's age
    (B) the size of the mouth opening
    (C) the shape of the patient's dental arches
    (D) patient's previous radiation exposure

41. The principle used in panoramic radiography is

    (A) long cone paralleling
    (B) laminagraphy
    (C) horizontal curvature
    (D) panoramography

42. A material or substance that does NOT stop or absorb x-rays is known as

    (A) radiographic
    (B) radiopaque
    (C) radiolucent
    (D) radiodontic

43. A material or substance that does stop or absorb x-rays is known as

    (A) radiographic
    (B) radiopaque
    (C) radiolucent
    (D) radiodontic

44. All of the tissues listed are radiopaque EXCEPT the

    (A) enamel
    (B) cortical plate
    (C) pulp chamber
    (D) alveolar bone

45. Which of these appears radiolucent?

    (A) caries
    (B) calculus
    (C) torus
    (D) root tips

46. What is the name of the diagonal radiopaque line visible at the lower part of the roots of the mandibular molars?

    (A) mandibular canal
    (B) external oblique ridge
    (C) inferior border of mandible
    (D) internal oblique line

47. What is the small circular radiolucency near the roots of the mandibular premolars called?

    (A) lingual foramen
    (B) mental foramen
    (C) mandibular foramen
    (D) incisive foramen

48. What term describes the U-shaped radiopaque structure often seen in maxillary molar films?

    (A) hamulus
    (B) tuberosity
    (C) zygoma
    (D) nasal septum

49. What is the thin radiopaque band between the maxillary incisors called?

    (A) median palatine suture
    (B) nasal septum
    (C) inverted Y
    (D) zygoma

50. What term describes the heavily radiopaque mid-point of the mandible?

    (A) zygoma
    (B) odontoma
    (C) hamulus
    (D) symphysis

51. What is the small circular radiolucency below the mandibular incisor roots called?

    (A) incisive foramen
    (B) lingual foramen
    (C) mental foramen
    (D) buccal foramen

52. What is the large radiolucent area shown on maxillary molar radiographs called?

    (A) maxillary sinus
    (B) maxillary septum
    (C) maxillary tuberosity
    (D) maxillary sequestrum

53. What is the long, narrow, and radiolucent area visible below the roots of the mandibular molars called?

    (A) inferior border
    (B) internal oblique line
    (C) external oblique line
    (D) mandibular canal

54. What is the radiopaque circular area below the apices of the mandibular incisors called?

    (A) genial tubercles
    (B) mental ridge
    (C) symphysis
    (D) lamina dura

55. Which of these structures is radiopaque?

    (A) pulp chamber
    (B) mucosa
    (C) periodontal ligament space
    (D) lamina dura

56. Which of these appears radiolucent?

    (A) granuloma
    (B) calculus
    (C) pulp stone
    (D) cementoma

57. The basic principle of the bisecting the angle technique is

    (A) central ray must be directed at right angles to the tooth
    (B) central ray must be directed at right angles to the film
    (C) central ray must be directed at right angles to an imaginary line that bisects the angle formed by the long axis of the tooth and the plane of film
    (D) central ray must be directed at a 45-degree angle to the embrasures

58. The basic principles of the paralleling technique are all of the following EXCEPT

    (A) film must be parallel to long axis of tooth
    (B) 8-inch short cone must be used
    (C) source of x-ray must be directed perpendicular to tooth and film
    (D) 16-inch extension or long cone must be used

59. When taking a full mouth series of intraoral x-rays, the sagittal plane of the patient's head should be

    (A) perpendicular to the floor
    (B) parallel to the floor
    (C) parallel to the tube
    (D) perpendicular to the central ray

60. The side of the nose is called the

    (A) tragus
    (B) zygoma
    (C) ala
    (D) maxilla

61. The ala–tragus line is parallel to the floor when taking

    (A) mandibular occlusal films
    (B) mandibular periapical films
    (C) extraoral films only
    (D) maxillary periapical films

62. The occlusal plane of the maxillary arch being radiographed should be

    (A) perpendicular to the floor
    (B) parallel to the floor
    (C) at an angle of 45 degrees to the floor
    (D) at an angle of 30 degrees to the floor

63. Vertical angulation in the bisecting technique for the same radiograph can differ in patients because of

    (A) the size of the teeth
    (B) anatomic differences
    (C) gagging
    (D) age

64. Periapical films should extend beyond the occlusal plane

    (A) ⅛ inch
    (B) ¼ inch
    (C) ⅜ inch
    (D) ½ inch

65. Firm placement of the film will help prevent

    (A) overlapping
    (B) foreshortening
    (C) gagging
    (D) elongation

66. A latent image is

    (A) an image taken with a long exposure
    (B) found on only fast films
    (C) composed of energized silver halide crystals
    (D) a very light image on the developed film

67. Cone cutting results from the central ray

    (A) not being aimed at the center of film
    (B) having incorrect horizontal angulation
    (C) having insufficient vertical angulation
    (D) being eliminated from a closed plastic cone

68. Black lines across the film may be the result of

    (A) double exposure
    (B) cone cutting

    (C) underexposure
    (D) excessive bending

69. Blurred films can result from

    (A) old film
    (B) movement of the patient
    (C) increased kVp
    (D) faulty x-ray unit

70. If a patient is reluctant to be radiographed, the auxiliary should

    (A) refer the patient to the dental hygienist
    (B) reschedule the patient
    (C) refer the patient to an x-ray laboratory
    (D) explain the procedure thoroughly to the patient

71. To visualize the two roots on the maxillary first premolar, the central ray should be directed

    (A) perpendicular to the buccal surface
    (B) perpendicular to the lingual surface
    (C) toward the occlusal surface
    (D) slightly from the mesial or distal surface

72. Exposure of a radiograph on a child

    (A) requires less time than an adult
    (B) requires more time than an adult
    (C) requires the same time as an adult
    (D) should never be attempted

73. Intensifying screens

    (A) are used in intraoral films
    (B) decrease exposure time of extraoral films
    (C) create additional x-rays
    (D) fuse with the film

74. As the target–film distance is increased, there is

    (A) more chance of overlapping
    (B) more chance of elongation
    (C) less distortion
    (D) more chance of foreshortening

75. A panorex film that exhibits distortion in the molar region and is lighter on one side of the film only indicates that

    (A) the patient's head was not tipped down at a 5-degree angle
    (B) the wrong caliper adjustment scale was read
    (C) the patient's chin was not positioned properly
    (D) a cotton roll was not placed between the anterior incisors

76. The usual number of films in a complete dentulous radiographic survey is

    (A) 10 to 12

(B) 18 to 20
(C) 24 to 26
(D) 26 to 28

77. In the paralleling technique, a device used to hold the film in the patient's mouth is

(A) a film holder
(B) a plastic dental instrument
(C) the patient's finger
(D) rubber bite block

78. Extraoral films are

(A) not sensitive to light
(B) less sensitive to light than intraoral films
(C) just as sensitive to light as intraoral films
(D) more sensitive to light than intraoral films

79. If the mA is increased while the kVp and the exposure time are kept constant, the resulting films will

(A) be lighter
(B) be darker
(C) remain the same
(D) have a herringbone pattern

80. Elongation is caused by

(A) insufficient vertical angulation
(B) too much vertical angulation
(C) insufficient horizontal angulation
(D) excessive bending of the film

81. Foreshortening is caused by

(A) insufficient vertical angulation
(B) too much vertical angulation
(C) insufficient horizontal angulation
(D) excessive bending of the film

82. If a film is exposed on the wrong side, the result will be

(A) darker films
(B) no image at all
(C) no effect
(D) a herringbone pattern

83. X-rays are most effectively stopped by

(A) copper
(B) glass
(C) lead
(D) tungsten

84. After a film is exposed, the target–film distance is doubled. The exposure time necessary to obtain a second film of equal density to the first film is

(A) the same as the first film
(B) twofold
(C) threefold
(D) fourfold

85. A patient with an extremely narrow maxillary arch presents placement problems in x-raying the premolar areas. In the bisection technique, which of the following placements would help solve this problem?

(A) use the parallel technique for this film
(B) use cross-section film placement
(C) force film into the midline of the palate and increase vertical angulation
(D) lay the film on a flat plane in contact with the opposite side of the palate to increase vertical angulation

86. Which of the following is used to describe the blackness of an exposed radiograph?

(A) density
(B) detail
(C) darkness
(D) development

87. The difference in density of various regions of a radiograph is called

(A) collimation
(B) contrast
(C) filtration
(D) definition

88. The dental auxiliary is asked to change the 8-inch short cone to the 16-inch long cone. At twice the distance, the intensity of the x-rays is now only

(A) ½ as great
(B) ¼ as great
(C) ⅙ as great
(D) ⅛ as great

89. For maximum penetration of x-rays, which of the following combinations would you select?

(A) 90 kVp and 10 mA
(B) 65 kVp and 10 mA
(C) 70 kVp and 90 mA
(D) 10 kVp and 65 mA

90. The dentist's new x-ray machine has inherent filtration of 2 mm of aluminum. The dentist is operating the x-ray machine above 70 kVp for diagnostic x-ray film. Which of the following amounts of added filtration will be necessary to meet the minimum total filtration required?

(A) 1.5 mm aluminum
(B) 0.5 mm aluminum
(C) 2.5 mm aluminum
(D) 2.0 mm aluminum

91. Appropriate infection control procedures during x-ray exposure should include

    (A) wiping the film holders with alcohol gauze
    (B) use of disposable cotton roll holders
    (C) placement of a lead screen around the patient
    (D) placement of a disposable plastic bag over the x-ray tubehead

92. When exposing the patient to only one periapical radiograph, the auxiliary

    (A) may diagnose the film
    (B) must enter this procedure in the dental chart
    (C) may take as many retakes as needed
    (D) does not need to use a lead apron on the patient

93. Cephalometric radiographs are used in which area of dentistry?

    (A) operative
    (B) pedodontics
    (C) orthodontics
    (D) periodontics

94. Extraoral films are placed in rigid frames called

    (A) film frames
    (B) skull plates
    (C) jaw plates
    (D) cassettes

95. The best sequence for exposing maxillary radiographs is

    (A) central incisors, right cuspid, left cuspid
    (B) central incisors, right cuspid, right bicuspid
    (C) central incisors, right biscupsid, right cuspid
    (D) central incisors, right molar, right bicuspid

96. Radiographs of edentulous portions of a patient's mouth

    (A) should be exposed routinely
    (B) should be exposed only on request of the patient
    (C) should be exposed only if the entire arch is edentulous
    (D) are unnecessary

97. A logical sequence for a full mouth survey of a patient with a complete dentition is

    (A) upper arch, bite-wings, lower arch
    (B) upper arch, lower arch, bite-wings
    (C) bite-wings, lower arch, upper arch
    (D) lower arch, bite-wings, upper arch

98. If the end of the x-ray cone approximates the tip of the patient's nose, the operator is exposing a radiograph of the

    (A) maxillary cuspid
    (B) maxillary central incisors
    (C) mandibular incisors
    (D) maxillary bicuspid

99. The developing solution

    (A) should always be left open
    (B) could be partially covered
    (C) should always be covered
    (D) should be covered only when films are being developed

100. Films left overnight in the fixer

    (A) will be clear
    (B) will be too dark to read
    (C) will not be affected
    (D) will disintegrate

101. During processing, when can radiographs safely be exposed to light?

    (A) after the final wash
    (B) after development
    (C) after the first wash
    (D) after being placed in the fixer

102. The thermometer used to measure the temperature of the processing solutions is located

    (A) in the developer
    (B) in the wash water
    (C) in the fixer
    (D) above the processing solutions on the wall

103. Film fog can occur if there is

    (A) extremely thick bone
    (B) a light leak in the darkroom
    (C) slow film
    (D) reversal of the film

104. Film is washed after removing it from the developing solution to

    (A) remove any debris on the film
    (B) speed up the developing process
    (C) stop the developing process
    (D) remove the precipitated silver salts

105. The fixing solution is

    (A) acidic
    (B) neutral
    (C) basic
    (D) first basic, then neutral after dilution

106. Two films are developed for the same length of time but at different temperatures. The film developed at the higher temperature will be

    (A) lighter
    (B) darker

(C) the same
(D) clear

107. If an unexposed film is processed, it will appear

(A) white
(B) black
(C) blue
(D) clear

108. Fixing the film

(A) removes the unaffected silver salts
(B) removes the affected silver salts
(C) softens the film
(D) peels the emulsion from the film base

109. The temperature of the radiographic processing solutions is adjusted by

(A) individual heaters
(B) chemical interaction
(C) a temperature-adjustable waterbath
(D) gas heaters

110. If a radiograph remains in the developing solution too long, the film will be

(A) lighter
(B) darker
(C) lighter only if the temperature is increased
(D) unaffected because time is not a factor

111. If a properly processed film is left overnight in the water, it will be

(A) dark
(B) light with faded image
(C) unchanged
(D) clear with no image

112. After the films are removed from the fixer, they are washed for

(A) 5–10 minutes
(B) 11–19 minutes
(C) 20–30 minutes
(D) 1 hour

113. For the developing chemicals to work, the solution must be

(A) acidic
(B) neutral
(C) basic
(D) very warm

114. A processed film reveals small white spots, indicating incomplete development. The error on the film during processing was caused by

(A) exposure to visible light and incomplete fixing

(B) films coming in contact with fixing solution before the proper processing procedure
(C) incomplete fixing and films not agitated in developer
(D) exposure to visible light and trapped air bubbles on film

115. Reticulation is

(A) cracking of the film emulsion
(B) an electric charge in the developing solution
(C) a latent image
(D) caused by excess radiation

116. The best way to dry processed film manually is to

(A) place films on a flat counter top with towels
(B) use the air syringe from the dental unit
(C) hang the films over the heat sterilizer
(D) hang film racks in the darkroom carefully so as not to allow wet films to contact each other

117. Films not fixed for a long enough period of time will appear

(A) to have black lines running through them
(B) to be brittle
(C) to have a brown tint
(D) white

118. The chemicals used in processing solutions are dissolved in

(A) cellulose acetate
(B) distilled water
(C) a thick emulsion
(D) potassium bromide

119. The strength of the safelight permitted in the darkroom depends on the

(A) size of the film
(B) secured lighting in the room
(C) sensitivity of the film
(D) tooth being radiographed

120. How often should the processing solutions be changed?

(A) each week
(B) every 3–4 weeks
(C) every 5–6 weeks
(D) every 7–8 weeks

121. The optimum time–temperature relationship for processing dental radiographs is

(A) 74°F for 4½ minutes
(B) 68°F for 4½ minutes
(C) 50°F for 5 minutes
(D) 70°F for 6 minutes

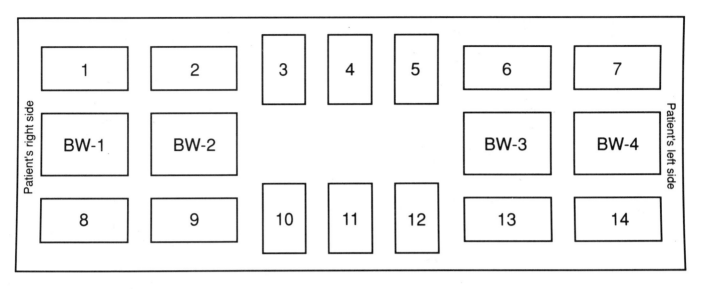

Figure 6–18.

DIRECTIONS: Figure 6–18 is a mount for radiographs, with each space assigned a number. Questions 122 through 139 have assorted films to be mounted. Based on anatomic landmarks, select the correct film placement for the mount. The bubble or raised dot on each film is toward you.

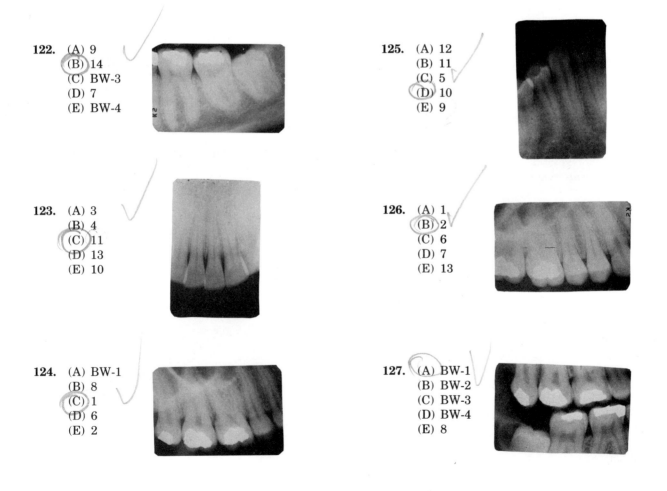

122. (A) 9
(B) 14
(C) BW-3
(D) 7
(E) BW-4

123. (A) 3
(B) 4
(C) 11
(D) 13
(E) 10

124. (A) BW-1
(B) 8
(C) 1
(D) 6
(E) 2

125. (A) 12
(B) 11
(C) 5
(D) 10
(E) 9

126. (A) 1
(B) 2
(C) 6
(D) 7
(E) 13

127. (A) BW-1
(B) BW-2
(C) BW-3
(D) BW-4
(E) 8

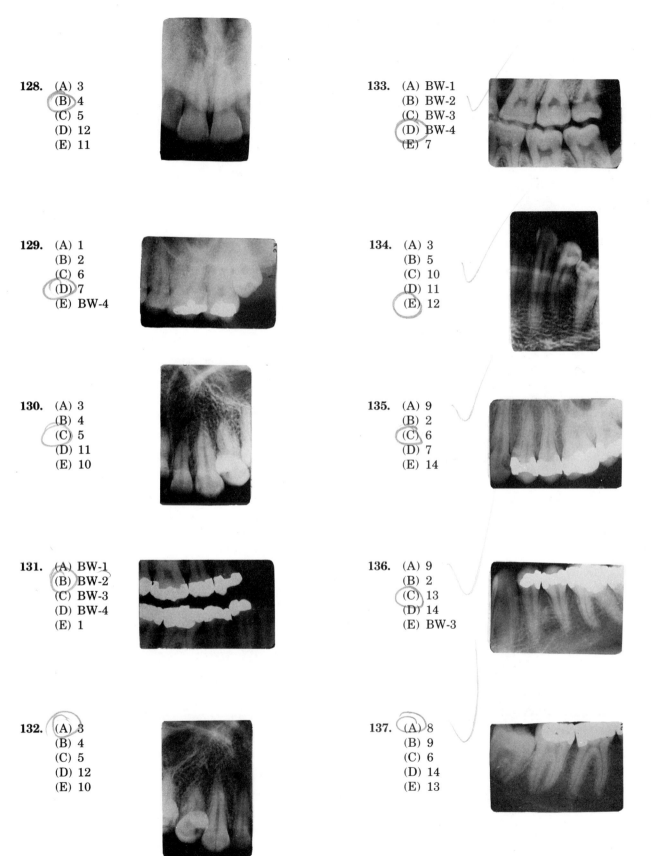

128. (A) 3
     (B) 4
     (C) 5
     (D) 12
     (E) 11

129. (A) 1
     (B) 2
     (C) 6
     (D) 7
     (E) BW-4

130. (A) 3
     (B) 4
     (C) 5
     (D) 11
     (E) 10

131. (A) BW-1
     (B) BW-2
     (C) BW-3
     (D) BW-4
     (E) 1

132. (A) 3
     (B) 4
     (C) 5
     (D) 12
     (E) 10

133. (A) BW-1
     (B) BW-2
     (C) BW-3
     (D) BW-4
     (E) 7

134. (A) 3
     (B) 5
     (C) 10
     (D) 11
     (E) 12

135. (A) 9
     (B) 2
     (C) 6
     (D) 7
     (E) 14

136. (A) 9
     (B) 2
     (C) 13
     (D) 14
     (E) BW-3

137. (A) 8
     (B) 9
     (C) 6
     (D) 14
     (E) 13

138. (A) BW-3
     (B) 2
     (C) 9
     (D) 7
     (E) 8

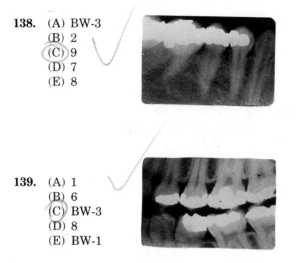

139. (A) 1
     (B) 6
     (C) BW-3
     (D) 8
     (E) BW-1

DIRECTIONS (Questions 140 through 151): For each of the items in this section, ONE or MORE of the numbered options is correct. Choose answer

    A   if only 1, 2, and 3 are correct
    B   if only 1 and 3 are correct
    C   if only 2 and 4 are correct
    D   if only 4 is correct
    E   if all are correct

140. Which of the following conditions cannot be identified radiographically?

     (1) herpetic lesions
     (2) root tips
     (3) frena
     (4) salivary stones

141. Extraoral films are used

     (1) to help diagnose fractures
     (2) when a patient cannot open his or her mouth
     (3) to help visualize pathologic conditions of the sinus
     (4) to evaluate the position of impacted teeth

142. A maxillary molar film reveals a triangular radiopaque landmark on the lower corner of the film. The landmark visible in this film is the

     (1) maxillary tuberosity
     (2) maxillary sinus
     (3) hamular process
     (4) coronoid process of mandible

143. The dental auxiliary's goal in radiation protection is zero occupational exposure. This is accomplished by

     (1) never holding the film for the patient
     (2) always being 6 feet away from the machine
     (3) working in a shielded area
     (4) wearing a film badge

144. In order to protect the patient from unnecessary x-ray exposure, the dental assistant should

     (1) drape the patient with lead-lined apron
     (2) use good chairside techniques that will avoid retakes
     (3) use high-speed film
     (4) use a closed-end pointed cone x-ray tube

145. Dark films will result from

     (1) underdeveloping
     (2) overdeveloping
     (3) underexposing
     (4) overexposing

146. Light films will result from

     (1) underdeveloping
     (2) overdeveloping
     (3) underexposure
     (4) overexposure

147. Overlapping is a result of

     (1) incorrect processing
     (2) patient movement
     (3) excessive bending of the film
     (4) incorrect horizontal angulation

148. Small silver halide crystals on the film result in

     (1) more radiation to the patient
     (2) better detail
     (3) slower film
     (4) film fogging

149. The generation of x-rays requires

     (1) electrons
     (2) heating of the cathode
     (3) a target
     (4) a lead screen

150. If a patient tends to gag easily during the x-ray procedure, the auxiliary should

     (1) allow patient to relax, then begin taking anterior films first
     (2) only expose those x-rays that do not cause a gag reflex
     (3) have the patient gargle with a mouth rinse
     (4) place cotton rolls on either side of the film to prevent discomfort

151. Secondary radiation emanates from the

     (1) patient's mouth
     (2) exposed film
     (3) closed end of cone
     (4) film holder

DIRECTIONS (Questions 152 through 161): Select the ONE BEST answer that identifies the error in radiographic technique.

152.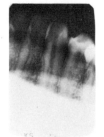

(A) overlapping
(B) cone cutting
(C) incorrect vertical angulation
(D) incorrect horizontal angulation

153.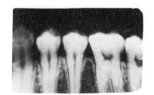

(A) cone cutting
(B) incorrect vertical angulation
(C) incorrect horizontal angulation
(D) incorrect film placement

154.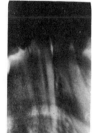

(A) incorrect vertical angulation
(B) incorrect horizontal angulation
(C) incorrect film placement
(D) cone cutting

155.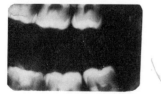

(A) overlapping
(B) cone cutting
(C) incorrect film placement
(D) incorrect horizontal angulation

156.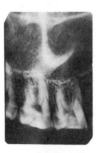

(A) cone cutting
(B) incorrect vertical angulation
(C) incorrect horizontal angulation
(D) incorrect film placement

157.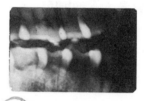

(A) incorrect horizontal angulation
(B) film is reversed
(C) underexposed
(D) cone cutting

158.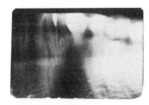

(A) film is reversed
(B) underexposed
(C) incorrect horizontal angulation
(D) cone cutting

159.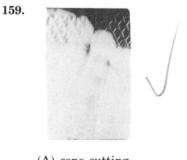

(A) cone cutting
(B) film is reversed
(C) underexposed
(D) incorrect vertical angulation

160.

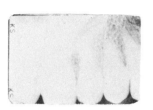

(A) overlapping
(B) incorrect film placement
(C) film is reversed
(D) underexposed

161.

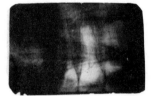

(A) incorrect processing
(B) film is reversed
(C) underexposed
(D) cone cutting

DIRECTIONS (Questions 162 through 170): For each of the items in this section, ONE or MORE of the numbered options is correct. Choose answer

A   if only 1, 2, and 3 are correct
B   if only 1 and 3 are correct
C   if only 2 and 4 are correct
D   if only 4 is correct
E   if all are correct

162. When seating the patient for a radiograph, the operator should

(1) tell the patient what is being done
(2) have the patient remove eyeglasses
(3) have the patient remove partials and dentures
(4) drape patient with a lead apron

163. Quality assurance is necessary to ensure that

(1) x-ray film is not outdated
(2) x-ray units are operating properly
(3) temperatures are accurate for processing
(4) test film runs are conducted periodically

164. Film racks should be

(1) made of plastic
(2) clean and dry
(3) kept in the watertank
(4) properly labeled

165. Exposure time is determined by

(1) kVp and mA
(2) vertical angulation
(3) film speed
(4) horizontal angulation

166. Radiographs taken of a pregnant patient must be done

(1) as quickly as possible to avoid extra exposure
(2) with two lead lap aprons in place
(3) never be done
(4) only under doctor's direct order in emergency situations

167. During x-ray exposure and processing procedures, appropriate infection control measures include

(1) use of barrier techniques for equipment and control switches
(2) use of disposable gloves
(3) use of sterile film holders
(4) proper disposal of contaminated gloves and outer film packet cover before day loader processing

168. Before exposing a panoramic radiograph on a patient, the dental assistant should request the removal of

(1) dentures
(2) eyeglasses
(3) removable appliances
(4) earrings

169. Which of these is (are) not a component of the XCP instruments?

(1) biteblock
(2) metal indicator rod
(3) plastic locator ring
(4) styrofoam shield

170. X-ray films appearing brownish after several months of storage are probably due to

(1) too much sunlight in the office
(2) improper fixing techniques
(3) coffee stains
(4) insufficient time in the wash

DIRECTIONS (Questions 1 through 175): Match the anatomic landmark in Column A with the appropriate x-ray interpretation in Column B.

COLUMN A

171. Incisive foramen
172. Coronoid process
173. Median palatine suture
174. External oblique line
175. Tuberosity

COLUMN B

A. radiopaque rounded end of the maxillary arch
B. radiolucency located between root apices of the maxillary centrals
C. radiopaque line on upper portion of mandibular molar roots
D. thin radiolucent line between maxillary incisors
E. fingerlike projection behind and below maxillary molars

DIRECTIONS (Questions 176 through 186): For each of the items in this section, ONE or MORE of the numbered options is correct. Choose answer

A if only 1, 2, and 3 are correct
B if only 1 and 3 are correct
C if only 2 and 4 are correct
D if only 4 is correct
E if all are correct

176. Which of the following are true of extraoral films?

(1) they are used when large areas of the facial structures need to be radiographed
(2) they may be loaded into cassettes
(3) they often are used when fractures of the mandible are suspected
(4) they may be used in conjunction with intensifying screens

177. Which of the following should be present in a diagnostically acceptable panoramic radiograph?

(1) the inferior border of the mandible is visible on both right and left sides of film
(2) no incisal overlap of anterior teeth
(3) patient symmetrically aligned so that condyles are equal distance from top of film
(4) uniform density with no contrast

178. Which of the following statements concerning automatic film processing units are true?

(1) the completely processed film can be obtained in about 5 minutes
(2) the same chemicals can be used as for manual processing
(3) they provide standardization of development
(4) they do not need to be cleaned

179. Of the following, the lead apron should be used on

(1) children
(2) women in the first trimester of pregnancy
(3) men to protect their reproductive cells
(4) patients over 50

180. Which of the following should be performed to control manual x-ray processing solutions properly?

(1) change solutions daily
(2) cover the tank when not in use
(3) stir solutions weekly
(4) adhere to time and temperature charts of processing solutions

181. Some of the somatic effects of long-term exposure to ionizing radiation include

(1) genetic deformities
(2) erythema
(3) alopecia
(4) blood dyscrasias

182. When mounting an edentulous film, anatomic indications of the maxillary molar area include the

(1) maxillary canal
(2) mental foramen
(3) internal oblique process
(4) hamular process

183. Which of the following could the dental assistant do when exposing radiographs of an edentulous patient who has a gagging problem?

(1) expose bite-wing radiographs
(2) use a panoramic radiograph
(3) use the bisecting angle technique because the film can be placed higher in the palate or deeper in the mandibular arch
(4) use an occlusal film for each arch

184. Low-energy x-rays are eliminated from the x-ray beam because they would

(1) not contribute to the radiographic image
(2) be absorbed by the patient's tissue
(3) contribute unnecessary radiation exposure to the patient
(4) increase the penetrating power of the beam

185. Which of the following would cause distortion of a completely processed radiograph?

(1) the fixing solution was replenished
(2) the film was excessively bent during exposure
(3) the developing solution was contaminated with fixer solution
(4) incorrect vertical or horizontal angulation

186. Which of the following controls on an x-ray unit should be checked before usage?

(1) milliamperage (mA)
(2) kilovoltage potential (kVp)
(3) on/off switch
(4) timer

DIRECTIONS (Questions 187 through 200): Each of the questions or incomplete statements in this section is followed by four suggested answers or completions. Select the ONE lettered answer or completion that is BEST in each case. Check your answers with the correct answers at the end of the chapter.

187. What is the name of the device used to stabilize the patient's head during special extraoral exposures?

    (A) laminagraph
    (B) cephalostat
    (C) antropometer
    (D) face bow

188. A panoramic film shows a blurred area in the center that was caused by the shifting of the chair. Which make of panoramic machine was used to make the exposure?

    (A) orthopantomagraphy
    (B) panelipse
    (C) orthoceph
    (D) panorex

189. The film size for a panoramic survey is

    (A) 8 × 10
    (B) 5 × 10
    (C) 5 × 12
    (D) 8 × 12

190. The film must be placed between the intensifying screens

    (A) with the blue side of the screen inside (with the film between)
    (B) with the white side of the screen inside (with the film between)
    (C) either side will produce acceptable results
    (D) no intensifying screen is needed to produce readable radiographs

191. Film used in extraoral radiography includes

    (A) intensifying screen film
    (B) double-coated film
    (C) screen or nonscreen film
    (D) opalescent film

192. When loading the film into the cassette before exposure (in extraoral radiography)

    (A) the film comes preloaded in the cassette
    (B) the procedure must be done in the darkroom
    (C) the film may be placed in the holder outside the darkroom
    (D) the film does not need an intensifying screen

193. The advantages of panographic radiography are all of the following EXCEPT

    (A) makes film exposure easier for patient
    (B) eliminates need for bite-wing x-rays
    (C) saves processing and mounting time
    (D) makes location of large pathologic conditions more readily identifiable

194. The pin on the drum that holds the film must be positioned in the slot

    (A) while securing the film in place
    (B) during exposure of the film
    (C) following exposure of the film
    (D) before releasing the patient

195. Which of these film sizes generally is used to make the posterior-anterior (facial) survey?

    (A) 8 × 4
    (B) 5 × 7
    (C) 5 × 12
    (D) 8 × 10

196. What type of exposure is needed to diagnose the TMJ area?

    (A) cephalometric
    (B) occlusal
    (C) panographic
    (D) lateral jaw survey

197. Which of these exposures helps with problems related to asymmetry?

    (A) posterior-anterior survey
    (B) occlusal
    (C) facial profile surveys
    (D) lateral jaws

198. Which type of film exposure is most helpful in location of a stone or calculus accumulation in Wharton's duct?

    (A) lateral jaw film
    (B) periapical film
    (C) panoramic film
    (D) occlusal film

199. Occlusal film placement is used for all of the following EXCEPT

    (A) to show size of cysts
    (B) to show shape of tori
    (C) to locate incipient caries
    (D) to locate fractures

200. All of the following is special equipment needed to expose extraoral radiographs EXCEPT

    (A) filtration
    (B) special machines
    (C) holders or cassettes
    (D) intensifying screens

Answers and Explanations

1. **(C)** The duties that can be performed legally by an assistant are determined by the Dental Practice Act of each state. It is the responsibility of a dental assistant to be aware of legal constraints.

2. **(D)** Reproductive cells are the most radiosensitive cells listed. Cells that undergo active division are the most radiosensitive. Cells ranked according to their radiosensitivity are sperm and ova, blood cells, epithelial cells, connective tissue cells, nerve cells, and muscle cells.

3. **(B)** The most penetrating x-rays have short wavelengths and high frequencies. They are called hard x-rays.

4. **(C)** X-rays are made up of bundles of energy called photons. Photons of x-ray frequency are capable of penetrating objects.

5. **(A)** The cathode is composed of a tungsten filament surrounded by a molybdenum focusing cup. The anode is composed of a tungsten target set inside a copper core.

6. **(D)** The milliamperage controls the heating of the cathode and thereby the density of the resultant electron cloud. Increasing the milliamperage will result in a denser cloud and increase in the number of x-rays produced.

7. **(B)** Collimation of the primary beam restricts its size and shape so it coincides as closely as possible with the size and shape of the film. As the collimated beam approaches the size of the film, there is an increased possibility of cone cutting.

8. **(C)** The lead diaphragm determines the size and shape of the x-ray beam as it leaves the x-ray head. The distance between the target and the film will determine the size of the beam at the film.

9. **(A)** The portion of the target struck by the electrons is called the focal spot. Heat produced when electrons strike the focal spot must be dissipated, or the x-ray tube might become damaged.

10. **(D)** Proper collimation of the primary beam results in a beam that closely approximates the size and shape of the film. This decreases the patient's exposure to radiation.

11. **(A)** The kVp determines the penetrating power of the x-ray beam. Increasing the kVp increases the electrical potential between the cathode and anode. This increases the force driving the electrons from the cathode to the anode, which results in an increase in the penetrating power of the resulting x-ray beam. Dental radiology uses 45 kVp to 95 kVp.

12. **(B)** The x-ray at the center of the primary beam is called the central ray.

13. **(D)** The housing of the x-ray tube is a glass envelope. The glass is lead lined except where the x-rays leave the tube.

14. **(B)** Filtration is the passing of the x-ray beam through an aluminum disc to eliminate the longer, weaker wavelength x-rays. Longer wavelength x-rays, also known as soft x-rays, do not have penetrating power and could be absorbed by the patient's cheek.

15. **(C)** Collimation limits the diameter of the x-ray beam to 2.75 to 3.0 inches at the patient's skin. Ideally, the x-ray beam should be just as large as the film being used.

16. **(A)** Scatter radiation is a type of secondary radiation created when the primary beam passes through an object.

17. **(B)** The penetrating power of primary radiation is greater than the penetrating power of the resulting secondary radiation produced. When the primary beam strikes an object, it gives up some energy, and

the resultant secondary radiation has less energy and less penetrating power.

18. **(B)** The initial sign of x-ray dermatitis is erythema (reddening).

19. **(C)** The latent period is the time period between the effects of cumulative radiation and visible tissue damage. Some severe reactions to radiation exposure may occur in a few days. Other side effects may not appear for 20 years or more.

20. **(C)** The amount of radiation a person receives is cumulative in the entire body. Therefore, people working with x-rays should take proper precautions to decrease their exposure.

21. **(A)** Maximum protection of the patient requires that the x-rays pass through a shielded open-ended cone. X-rays passing through a closed short cone produce scatter radiation.

22. **(B)** An easy way to tell the amount of radiation one is receiving is to wear a radiation film badge. The badge is worn for a period of time, after which the radiation exposure can be measured. If the occupational dose is too high, measures must be taken to correct the problem.

23. **(A)** The maximum whole body dose considered permissible is 0.1 rem/week (100 mR/week). Ideally, the operator should receive zero occupational radiation.

24. **(D)** The operator must avoid all radiation. He or she is most frequently exposed to secondary radiation. Natural sunlight need not be avoided.

25. **(A)** In order to be protected from secondary radiation, the operator should stand at least 6 feet away from the x-ray head when exposing film.

26. **(B)** To prevent gonadal exposure to x-rays, the patient should wear a lead apron. X-rays will not pass through lead. Therefore, the gonadal tissue, which is very sensitive to radiation, will be protected.

27. **(C)** If not in use, the leaded apron must be stored unfolded, preferably over a support rod. Repeated folding of the lead apron and collar will damage the material.

28. **(C)** The characteristic of x-rays that makes them both beneficial and hazardous is their ability to destroy tissue. Radiation is used in medicine both as a diagnostic tool and to intentionally destroy certain tissue (such as carcinomas).

29. **(B)** The best technique to decrease radiation exposure is to use the fastest film possible.

30. **(C)** Film speed is determined by the size of the silver bromide crystals. Larger crystals produce faster film. Faster film requires less total radiation for exposure. Film speed ranges from A to F. D and F are the fastest.

31. **(A)** The radiographic film is a cellulose acetate base thinly covered on both sides with a gelatin emulsion of silver bromide salts.

32. **(D)** The button or dot is used to orient the films when mounting. All films should be oriented with the button in the same direction when mounting.

33. **(B)** The purpose of the lead foil in dental film is to prevent fogging or a darkening of the film, which may be caused from secondary radiation.

34. **(C)** Bite-wing films are used for diagnosis of interproximal caries, visualizing the height of interproximal bone, and determining the proximal adaptation of restorations.

35. **(A)** Water's film is an extraoral film used to help visualize the sinus. Extraoral films are large films that are positioned beside the patient's face. They are used to visualize large portions of the skull, mandible, or maxilla.

36. **(D)** X-ray films should be kept by the dentist indefinitely. The x-ray films are the property of the dentist and are part of the patient's permanent record. X-ray films may be used as evidence in a court of law.

37. **(A)** Only those films necessary for proper diagnosis will be exposed. The patient should be informed that the amount of dental radiation during exposure is minimal and that he or she is protected by a lead apron against scattered radiation.

38. **(D)** Periapical films are used to show the entire tooth and the supporting structures. They come in three sizes: small for children, regular for adults, and narrow for anterior teeth.

39. **(B)** Root tip fractures are not visible on interproximal or bite-wing films. A periapical film is required to assess a root tip fracture.

40. **(D)** A history of the patient's previous radiation exposure is not a factor when considering film size. Age and size of dental arch must be evaluated before selecting appropriate film size.

41. **(B)** The principle used in panoramic radiography is laminagraphy. Laminagraphy is the focusing of the x-ray beam at a point that will appear on the resulting film. Other objects in the beam's path are out of focus and do not appear on the radiograph.

42. **(C)** Radiolucency depends on the density of an object. The less dense an object, the more radiolucent it is, and the darker it will appear on radiographs.

43. **(B)** Radiopaque structures appear white. The denser a structure, the more radiopaque it will appear. The most radiopaque structure of a tooth is the enamel.

44. **(C)** The pulp chamber is radiolucent and appears dark on an x-ray.

45. **(A)** Caries appears radiolucent on an x-ray. Calculus, tori, and root tips are denser structures and appear radiopaque.

46. **(D)** The diagonal radiopaque line that is visible on the lower part of the roots of the mandibular molars is the internal oblique line.

47. **(B)** The small circular radiolucency near the roots of the mandibular premolars is called the mental foramen.

48. **(C)** The U-shaped radiopaque structure often seen in the maxillary molar area is the zygoma.

49. **(B)** The thin radiopaque band between the maxillary incisors is called the nasal septum.

50. **(D)** The heavy radiopaque midpoint of the mandible is called the symphysis.

51. **(B)** The small circular radiolucency below the mandibular incisor roots is called the lingual foramen.

52. **(A)** The large radiolucent areas shown above the maxillary molars and appearing as white lines are called the maxillary sinuses.

53. **(D)** The mandibular canal appears long, narrow, and radiolucent below the roots of the mandibular molars.

54. **(A)** The radiopaque circular area below the apices of the mandibular incisors is called the genial tubercles.

55. **(D)** The lamina dura appears radiopaque.

56. **(A)** A granuloma is less dense and will appear radiolucent.

57. **(C)** The bisecting the angle technique requires that the central ray be perpendicular to the line bisecting the angle formed by the film and the tooth.

58. **(B)** The paralleling technique requires that the film be parallel to the tooth and that a 16-inch cone be used. The central ray is directed perpendicular to the

tooth and film. The paralleling technique does not use the 8-inch short cone.

59. **(A)** The sagittal plane of the patient's head should be perpendicular to the floor. The vertical angulation on the x-ray head is based on this position.

60. **(C)** The side of the nose, adjoining the nostrils, is known as the ala. A line drawn between the ala of the nose and the tragus of the ear parallels the maxillary teeth and is used as a guide when taking x-rays.

61. **(D)** The ala–tragus line is parallel to the floor when taking maxillary periapical films, bite-wing films, and maxillary occlusal films.

62. **(B)** When positioning the patient, the occlusal plane of the arch being radiographed should be parallel to the floor.

63. **(B)** Vertical angulation may be altered from patient to patient depending on anatomic structure differences, such as the height of the vault of the palate.

64. **(A)** The periapical films are extended ⅛ inch beyond the occlusal surface or incisal edge. The resulting film should also show 3 mm beyond the root apex.

65. **(C)** Firm placement of the film will help prevent gagging by avoiding movement of the film over gag-sensitive areas of the palate.

66. **(C)** The latent image is not truly an image but a potential image composed of energized silver halide crystals. The latent image will become a visible image after processing the exposed film.

67. **(A)** Cone cutting is caused by the central ray not being aimed at the center of the film. This results in part of the film not being exposed to radiation.

68. **(D)** Black lines across the film are indicative of excessive bending that has cracked the emulsion.

69. **(B)** A blurred film will result if the patient moves while dental film is being exposed.

70. **(D)** If a patient is reluctant to be radiographed, the auxiliary should explain the procedure thoroughly before taking the radiographs. Emphasis on the use of safety devices, such as the lead apron and collar, to protect the body from unnecessary scatter radiation, the use of fast film to limit exposure time, and the low dosage of x-rays emitted for dental films may be presented. The doctor depends on the dental x-rays for thorough treatment planning and diagnosis.

71. **(D)** The maxillary first bicuspid has two roots that lie beside each other in a buccal palatal orientation. To radiographically separate the roots, which may be necessary in root canal therapy, the horizontal angulation should have the central beam slightly mesial or distal to the ideal angulation. The ideal horizontal angulation, with the central ray perpendicular to the buccal surface, would cause the roots to be superimposed on one another.

72. **(A)** Less time is necessary for radiograph exposures on children because the tissues the radiation must pass through are not as dense as those of adults.

73. **(B)** Intensifying screens decrease exposure time of extraoral radiographs by creating an illuminating pattern of the object through which the x-ray has passed. The illuminating pattern continues to expose the film after the radiation exposure has stopped.

74. **(C)** As the target–film distance increases, there is less distortion because the x-rays are more parallel as they strike the object and film. If the target–film distance is increased, the exposure time must be increased to obtain a properly exposed film.

75. **(C)** To prevent distortion of panorex films, the patient's chin must be properly placed in the chin rest so that the head is positioned symmetrically.

76. **(B)** The full mouth series of a dentulous person is composed of 18 to 20 films. An 18-film series would consist of films of the maxillary and mandibular central and lateral incisors, right and left canines, right and left premolars, right and left molars, and bite-wings of the right and left premolars and right and left molars.

77. **(A)** Devices used to hold the film in the paralleling technique include a film holder and hemostats.

78. **(D)** Extraoral films are more light sensitive than are intraoral films.

79. **(B)** Increasing the mA increases the electron density and subsequently the quantity of the resulting x-rays. An increase in the quantity of x-rays will result in more x-rays affecting the film and subsequently darker film.

80. **(A)** Elongation can be caused by insufficient vertical angulation, improper positioning of the patient's head, or improper film placement.

81. **(B)** Foreshortening can be caused by too much vertical angulation, improper positioning of the patient's head, or improper film placement.

82. **(D)** A herringbone pattern results if the film is exposed when it is reversed in the patient's mouth. This pattern is caused by the radiation passing through the lead foil, which has this pattern. The resultant film is light and cannot be used for diagnostic purposes.

83. **(C)** X-rays are most effectively stopped by lead. However, all matter will attenuate x-rays to varying degrees.

84. **(D)** When the target–film distance is doubled, the exposure time must be increased fourfold to maintain equal film density. This is an example of the inverse-square law of radiation, which states that radiation intensity is inversely proportional to the square of the distances.

85. **(D)** An extremely narrow maxillary arch will require special film adaptation, and appropriate adjustments should be made to provide accuracy and minimal patient discomfort.

86. **(A)** The term density is used to describe the blackness of an exposed radiograph. An overexposed film will appear very dark (high density), and an underexposed film will reveal much lightness (low density).

87. **(B)** The difference in density of various regions of a radiograph is called contrast. Contrast refers to how the dark and light areas of a film are differentiated. Definition refers to the sharpness or clarity of the images outlined on the film.

88. **(B)** The intensity of the x-rays is now only ¼ as great based on the inverse-square law, which states that the intensity of the light will vary inversely as the square of the distance from its source. If the mA and kVp remain unchanged but the target–film distance is doubled, the intensity of radiation is ¼ the intensity at the original distance.

89. **(A)** For maximum penetration of x-rays, a higher kVp is selected. When the kVp is increased, the x-ray wavelength is shortened and the x-ray beam emits a higher energy source (photons), allowing effective penetration of thicker structures with greater density. In order to maintain proper radiographic contrast and density, the mA must be reduced whenever the kVp is increased.

90. **(B)** The dental x-ray unit must be operated under certain federal and state safety specifications. Filtration of 2.5 mm aluminum is required for all x-ray units operating at 70 kVp or higher. Filtration of 1.5 mm aluminum is required for x-ray units operating below 70 kVp. The process of filtration by use of an aluminum disc eliminates longer, weaker wave-

length x-rays so that the patient will receive only useful x-ray beams for maximum exposure.

91. **(D)** Appropriate infection control procedures during x-ray exposure includes the placement of a disposable plastic bag over the x-ray tube head. The auxiliary should use protective barriers, including gloves, glasses, and face mask.

92. **(B)** Every clinical procedure involving direct patient care should be recorded in the patient's dental chart. Individual periapical films must be dated and labeled before mounting.

93. **(C)** Cephalometric films are extraoral films used in orthodontics to relate anatomic landmarks of the mandible and maxilla to the rest of the skull and to make cephalometric tracings.

94. **(D)** Extraoral films are sheets of film placed in rigid metal–plastic frames called cassettes. To decrease the amount of radiation needed for an exposure, the cassette usually contains an intensifying screen.

95. **(B)** The best sequence for maxillary radiographs is to begin with film easy for the patient to hold and continue in a sequence that will avoid any possible omissions. The best choice is to begin with the central incisors and continue posteriorly on one side and then repeat the pattern on the other side.

96. **(A)** Radiographs of edentulous areas should be exposed routinely to check for any pathologic conditions in the area (eg, retained root tips, foreign bodies).

97. **(A)** A logical sequence for a full mouth survey is one where the patient's position is changed as infrequently as possible. First, the maxillary periapical radiographs and bite-wings are taken with the ala–tragus line parallel to the floor. Then, the patient's head position is altered so that the occlusal plane of the mandibular teeth is parallel to the floor, and mandibular radiographs are exposed.

98. **(B)** When the end of the cone approximates the tip of the patient's nose, a radiograph of the patient's central incisors is being exposed. The vertical angulation is about +50 degrees.

99. **(C)** Developing solution has an affinity for oxygen. Therefore, if it is left uncovered, the chemicals will oxidize and lose their strength.

100. **(C)** Films cannot be overfixed and can be left in the fixer indefinitely.

101. **(D)** It is safe to expose radiographs to light after they have been placed in the fixer. The radiographs can be read at this time and then placed back into the fixer to complete the processing.

102. **(A)** The thermometer used to measure the temperature of the processing solutions is located in the developing solution. The temperature of the developer will determine how long the films will be kept in this solution. Until a temperature equilibrium is reached, the waterbath is warmer than the developing solution. If the thermometer was kept in the waterbath, the resulting films, developed before equilibrium was reached, would be underdeveloped.

103. **(B)** Film fog appears as a dull gray finish on the processed film. Some causes are light leak in the darkroom, old film, or exposure of film to secondary or stray radiation.

104. **(C)** The film is washed after it is removed from the developer and before it is put in the fixer in order to wash off the developing solution and stop the developing process. Washing also removes all chemicals from the film so the fixing solution is not contaminated.

105. **(A)** The fixing solution is acidic. The following chemicals make up the fixer: sodium thiosulfate, which dissolves undeveloped silver salts, alum to shrink and harden the gelatin emulsion, sodium sulfate, a preservative against oxidation, acetic acid to increase action of the preservative, and distilled water, the medium in which the chemical activity takes place.

106. **(B)** Higher temperature will cause an increase in precipitation of the silver halide, resulting in a darker film.

107. **(D)** When a film is placed in the fixing solution unaffected (or unprecipitated), silver bromide crystals are removed. Therefore, the emulsion of an unexposed film will be removed completely, and the film will be clear.

108. **(A)** Fixing the film removes the unaffected silver halides. Areas in which these halides are removed will appear lighter in the final film. Fixing also rehardens the emulsion.

109. **(C)** The temperature of the processing solution usually is adjusted by immersing containers of the processing solution in a temperature-adjustable waterbath.

110. **(B)** The longer film remains in the developer, the more silver halide will precipitate and, therefore, the darker the film will become.

111. **(D)** Processed films left in the water overnight will lose all of their image and appear clear. Films should *never* be left in the water overnight.

112. **(C)** After fixing, the film is washed for 20 to 30 minutes and then dried. If the films are washed too long, they will become lighter because some of the precipitated silver bromide will wash off. If the films are not washed long enough, some residue from the fixer may remain, and the films will have a brown tint.

113. **(C)** In order to develop films, the developing solution must have a basic pH. The following chemicals make up the developer: hydroquinone, an oxidizing agent that gives the film contrast, Elon, another oxidizing agent to give film detail, sodium sulfite, a preservative to lengthen the life of the solution, sodium carbonate to make the solution basic, potassium bromide to make the aforementioned chemicals act selectively, and distilled water, the medium in which the chemical activity takes place.

114. **(B)** White spots may appear on a processed film if contaminated with fixing solution before the developing phase of processing. The silver halide crystals are unable to react with the developing solution properly, causing a whitened area to appear on the processed film.

115. **(A)** Reticulation is the cracking of the film emulsion due to large temperature differences between the processing solutions.

116. **(D)** The processed films should be dried by suspending them in air. A fan may be used to speed up the drying process. However, the films should not be allowed to touch each other or anything else until they are dry.

117. **(C)** Film not fixed for a long enough period of time (about 10 minutes) will have a brown tint. Radiographs may be read after a short period of fixing (wet reading) but must be returned to the fixing solution to ensure complete removal of the unaffected silver bromide crystals.

118. **(B)** The chemicals used in processing solutions are dissolved in distilled water. Other types of water contain chemicals that can interfere with the proper processing of radiographs.

119. **(C)** The strength of the safelight in the darkroom is dependent on the sensitivity of the film. The faster the film, the more light sensitive the film and, therefore, the less the strength of the safelight.

120. **(B)** The processing solutions should be changed at least every 3 to 4 weeks, depending on usage. The solutions lose strength through exposure to air, heavy usage, and contamination. Regular quality assurance film test runs should be conducted to ensure that processing solutions are effective.

121. **(B)** The optimum time–temperature for processing films varies with manufacturer's specifications. An accepted time–temperature range is 68°F for 4½ minutes.

122. **(B)**

123. **(C)**

124. **(C)**

125. **(D)**

126. **(B)**

127. **(A)**

128. **(B)**

129. **(D)**

130. **(C)**

131. **(B)**

132. **(A)**

133. **(D)**

134. **(E)**

135. **(C)**

136. **(C)**

137. **(A)**

138. **(C)**

139. **(C)**

140. **(B)** Soft tissue conditions cannot be identified radiographically unless they are lesions within hard tissues. Therefore, herpetic lesions and frena cannot be identified radiographically. A soft tissue lesion, such as a granuloma, within bone will appear radiographically radiolucent compared with its more radiopaque surrounding.

141. **(E)** Extraoral films are used to help visualize fractures, pathologic conditions of the sinus, the temporomandibular joint, the position of impacted teeth, and large pathologic lesions. They are used also when a patient cannot open his or her mouth.

142. (D) The coronoid process appears radiopaque in the lower distal portion of a maxillary molar film.

143. (E) Occupational safety measures for the dental auxiliary operating radiographic equipment include never holding the x-ray film in the patient's mouth during exposure, always working in a shielded area (lead lined), standing behind protective shielded areas at least 6 feet away from the target area, and regular monitoring of an x-ray film badge.

144. (A) To protect the patient from unnecessary x-ray exposure, the dental auxiliary should drape the patient with a lead-lined apron, use technique factors that avoid retakes resulting in low patient exposure, and use fast films and x-ray machines with a collimator.

145. (C) Dark films can result from overexposure (too much radiation contacts the film because of an increase in the quantity of radiation or the exposure time) or overdevelopment (more silver halide crystals are precipitated if the developing solution is too warm or if the films are left in the solution too long).

146. (B) Light films may result from underexposing (not enough radiation reaches the film because of insufficient quantity or insufficient exposure), underdeveloping (insufficient amounts of affected silver halide are precipitated; this can be caused by a cold developing solution or keeping the films in the developing solution too short a period of time), or overwashing, resulting in lighter films because affected silver halide crystals will be washed off.

147. (D) Overlapping occurs if the central ray is not parallel to the proximal contacts in the horizontal plane. If overlapping occurs, parts of adjacent teeth are superimposed on each other, and the films cannot be used diagnostically.

148. (A) Small silver halide crystals (grains) on the film result in a slow film that requires a long exposure time but results in a radiograph with fine detail. Slow film does not offer a sufficient increase in diagnostic value over fast film to justify its use.

149. (A) The sequence of events that leads to x-ray generation is first heating the cathode to produce an electron cloud. The density of the cloud produced depends on the milliampere (mA). Second is the creation of an electric potential between the cathode and anode (target). The speed of the crossing depends on the kilovolt (kVp). Third, the collision of the electrons with the anode produces x-rays (photons).

150. (B) If a patient tends to gag easily during the x-ray procedure, the auxiliary should allow the patient to relax, then begin taking anterior films first. The patient may also be allowed to gargle with mouthwash to help alleviate a gag reflex.

151. (A) Secondary radiation is radiation resulting from the interaction of the primary beam and any object in contacts.

152. (B)

153. (D)

154. (A)

155. (C)

156. (D)

157. (A)

158. (C)

159. (B)

160. (D)

161. (A)

162. (E) When seating the patient for a radiograph, the operator should explain the procedure to the patient and then ask the patient to remove any prosthetic appliances, such as partials or dentures. Eyeglasses may be removed as well. Drape the patient with a lead-lined apron and thyroid lead collar.

163. (E) Methods of ensuring high-quality x-ray film exposures with minimum radiation exposure for patient and operator include instruments of quality assurance, such as regular monitoring and testing of equipment to prevent malfunctions, regular maintenance of processing solutions, including regulation of solution temperatures, and regular test film runs.

164. (C) X-ray racks should contain enough clips to hold a full series of films, be numbered or lettered for patient identification, and be clean and dry so as not to contaminate the processing solutions or affect the films.

165. (B) The exposure time is determined by the mA, the kVp, the density of the bone and structures the primary beam must pass through, the film speed, and the focal (target) film distance.

166. (D) Radiographs taken of a pregnant patient must

be kept at a minimum and performed only in emergency situations under the doctor's direct order.

167. **(E)** Infection control measures must be employed during radiographic procedures. They include protective barriers for the operator and appropriate sterilization and disinfection of equipment and x-ray armamentarium. Special procedures are followed to prevent contamination of day loader processing units. When developing films, contaminated film packets must be disposed of properly and kept from contaminating other surfaces and objects by isolating in a separate paper cup.

168. **(E)** Before exposing a panoramic radiograph on a patient, the auxiliary should ask the patient to remove any partials or dentures, eyeglasses, and earrings.

169. **(D)** The styrofoam shield is not part of the XCP armamentarium. The extension cone paralleling instruments include a plastic bite block, a long metal indicator rod, and a round plastic locater ring.

170. **(C)** X-ray films may appear brownish in color due to improper fixing techniques and insufficient time in the wash. Other causes may include weak fixing solutions and outdated film.

171. **(B)**

172. **(E)**

173. **(D)**

174. **(C)**

175. **(A)**

176. **(E)** Extraoral radiographs are taken when the area of concern cannot be diagnosed adequately with intraoral radiographic techniques. They are used when large areas of the facial structures need to be radiographed. Situations requiring extraoral radiographs may include the use of cassettes and intensifying screens, as in panoramic radiography. Extraoral exposures allow the clinician to view impacted teeth, sinuses, cysts, jaw fractures, occlusal relationships, and lateral projections of the TMJ area.

177. **(A)** A diagnostically acceptable panoramic radiograph displays both right and left sides of the inferior border of the mandible and reveals no excessive overlapping of the teeth. If the patient is symmetrically aligned, the right and left condyles will be exposed at an equal distance from the top of the film.

178. **(B)** Automatic film processing units require special types of chemical solutions unlike the manual processing tanks. The automatic processing units must be cleaned periodically and monitored to maintain optimum processed film quality. The automatic processor units provide rapid development of the exposed film and developing standardization.

179. **(E)** The lead apron is a requirement for all patients who are being exposed to dental x-rays.

180. **(C)** Quality control of processing solutions is necessary to ensure consistent quality of film processing techniques. When not in use, processing tanks must be covered to prevent dehydration or contamination. Time and temperature charts for processing solutions must be followed strictly during manual processing procedures. A thermometer should be available in the wash tank and checked before developing exposed x-ray film.

181. **(E)** Long-term effects of overexposure to ionizing radiation may cause necrotic reactions to living cells. Dangers of overexposure may cause cancer, blood dyscrasia, alopecia (hair loss), erythema, and genetic deformities.

182. **(D)** A radiopaque structure present in the maxillary molar region is the hamular process.

183. **(C)** For patients with a high gag reflex, the auxiliary may have to take a panoramic x-ray or an occlusal film.

184. **(A)** Low-intensity wavelengths of the x-ray beam are not diagnostically useful in film exposures and would contribute unnecessary radiation exposure to the patient.

185. **(C)** Distortion of a processed film will occur if a film is excessively bent during exposure or from incorrect horizontal or vertical angulation.

186. **(E)** Daily and weekly monitoring of x-ray equipment is necessary for quality assurance. Before use, all control devices, such as the timer, mA and kVp settings, and on/off switch, should be inspected.

187. **(B)** The cephalostat is used to stabilize the patient's head during special extraoral exposures. The cephalostat holds the patient's head parallel and at right angles to the x-ray beam.

188. **(D)** The panorex machine requires movement of the chair to complete the film exposure of the other half of x-ray film, resulting in a white unexposed strip extending vertically down the center of the exposed film. The panorex extraoral radiograph

shows the complete maxillary and mandibular arch in one exposure.

189. **(C)** The film size for a panoramic survey is 5 × 12.

190. **(B)** The unexposed film is placed at the base of the opened intensifying screen. The white side of the intensifying screen must be on the inside, with the film in between. The intensifying screen allows production of a film with greater diagnostic quality through a minimum amount of radiation.

191. **(C)** Screen and nonscreen film is used for extraoral radiographs. Screen film is designed to be used in a cassette holder with an intensifying screen, and nonscreen film is designed for use in a cardboard exposure holder.

192. **(B)** When loading extraoral film into the cassette, the procedure must always be done in the darkroom, since the x-ray film is light sensitive.

193. **(B)** Panoramic radiography does not eliminate the need for bite-wing x-rays because the panoramic x-ray is an extraoral film. It is exposed outside the patient's mouth, and there is loss of detail in the radiograph. Interproximal caries can best be detected by intraoral bite-wing film exposures.

194. **(A)** The pin on the drum that holds the film must be positioned in the slot while securing the film in place.

195. **(D)** The posterior-anterior facial survey requires an 8 × 10 film size.

196. **(D)** The lateral jaw survey is used to diagnose the TMJ area. A 5 × 7 inch film is used and placed extraorally along the mandible and centered over the first molars.

197. **(C)** The facial profile survey is used to diagnose facial asymmetry problems. The radiograph is commonly used in orthodontic procedures.

198. **(D)** The occlusal exposure is beneficial in locating a salivary duct stone, or calculus accumulation along the floor of the mouth. The occlusal intraoral x-ray allows for a broader view of the entire arch.

199. **(C)** Occlusal films are not used to diagnose and locate incipient caries.

200. **(A)** Filtration is not considered special equipment for extraoral radiographs. Filters are made of metal, aluminum, or copper and are placed inside the x-ray cone to absorb the longer-wavelength unnecessary rays emitted from the primary beam.

BIBLIOGRAPHY

Atchison KA. *Radiographic Safety*. Western Dental Education Center Correspondence Course. Los Angeles: Department of Veteran Affairs, West Los Angeles VA Medical Center, 1987.

Barr JH, Stephens RG. *Dental Radiography*. Philadelphia: WB Saunders Co, 1980.

Butsumyo D, Deboom G, Lynne S, Parrot K. *Principles and Practice of Dental Radiography*. Los Angeles: Western Dental Education Center Correspondence Course. Department of Veteran Affairs, West Los Angeles VA Medical Center, 1988.

deLyre WR, Johnson N. *Essentials of Dental Radiology for Dental Assistants and Hygienists,* 4th ed. Norwalk, Conn: Appleton & Lange, 1989.

Eastman Kodak Company. *X-rays in Dentistry*. Rochester, NY, 1977.

Eastman Kodak Company. *Quality Assurance in Dental Radiography*. Rochester, NY, 1990.

Eastman Kodak Company. *Radiation Safety in Dental Radiography*. Rochester, NY, 1990.

Eastman Kodak Company. *Successful Panoramic Radiography*. Rochester, NY, 1990.

Frommer HH. *Radiology for Dental Auxiliaries*, 4th ed. St. Louis: CV Mosby Co, 1987.

Langland OE, Sippy FH. *Textbook of Dental Radiography*, 2nd ed. Springfield, Ill: Charles C Thomas Publishers, 1984.

Manson-Hing LR. *Fundamentals of Dental Radiography*, 3rd ed. Philadelphia: Lea & Febiger Publishers, 1990.

O'Brien R. *Dental Radiography: An Introduction for Dental Hygienists and Assistants*, 4th ed. Philadelphia: WB Saunders Co, 1982.

Torres H, Ehrlich A. *Modern Dental Assisting,* 4th ed. Philadelphia: WB Saunders Co, 1990.

Wuehrmann A, Manson-Hing LR. *Dental Radiology*, 5th ed. St. Louis: CV Mosby Co, 1981.

CHAPTER 7

Dental Materials

INTRODUCTION

The science of dental materials includes a wide range of natural and synthetic substances and products used in the delivery of oral health care. Auxiliaries play an essential role in the preparation, manipulation, and application of dental materials in the dental office. Consequently, the importance of a thorough understanding of the physical and biologic properties of dental materials is necessary for the dental auxiliary in order to perform effectively and accurately when preparing and handling dental materials. This chapter provides a synopsis of dental restorative materials, dental cements, gypsum products, impression materials, gold alloys, and gold casting procedures.

PROPERTIES OF MATTER

The science of dental materials requires a basic understanding of the properties of matter. All dental materials are made up of atomic matter that directly affects the chemical and physical working properties of the material.

Matter exists in three different states: solid, liquid, and gas. By altering temperature and pressure, most materials can be changed to any of the three states. Temperature is a measure of the intensity of heat. The amount of heat evolved or absorbed during a chemical reaction is called the *heat of reaction*. If heat is evolved, or given off, the reaction is described as *exothermic*. If heat is absorbed, the reaction is *endothermic*. The setting of dental stone and acrylic exhibits exothermic reactions. Caution must be exercised when using these materials intraorally to avoid damaging the pulpal tissues and oral mucosa.

Heat is measured in either Fahrenheit or Celsius degrees. However, temperature expressed by one system can be converted easily to the other.

To convert degrees Fahrenheit to degrees Celsius, the following formula is used.

$$°C = 5/9 \ (°F - 32)$$

To convert degrees Celsius to degrees Fahrenheit, the following formula is used.

$$°F = 9/5 \ (°C + 32)$$

GYPSUM PRODUCTS: PLASTER AND STONE

Gypsum products are used in dentistry to form casts and dies that are positive reproductions of patients' hard and soft oral tissues. These materials can also be used intraorally as impression materials for taking full denture impressions or soldering registrations for casting. However, intraoral use of gypsum products is diminishing, since other materials can give equal accuracy and detail and are easier to use intraorally.

Plasters and stones are made by grinding gypsum under high temperatures (230–250°F) to drive off part of the water of crystallization. This process is called calcining. The main constituent of all plasters or stones is calcium sulfate hemihydrate. The degree of refinement of the calcium sulfate hemihydrate is contingent on whether plaster or stone is desired. Particles in plaster are more irregular and spongy, whereas stone has more dense particles in more crystalline forms. The difference in particle shape between plasters and stones reflects the difference in properties. Plasters are not as strong as stones, although both are easy to manipulate.

Stone can be further classified into class I and II stones. Class I stone contains more regular particles and is used mainly for pouring casts. Class II stone, also known as improved stone, contains a greater number of random-shaped particles and, as a result, is a harder material. Improved stone is used primarily to make dies.

Gypsum products produce an exothermic reaction, that is, heat is released. The amount of water mixed with the plaster or stone is very important and is expressed as the water to powder (w/p) ratio. For example, the more water added, the longer the setting time and the weaker the result. Setting time is affected also by the length and speed of mixing. The longer and more rapid the mix, the shorter the setting time. Setting time can be accelerated or retarded by using chemical additives. Sodium tetraborate (Borax) will retard setting time, whereas adding salts, such as sodium chloride or potassium sulfate, in small quantities will accelerate the set.

Accurate models demand that gypsum products, when set, not change their shape. Consequently, the dimensional stability of these products is important. Improper manipulation can cause changes in dimension that can result in an inaccurate model from an accurate impression.

Plasters and stone are mixed in a flexible rubber bowl with a stiff spatula. A premeasured amount of water is added to the gypsum product. One difficulty encountered with mixing is the incorporation of air bubbles. These bubbles, however, can be removed by using an automatic vibrator and vibrating the mix until no more bubbles come to the surface. The mix can then be poured or shaped as needed.

When completely set and hardened, gypsum materials may be trimmed with a laboratory model trimmer. Cast study models are trimmed geometrically and may be polished for esthetics before the patient case presentation appointment.

Special precautions must be taken by the dental auxiliary when working with gypsum products, including the use of protective eyewear during the trimming procedures and while handling the dry powder gypsum plaster or stones. A mask is recommended to prevent inhalation of the fine gypsum powders during manipulation. Auxiliaries should work in well-ventilated laboratory areas to minimize prolonged exposure to the gypsum materials.

RESTORATIVE MATERIALS

Direct restorative materials are used to replace tooth structure that has been naturally or mechanically removed. The restorative materials are used for permanent restorations.

Dental amalgam, a combination of mercury with a silver-tin alloy containing small amounts of copper and zinc, is the material of choice for approximately 75% of all dental restorations. Each constituent of the material adds properties to the final product. Silver adds strength and decreases flow. Tin tends to reduce expansion, but it also reduces strength. Zinc acts as a deoxidizer. Copper improves strength and hardness. Mercury wets the alloy particles and chemically reacts with the alloy to begin the hardening process. Mercury is mixed with the metallic alloy, which is produced in different forms ranging from a fine powder to a compressed pellet or sphere. The process of mixing together silver alloy particles with liquid mercury is called trituration. Trituration may occur by using a mechanical amalgamator. Premeasured and premixed capsules eliminate direct contact with free mercury and are available for use with the amalgamator. The resulting amalgam is plastic and can be inserted, condensed, and carved easily in the cavity preparation.

Undertrituration or overtrituration diminishes the properties of amalgam. Undertriturated amalgam becomes crumbly and is difficult to manipulate. Its strength also is diminished. Overtriturated amalgam is runny in consistency and is difficult to manipulate.

Amalgam is widely used for its high compressive strength, relative inexpensiveness, ease of manipulation, and tendency to reduce marginal leakage.

Mercury toxicity awareness can reduce potential re-lated occupational hazards from mercury contamination in the dental office. Mercury contamination may occur from accidental spills and direct contact with the liquid metal. Heating of contaminated amalgam carrier instruments and inhaling the mercury vapors are other methods of mercury toxicity. Mulling the amalgam in bare hands, improper disposal methods of unwanted mercury scraps, mechanical amalgamator leakage, and working in a non-ventilated area with metal exposure also are occupational hazards.

Symptoms of mercury toxicity may range from chronic headaches and fatigue to more serious health problems related to kidney dysfunctions, tremors, speech disorders, and death. Special precautions must be taken by the dental auxiliary when handling mercury to avoid potential health risks.

Mercury toxicity preventive measures include

1. Avoid handling fresh alloy and direct contact with mercury.
2. Properly dispose of scrap mercury, preferably in a closed container with a liquid solution.
3. Work in a well-ventilated area of the office when handling mercury materials. Use gloves.
4. Pick up spilled mercury immediately with special office emergency spill kits.
5. Use tightly sealed capsules during amalgamation.
6. When removing old amalgam restorations, use the high-speed evacuator and a water spray. Masks and face shields should be worn.

COMPOSITE RESIN MATERIALS

Composite resins are used primarily for anterior restorations. In addition, composite resins can be used to correct anomalies of enamel development and other esthetic problems and to bond orthodontic brackets. Composites contain a monomer or an aromatic dimethacrylate (most commonly BIS-GMA), an accelerator, organic peroxide, and a filler, such as quartz or glass. Catalysts that quicken setting time vary according to the system used. These systems include self-curing, ultraviolet light curing, and visible light curing. Composite is moderately strong and can be easily manipulated. However, it can be abraded and lose its finish easily.

If the composite is a paste/paste self-curing system, it is mixed by placing equal portions of catalyst and base on a small mixing pad. Different sides of double-ended plastic spatulas are used to avoid contaminating the materials. The two pastes are incorporated into a homogeneous mixture. Etching the enamel walls of the preparation with phosphoric acid before insertion of the composite improves retention and diminishes marginal leakage. Placement of the mixed composite resin material is done with a plastic placement instrument. A celluloid matrix strip is used if indicated for Class III restorations. Composite resin restorative materials should not be manipulated with metal instruments.

PIT AND FISSURE SEALANTS

Pit and fissure sealants are synthetic resins that play an important role in preventive dental procedures. The resin is an organic polymer that bonds to the enamel surface by penetrating into the enamel pores created on the tooth as a result of acid etching techniques with phosphoric acid. The resin material is an unfilled BIS-GMA resin that reacts with a light-cured polymerization system or the peroxide-amine technique of polymerization. Pit and fissure resins exhibit properties of low viscosity, which allow the material to flow easily over the tooth. Sealants are subject to occlusal wear and must be examined at regular recall intervals.

BONDING

Enamel bonding agents are used to repair ortho brackets and fractured anterior teeth and for esthetics. The synthetic type of bonding resin exhibits similar chemical and physical properties as the composite resins and the pit and fissure sealants. Before placement of a bonding agent, it is necessary to acid etch the tooth surface.

ACRYLIC RESINS

Acrylic resins are polymeric restorative materials used in anterior teeth. The resins come in a powder and liquid form. The liquid is a monomer comprising methyl methylacrylate (hydroquinone), an accelerator, and an organic sulfonic acid. The powder is a polymer of polymethyl methacrylate, benzoyl peroxide (a catalyst), and metal oxides. The material has an ability to withstand fracture and is available in a wide range of shades. Disadvantages include a low resistance to wear and inability to prevent recurring caries. In addition, the restoration can change shape over time and alternately expands and contracts. This results in an exchange of fluids in the margins, the process known as percolation.

There are two techniques of applying direct acrylic resins to a tooth preparation: brush or Nealon and bulk techniques. In the brush technique, liquid and powder are placed into separate dappen dishes. A sable brush is dipped into the liquid and then into the powder, and the acrylic bead is placed into the tooth preparation. This method is repeated until the tooth is fully restored.

In the bulk technique, powder and liquid are mixed in a single dappen dish until a doughlike consistency is obtained. The mix is placed in the tooth preparation with a plastic instrument and is held in place with a matrix until it is set.

DIRECT GOLD RESTORATIONS

Direct gold restorations are used in many areas of the oral cavity. The use of gold is costly, time consuming, and often unesthetic and, as a result, is diminishing. Direct gold restorative materials come in several forms: gold foil, mat gold, and powdered gold.

Working the gold into the preparation is facilitated by the malleability, ductility, and welding ability of the material. It adapts to the walls of a preparation very well, making recurrent caries formation less likely than with other materials. Gold foil does not corrode or tarnish. The time involved in condensation of a gold foil restoration is extensive, since the material must be condensed layer by layer (cold welded), and as a result, it can present difficulties for the patient.

In order for the gold to be pure (without moisture or the presence of ammonia used in manufacturing), each particle of gold must be annealed before it is placed into the cavity preparation. This process can be done on an annealing tray placed over a flame or on a hot plate. After the gold particle (eg, pellet, powder) has been annealed, it is then placed into the correct spot by the dentist and condensed into the preparation. After adequate condensation, the restoration is polished.

SILICATE CEMENT

Silicate cement is an anterior restorative material supplied in a powder/liquid form. The silicate powder is a glass product, containing silica, aluminum, sodium or calcium phosphate, calcium fluoride, and sodium-aluminum fluoride. The liquid is a phosphoric acid solution containing phosphoric acid, aluminum and zinc phosphates, and water. Silicate cements are anticariogenic because of the active fluorides in the cement. However, they are no longer widely used because they have a high degree of solubility, abrasion, and dehydration in oral fluids, which tend to reduce the life of the restoration.

DENTAL CEMENTS

Cements in dentistry are used as luting agents for permanent restorations and orthodontic bands, as temporary restorations, and as thermal insulators for the pulp under metallic restorations. Varnishes and liners, also included under the classification of cements, are used in thin layers on the dentin to prevent irritating chemicals from reaching pulpal tissues. Zinc phosphate cement is a powder/liquid system. The powder is composed of zinc oxide and magnesium oxide, and the liquid contains phosphoric acid, water, and a small amount of aluminum phosphate. Zinc phosphate cements are high in acidity and can cause pulpal damage if not mixed properly. As is true of all cements, they are soluble in oral fluids and will not adhere to tooth structure under moist conditions.

Advantages of zinc phosphate cement are its properties of malleability and high compressive strength. Setting time can be controlled, allowing the dentist flexibility to use the material for various procedures simultaneously, such as cementation of several orthodontic bands from one single mix.

Zinc phosphate cement is mixed on a dry, cool glass slab with a metal spatula. Drops of the liquid are placed on the glass slab, and small increments of powder are incorporated using a rotary motion with the spatula held flat against the glass slab. The material is mixed over a large area of the glass slab in order to dissipate heat. The correct consistency for cementation can be determined by checking the flow of the mix. A thinner mix is desired for final luting procedures, and a thicker mix is used for insulating bases under restorations.

GLASS IONOMER CEMENTS

Glass ionomer cements may be used for permanent luting procedures of dental crowns and fixed bridgework. The composition of the glass ionomer cement powder is an aluminosilicate glass structure, and the liquid composition is a polycarboxylate copolymer in an aqueous solution. Glass ionomer cements exhibit high compressive strength, and are more resistant to the effects of erosion in the oral cavity. The glass ionomer cements also have the ability to form a stronger adhesive bond to dentin and enamel, creating a tighter seal and inhibiting secondary decay. Glass ionomer cements are cariostatic because of their ability to release fluoride ions incorporated in the powder composition of the ionomer cements used for permanent restorations of anterior teeth.

Glass ionomer cements can be mixed on a cool glass slab or on a nonabsorbent paper pad. The powder is incorporated into the liquid rapidly while spatulating. Unlike zinc phosphate cements, which incorporate several small increments of powder over a longer spatulation period, the glass ionomers incorporate three to four large increments of powder over a 45-second time period of mixing. Strict adherence to preventing moisture contamination before final cementation procedures must be followed when working with the glass ionomers. Premature moisture contact may contribute to tooth hypersensitivity and microleakage.

ZINC OXIDE-EUGENOL

Zinc oxide-eugenol (ZOE) usually is dispensed in a powder/liquid system. The powder is composed of zinc oxide, which can contain a small amount of fillers and zinc salts, and the liquid is eugenol (oil of cloves). This cement has a sedative effect on the pulpal tissues and is used to ameliorate pain from toothaches. ZOE is easy to manipulate, and setting can be controlled by accelerators, decreasing moisture, or altering the powder/liquid ratio. ZOE has low compressive strength and is highly soluble in oral fluids. Consequently, it is not used in final restorations. ZOE may be used as an insulating base under restorations and for cementation of temporary crowns or as a sedative temporary dressing.

ZOE is mixed by adding the powder to the liquid in small amounts and vigorously spatulating the mix with a metal spatula on an oil-impervious paper pad or glass slab until the desired thickness is obtained. As with all cements, the more powder used, the stronger the material.

Improved zinc oxide-eugenol also comes in a strengthened form, reinforced with ethoxybenzoic acid (EBA). It is a powder/liquid system that is easy to manipulate, flows readily under pressure, and has a long working time. It achieves adequate strength only if there is a high powder/liquid ratio. The material is mixed on a glass slab, and powder is added to the liquid. The mix is then spatulated vigorously under pressure for 2 minutes to achieve fluidity. Lowering the temperature of the glass slab will slow the cement to set. EBA cements are used for luting of permanent castings, such as inlays, crowns, and bridges.

POLYCARBOXYLATE CEMENT

Polycarboxylate cement, also referred to as carboxylate and polyacrylate, is a powder/liquid system used for luting or insulating pulpal tissue. The powder consists mainly of zinc oxide, with some magnesium oxide and aluminum oxide. The liquid contains polyacrylic and organic acids in an aqueous solution. This cement is not irritating to pulpal tissue, has relatively low solubility in oral fluids, and adheres best to clean enamel. One disadvantage is its short working time (maximum 3½ minutes) and setting time (5–8 minutes).

Polycarboxylate cement can be mixed on a paper pad or glass slab. When mixed on a cool glass slab, working time may be increased. The powder is incorporated into the liquid in large increments and spatulated quickly until homogeneous. Failure to mix the cement rapidly will produce a mix with a dull appearance and tacky consistency unsuitable for cementation procedures of permanent castings.

VARNISHES AND LINERS

Varnishes and liners are used to insulate pulpal tissue. Varnish is a coating material, consisting mainly of a natural gum or a synthetic resin in an organic solvent solution. Varnishes block irritating chemicals contained in restorative materials from entering the dentinal tubules and affecting the pulp.

The technique for using varnish involves dipping a cotton pledget into the varnish, removing the excess, and coating the walls of the cavity. Application of the varnish may be done also with a fine brush. At least two coatings of varnish should be applied to cover all walls of the cavity preparation. Setting time is approximately 15 to 30 seconds.

CALCIUM HYDROXIDE

(Daycal)

Calcium hydroxide is a liner available in liquid/paste or paste/paste form. The paste hardens and forms a thin layer over the dentin. It stimulates the formation of secondary dentin, which acts as additional protection for the pulp. It also forms a barrier against irritants from marginal leakage of restorative materials. This material must be used only on dentin, since placement on enamel walls of cavity preparations can contribute to marginal leakage of final restorations as a result of its high degree of solubility in oral fluids.

Calcium hydroxide is missed on a paper pad with a small, metal, ball-shaped applicator. Equal amounts of the base and catalyst are extruded onto the mixing pad and rapidly mixed until homogeneous. The cavity liner may be applied with the same instrument used for mixing or with an explorer.

DENTAL PORCELAIN

Dental porcelain is an esthetic material widely used in final restorations. It is highly compatible with oral tissues and is resistant to abrasion. It is used in the fabrication of artificial teeth in dentures, for crowns, and as a veneer fused to metal copings. Porcelains are classified by the temperature at which they mature. All are made of particles of feldspar and quartz. The feldspar serves as a matrix for the quartz, and the quartz is a strengthener and filler.

Porcelain is highly resistant to the forces of compression but also highly susceptible to bending forces. Consequently, restorations and tooth preparations must be designed to deemphasize exposure to unnecessary bending forces in the oral cavity.

Porcelain is produced as a powder that is mixed with water to form a pastelike substance that can be molded or condensed into the desired shape. The substance is then fired in a furnace and subsequently is glazed to polish the surface and improve the strength of the restoration. It is important to use minimum amounts of water to avoid shrinkage during the condensation or firing processes.

The finished restoration can then be placed into the mouth. Restorations totally fabricated from porcelain are used primarily in the anterior portion of the mouth. When used for posterior restorations, the material is fused to a cast alloy coping that fits the prepared tooth or teeth.

IMPRESSION MATERIALS

Impression materials are used in dentistry to obtain accurate, detailed negative images of hard and soft oral tissues. There are two major categories of impression materials, elastic and plastic, that can be subdivided further into chemosetting impression materials and thermosetting impression materials. Elastic materials are capable of being deformed under stress and returning to their original shape after setting. Plastic impression materials are categorized as those that are unable to return to their original shape after deformation. They are model plastic (compound), dental wax, zinc oxide-eugenol paste, and impression plaster.

Elastic Impression Materials

Reversible or agar hydrocolloid is a thermoelastic material in which an impression is recorded through the physical change of agar from a sol to a gel. Agar hydrocolloid is packaged in tubes and is composed of 80% to 85% water, 12% to 15% agar, a small percentage of sodium tetraborate (Borax), which adds strength, and 2% potassium sulfate, which enhances proper setting. The material is prepared by placing it in a waterbath conditioner at 212°F. It is stored at 150°F in a second bath. Before the impression is taken, it is placed in water-cooled trays and immersed in a third tempering bath to bring the material to a tolerable temperature for contact with the oral tissues.

Agar hydrocolloids are extremely accurate materials and are used for final impressions to make models for the fabrication of partial dentures, crowns, bridges, and inlays. The material has a low tear strength and the potential for high-dimensional change resulting from imbibition (the taking up of water). To minimize dimensional distortions, the impression should be poured immediately.

Irreversible or alginate hydrocolloid is a material that produces an impression through the process of chemical change. Mixing the soluble sodium alginate, which also contains calcium sulfate, with water results in the formation of an insoluble calcium alginate gel. Trisodium phosphate in the powder acts as a retardant, permitting more working time. The remaining ingredients include diatomaceous earth, which acts as a filler, a complex fluoride compound, which helps create adequate surface strength for the gypsum model materials, a coloring agent, and flavor additives.

The material is manipulated by first placing the powder, measured in scoops, into a rubber mixing bowl. A measured amount of water at room temperature (70°F) is then added, and the mix is spatulated in a whipping motion until a homogeneous sol is formed. The temperature of the water is extremely important, since higher temperatures shorten working and setting times. The mix is placed immediately in a fitted perforated or rim-locked tray.

Alginate is not as accurate in recording fine detail as other impression materials (eg, reversible hydrocolloids), and as a result, it is used to take impressions for study models used in diagnosis and the fabrication of orthodontic appliances and night guards. The material can be used to take final impressions for partial dentures. Alginate is easy to manipulate, in addition to being inexpensive. It has a low tear strength and is not dimensionally stable because of syneresis (loss of water) and imbibition. Alginate impressions should be poured immediately.

Elastomers

Elastomers are elastic impression materials manufactured from synthetic rubber and appearing soft and rubberlike when set.

Polysulfide impression material, also known as mercaptan, produces an impression through the chemical process of polymerization, which is the chemical reaction whereby single units (monomers) link to form larger units (polymers).

The material is supplied in two tubes of paste. One tube, the base, contains the basic reactive substance, a low-molecular-weight polysulfide polymer, and fillers. The other tube, the accelerator, contains lead peroxide and sulfur, which actually cause the vulcanization reaction that forms a longer-chain rubber material.

The material is mixed by spatulating equal lengths of base and accelerator on a paper pad for 45 to 60 seconds. The material, homogenized in color, is then placed in a preformed custom or stock tray and inserted into the patient's mouth. The material sets in about 6 to 8 minutes and is very accurate. It is used to take final impressions for models on which crowns, bridges, inlays, and partial dentures are fabricated. The material's disadvantages are its offensive smell, staining ability, and inconsistent setting time, which is shortened by increased temperature and humidity.

Silicone impression material is similar to polysulfide material in many ways. It sets via a polymerization reaction in 6 to 8 minutes and is supplied in two tubes (a base and a catalyst). It is carried to the mouth in the same type of tray as polysulfide and is used for the same purposes. The base, a paste, contains a polymer, dimethylsilocaine, and an organic filler. The catalyst, usually a liquid, contains an octoate that initiates the reaction. The base is dispensed onto a paper pad, and the catalyst is added. The material is spatulated for about a minute until a homogeneous color results. Its color and odor are among its advantages, and its disadvantages include a shorter shelf-life than that of other impression materials. Silicone is available also in a putty/wash system. The putty is mixed with a liquid catalyst. The putty contains up to 70% fillers as compared with the 45% of the regular-bodied silicone. After the putty has set, a wash material (a fluid silicone base mixed with the same liquid catalyst) is smoothed over the putty impression and placed over the teeth. This process results in an accurate, detailed impression.

Polyether impression materials are the third impression material in the elastomeric group and are similar to polysulfide and silicone in their polymerization reaction. However, when polyether is used, the impression can be recorded in a single step without a second wash impression. The material is supplied in two tubes. The base contains a polyether polymer, and the accelerator is a sulfonic acid ester. The materials are dispensed in equal lengths onto a paper mixing pad and spatulated for about 45 to 60 seconds until a homogeneous color is attained. Setting time is 2½ to 3 minutes. Polyether materials are highly accurate and are used for the same purposes as other elastic impression materials. A factor to be considered when using these materials is the difficulty of removing set impressions from the patient's mouth because

polyether impression materials exhibit a high degree of stiffness. A body modifier or thinner may be incorporated to reduce the stiffness. The polyether chemistry of this material may cause hypersensitivity in certain individuals.

Plastic Impression Materials

Thermal modeling plastic, or *dental compound,* is a material that produces an impression through a physical change of shape at a specific temperature. It is comprised of various thermoplastic resins, waxes, fillers, and coloring agents. Thermal modeling plastics are used to take preliminary impressions for full or partial dentures and for final impressions of single crown preparations. When denture impressions are desired, compound shaped wafers or cakes are used. When single crown impressions are desired, compound sticks are used. Dental compound has low thermal conductivity and should be heated slowly and evenly.

When preparing the material for a preliminary impression, it should be softened in a waterbath at 130°F until it can be kneaded. The compound should not remain in the water for too long a period because some of the necessary ingredients dissolve and a grainy material results. Similarly, when stick compound is warmed over a flame, it should be heated in a manner that prevents melting or dripping in order to maintain suitable flow properties. The materials are impressed against the mouth tissues while still warm and flowing (113°F). By the time the material reaches mouth temperature (98.6°F), it exhibits very little flow. Corrective washes (or final impressions) are taken over denture impressions.

Dental waxes are thermoplastic materials that come in many forms and are used for various procedures. They are categorized into three groups: pattern waxes, processing waxes, and impression waxes. These dental waxes are composed of a combination of materials that form organic polymers. Ingredients include resins, oils, fat, gums, pigments, and natural and synthetic waxes.

Pattern waxes are used to form the patterns from which metal or resin restorations are cast. Examples of pattern waxes are inlay wax, used to produce patterns for inlays, crowns, and pontics, and casting wax, used to create the pattern for the metal framework of a removable prosthesis.

Processing waxes are waxes used in the laboratory. Examples include boxing wax, used to prepare gypsum models, sticky wax, used to reattach plaster impressions, and periphery wax, used to adjust trays to the appropriate size.

Impression wax manufactured in various arch shapes is used when taking full denture impressions. Examples include corrective impression wax, used to record or fill specific areas of impressions made from other materials when minute detail is desired, and bite registration wax and wafer impression wax, used to record occlusal registration.

Zinc oxide-eugenol impression pastes are used for secondary impressions. ZOE functions as a final wash and is inserted into a preliminary impression tray. It is used most often for full denture impressions in a preformed tray. The material is dispensed in a paste/paste system and mixed on oil-impervious paper. Initial setting time is approximately 3 to 6 minutes, and final set ranges from 10 to 15 minutes. Setting time can be accelerated using a zinc acetate salt or a drop of water. Although the material is dimensionally stable, ZOE impression paste can irritate oral tissues because of its eugenol constituent, which can cause burning or stinging.

ACRYLIC DENTURE BASE RESINS

Denture bases are made from acrylic resins because of the material's dimensional stability, esthetic appearance, ability to absorb shock, and weight. Self-curing acrylic resins can be worked and set at room temperature and often are used to repair dentures that have broken. Acrylic resins are used also to rebase and reline dentures. Because the oral tissues on which the dentures rest change with time, dentures must sometimes be adapted to accommodate these changes. When dentures are rebased, the old base is used as an impression tray. The former base is replaced with one made from a new impression. The same teeth are used for the new base.

When minor changes occur in the oral tissues, a denture can be relined rather than rebased. The existing base is used to take an impression, and the appropriate amount of acrylic is added to accommodate the changes.

Acrylic resin also is used to make custom trays for impressions. These trays produce high-quality impressions because they are accurate replications of individual oral tissues. Temporary crowns are fabricated from acrylic resin, and permanent crowns often are faced with acrylic veneers.

CAST GOLD RESTORATIONS

Often, in a severely deteriorated tooth that is missing a considerable amount of structure, direct filling materials, such as amalgam, cannot be used because they would be unable to withstand masticatory forces. Rather, stronger cast restorations are fabricated.

The use of pure metal in dentistry is quite limited. The most commonly used materials are combinations of two or more metals, known as alloys. Casting gold alloys can contain gold, silver, copper, palladium, platinum, and zinc. Gold resists tarnish and corrosion and contributes ductility and malleability to the alloy. Silver reduces the deep yellow color of gold and red tint of copper by its natural gray color. Copper increases the strength and hardness of the alloy and generally reduces the melting point. Platinum increases the strength, hardness, and resistance to tarnish and corrosion. Like silver, it also helps whiten the color. Palladium increases the melting point, hardens the compound, and whitens the alloy. Zinc acts as a scavenger, reacting with any oxides first, and increases

TABLE 7–1. CLASSIFICATION OF CASTING GOLD ALLOYS

Type I alloys are soft and are used for simple inlays

Type II alloys are harder and can be used for two and three surface inlays and are the most common alloys used for operative procedures

Type III alloys are used for fixed prostheses, crown and bridge abutments

Type IV alloys are extra hard and are used for denture frameworks

the castibility of the alloy. It also reduces the melting point.

Gold alloys are cast into inlays, crowns, bridges, and partial denture frameworks. The base metal alloys, such as cobalt chromium, are used in constructing partial denture frameworks.

Gold alloy materials are classified according to gold content and hardness, which correlates to material strength. There are four types of dental gold alloys (Table 7–1).

GOLD CASTING PROCEDURES

The objective of the casting procedure is to provide an accurate metallic duplication of missing tooth structures. The first procedure in the casting of an inlay or a crown is preparation of a wax pattern. This pattern is carved directly on the prepared tooth or on a die representing a reproduction of the tooth and prepared cavity. If the pattern is made on the tooth itself, the technique is termed direct. Similarly, if the pattern is made on a die, the technique is termed indirect.

The wax pattern forms the outline of the mold into which the molten gold alloy is cast. It is, therefore, imperative that the pattern accurately represent the missing tooth structure.

After the pattern is removed from the prepared cavity, it is attached to a sprue former. The sprue former provides an ingate into the investment through which the molten alloy can enter the mold. The size of the sprue former depends on the type and size of the pattern, the type of casting machine used, and the dimensions of the flask or ring in which the casting is made.

The wax pattern is then surrounded by a gypsum material, known as investment. The investment serves as a binder to hold the other ingredients together and provides rigidity. Since gold alloy contracts on setting, expansion of investment is desirable for compensation. The setting expansion or thermal expansion can be controlled by altering the proportion of water in the investment mix. Thus, the appropriate amount of expansion to compensate for the shrinkage of gold can be attained.

After the investment has hardened for at least 30 minutes, the sprue former is removed, and the sprue, if it is plastic or wax, is left in the investment. The casting ring containing the invested pattern is heated slowly to the temperature at which the maximal thermal expansion of the investment is obtained (usually 700°C or 1292°F), and the wax pattern is eliminated by the heat. The investment should be heated for at least 1 hour. After the casting temperature has been attained, the casting can be made.

After the casting has been completed, when the metal is dull red, the ring is immersed in water. The casting is brushed free of debris. However, surface film may make the casting appear dark. A process called pickling, that is heating the discolored casting in a 50% solution of hydrochloric acid, removes the film. The casting is thoroughly washed, then inspected for defects. The casting is then ready to be finished and polished for seating.

ABRASIVE MATERIALS

Dental restorations usually are rough and irregular after construction. In order to improve their appearance and comfort and to increase their resistance to tarnish and corrosion, they are abraded and polished. Abrasive materials capable of cutting or scratching are used to smooth the surfaces. Initially, coarse abrasives are used, followed sequentially by progressively finer materials. As a result of this process, the scratches become undetectable, and the restoration's surfaces become smooth.

The polishing process may take place either intraorally or in a laboratory. If the polishing is done in the mouth, caution must be taken to prevent overheating the tooth and consequently damaging vital tissues. It is also important to choose abrasive agents that will not stain either the tooth or the restoration. Common abrasive materials used in dentistry include diamond stones, wheels, and discs, carborundum wheels and discs, aluminum oxide discs, and quartz sandpaper discs. Most of these agents are available in graduated degrees of abrasiveness.

Questions

1. Dental materials that meet all criteria of specification standards established by the American Dental Association are labeled

   (A) Certified Dental Materials
   (B) Popular Dental Materials
   (C) Approved Dental Materials
   (D) Improved Dental Materials

2. What is the most frequently used restorative material?

   (A) composite
   (B) gold
   (C) amalgam
   (D) porcelain

3. Which material is used primarily to stop noxious chemicals from reaching the pulp?

   (A) calcium hydroxide
   (B) zinc oxide-eugenol
   (C) varnish
   (D) zinc phosphate cement

4. Calcium hydroxide is used as a base primarily to

   (A) protect the pulp from bacterial invasion
   (B) insulate the pulp thermally
   (C) insulate the pulp chemically
   (D) promote secondary dentin formation

5. The effect of zinc oxide-eugenol on the pulp

   (A) is irritating
   (B) encourages pulpal fibrosis
   (C) is sedating
   (D) has no effect

6. Which chemical accelerates the setting time of zinc oxide-eugenol cement?

   (A) roxin
   (B) oil of cloves
   (C) zinc oxide
   (D) zinc acetate

7. What is the consistency of zinc oxide-eugenol cement, used as a temporary restoration?

   (A) fluid and thin
   (B) puttylike
   (C) firm
   (D) smooth and creamy

8. Glass ionomer cement is used as a

   (A) sedative base
   (B) cavity liner
   (C) temporary restoration
   (D) luting agent

9. Excess zinc phosphate cement powder left on the mixing slab is

   (A) discarded
   (B) returned to the bottle
   (C) placed under the cement base in the cavity preparation
   (D) placed over the cement base in the cavity preparation

10. Preventive sealant resins are placed on the

    (A) occlusal surface of the tooth
    (B) proximal surface of the tooth
    (C) gingival third of the tooth
    (D) cusp tips

11. The chemical used to etch enamel is

    (A) zinc oxide
    (B) methyl methacrylate
    (C) phosphoric acid
    (D) eugenol

12. What is the main component of composite restorative materials?

    (A) methyl methacrylate
    (B) zinc oxide
    (C) calcium hydroxide
    (D) inorganic filler

13. The type of spatula used to mix composite is

    (A) plastic
    (B) stainless steel
    (C) iron
    (D) glass

14. The process of chemically combining monomer and polymer is called

    (A) plating
    (B) mesmerizing
    (C) polymerization
    (D) vulcanization

15. The main component of acrylic monomer is

    (A) quartz filler
    (B) methyl methacrylate
    (C) liquid acrylic
    (D) sulfuric acid

16. Acrylic is applied to the cavity preparation

    (A) in small increments
    (B) with an amalgam carrier
    (C) with a celluloid matrix strip
    (D) with a plastic tray

17. To process denture base acrylic, it is necessary to

    (A) use only acrylic teeth
    (B) shake the material for 5 minutes
    (C) add extra accelerator
    (D) heat the material

18. When constructing a custom acrylic tray, placing it in warm water will

    (A) increase its strength
    (B) delay the setting
    (C) speed polymerization
    (D) spring the material past any undercuts on the model

19. When constructing a custom acrylic tray, it is best to remove most of the excess material with

    (A) a lathe after the acrylic has set
    (B) a knife before the acrylic has set
    (C) high-speed burs after the material sets
    (D) high-speed burs before the material sets

20. What is the most esthetic material that can be used in fabricating an anterior bridge?

    (A) acrylic
    (B) gold
    (C) cobalt-chrome
    (D) porcelain fused to metal

21. Noble metals

    (A) will not conduct an electrical current
    (B) will not tarnish or corrode in oral fluids
    (C) must be used in all oral restorations
    (D) are all very soft

22. The main component of dental porcelain is

    (A) clay
    (B) silica
    (C) feldspar
    (D) borax

23. The primary reason for using an individual porcelain jacket is

    (A) esthetics
    (B) edge strength
    (C) crushing strength
    (D) the amount of overjet

24. Chromium-cobalt alloys are used in dentistry for implants and

    (A) posts to reinforce teeth
    (B) intercoronal restorations
    (C) orthodontic appliances
    (D) frameworks for partial dentures

25. Stainless steel is used most in dentistry

    (A) to strengthen amalgam
    (B) in orthodontic wires
    (C) to construct clasps for partial dentures
    (D) to replace internal gold restorations

26. The material used in its pure form in dentistry is

    (A) amalgam
    (B) composite
    (C) gold
    (D) silver

27. The largest component of amalgam alloy is

    (A) silver
    (B) tin
    (C) zinc
    (D) copper

28. Why is zinc sometimes not incorporated in the amalgam alloy?

    (A) zinc only acts as a filler
    (B) zinc weakens Class II restorations
    (C) zinc causes the amalgam to pit if the restoration is polished
    (D) zinc causes delayed expansion of the amalgam restoration if any water is present while the amalgam is setting

29. Which technique of combining mercury with amalgam alloy ensures consistent excellent results?

    (A) amalgam fillings
    (B) amalgam pellets
    (C) premeasured capsules
    (D) use of an amalgamator

30. Insufficient mercury in an amalgam mix results in

    (A) an increase in thermal conductivity
    (B) a grainy texture
    (C) gray staining of the gingiva
    (D) excessive percolation

31. The crushing strength of amalgam is

    (A) 15,000 psi
    (B) 30,000 psi
    (C) 45,000 psi
    (D) 60,000 psi

32. Amalgamation is the process of

    (A) combining mercury with amalgam alloy
    (B) plugging amalgam into the preparation
    (C) dispensing the amalgam
    (D) burnishing the amalgam against the matrix band

33. The purpose of trituration is to

    (A) increase galvanization
    (B) cause a final expansion in amalgam restorations
    (C) decrease the thermal conductivity of amalgam restoration
    (D) expose each amalgam particle to mercury

34. Undertrituration of amalgam will result in

    (A) excessive expansion
    (B) excessive contraction
    (C) slight contraction
    (D) no effect

35. As amalgam is condensed, excess mercury

    (A) decreases the setting time
    (B) is brought to the surface
    (C) will dissolve the matrix band
    (D) liquifies the alloy particles

36. If amalgam is carved after it has started to set, what will occur?

    (A) corrosion
    (B) chipping
    (C) discoloration
    (D) expansion

37. The most frequent complaint of patients shortly after amalgam restorations are placed is

    (A) pain on percussion
    (B) an open contact point
    (C) cold sensitivity
    (D) numbness around the gingiva

38. Tarnishing and corrosion of amalgam can be reduced by

    (A) polishing the amalgam
    (B) using a zinc oxide base
    (C) increasing the tin content of amalgam alloy
    (D) decreasing the size of the amalgam fillings

39. Overheating amalgam restorations during polishing can result in

    (A) creating a restoration high in occlusion
    (B) shrinkage in the restoration
    (C) pulpal damage
    (D) an aphthous ulcer

40. Pins are used in restorative dentistry to

    (A) increase the crushing strength of the restorative material
    (B) hold a tooth together
    (C) fracture the enamel
    (D) increase retention

41. Gold foil is annealed

    (A) to form gold oxides
    (B) to remove volatile surface impurities
    (C) to soften the gold
    (D) to harden the gold

42. Casting gold is used for

    (A) ortho wire
    (B) partial clasps
    (C) inlays
    (D) splints

43. Flux is used during casting to

    (A) remove the oxides formed on the gold alloy
    (B) lower the melting point
    (C) replace casting wax
    (D) speed the burnout process

44. Pickling

    (A) is accomplished by soaking the casting in baking soda
    (B) causes porosity in gold
    (C) removes surface oxides from gold castings
    (D) removes investment from gold castings

45. Why is it a disadvantage if filling materials are radiolucent?

    (A) they are always good thermal conductors
    (B) they irritate the pulp
    (C) they always cause galvanic shock
    (D) it is difficult to differentiate between the restoration and recurrent decay on a radiograph

46. Which material most closely approximates the compressive strength of amalgam?

    (A) acrylic
    (B) composite
    (C) sealants
    (D) silicate

47. What is the main component of zinc polyacrylate cement powder?

    (A) zinc acetate
    (B) zinc oxide
    (C) methyl methacrylate
    (D) polyacrylic acid

48. If water evaporates from the liquid portion of zinc phosphate cement, the setting time is

    (A) shortened
    (B) not affected
    (C) lengthened
    (D) indefinite

49. Increasing the powder/liquid ratio of zinc phosphate cement will result in

    (A) an increase in pulpal irritation
    (B) decreased solubility
    (C) decreased crushing strength
    (D) heterogeneous mix

50. Which cement is irritating to the pulp?

    (A) carboxylate cement
    (B) zinc oxide-eugenol cement
    (C) zinc phosphate
    (D) ethoxybenzoic acid

51. Which cement has the highest crushing strength?

    (A) zinc phosphate
    (B) zinc oxide-eugenol
    (C) calcium hydroxide
    (D) all cements have the same crushing strength

52. Dew point is the

    (A) melting point of thermoplastic materials
    (B) creamy consistency of cements
    (C) setting temperature of zinc oxide-eugenol cement
    (D) temperature at which water vapor condenses

53. If dentures are cleaned in boiling water, they

    (A) become sticky
    (B) warp
    (C) melt
    (D) galvanize

54. To repair a fractured temporary fixed bridge

    (A) the bridge is seated in the patient's mouth, and small additions of acrylic are brushed on the fractured area
    (B) the bridge is seated in the patient's mouth, and a large amount of acrylic is mixed and adapted around the entire bridge
    (C) the bridge is removed from the patient's mouth, sticky wax is added to hold fractured pieces together, and small amounts of acrylic are then added
    (D) the bridge is removed from the patient's mouth, the fractured pieces are embedded in fast-setting plaster, and small amounts of acrylic are added

55. To repair a fractured maxillary denture

    (A) the fractured denture is placed in the patient's mouth, and small amounts of acrylic are added to the fracture site
    (B) the fractured denture is placed in the patient's mouth, the edges are luted together with sticky wax, and small amounts of acrylic are added to the fractured site
    (C) the fractured denture is luted together with sticky wax out of patient's mouth, the fractured denture is embedded, and acrylic is added to the fracture site
    (D) none of the above

56. To replace an intact tooth broken from a denture

   (A) the site on the denture is roughened, some quick-cure acrylic is added, and the tooth is reset
   (B) the tooth is luted to the denture with sticky wax, and the area is embedded in quick-setting plaster and boiled for 10 minutes
   (C) the lingual portion of the tooth is cut off, and the tooth is held in position while a loose mix of acrylic is vibrated into the area
   (D) none of the above

57. An impression is a

   (A) negative reproduction of oral tissues
   (B) flexible model
   (C) metallic casting
   (D) positive reproduction of a prepared tooth

58. Impression materials can be classified according to

   (A) cost
   (B) nature of the material as it is being removed from the mouth
   (C) setting time
   (D) accuracy

59. The impression material capable of change from gel to sol to gel is

   (A) compound
   (B) silicone
   (C) reversible hydrocolloid
   (D) irreversible hydrocolloid

60. Imbibition is the

   (A) loss of water by hydrocolloid impressions
   (B) increase in model size due to expansion
   (C) decrease in model size due to evaporation of water
   (D) uptake of water by hydrocolloid impressions

61. Syneresis is the

   (A) uptake of water by hydrocolloid impressions
   (B) uptake of water by gypsum products
   (C) loss of water by hydrocolloid impressions
   (D) expansion of elastic impression materials

62. Undermixing irreversible hydrocolloid impression material results in

   (A) finer surface detail
   (B) an increased setting time
   (C) an increased tear strength
   (D) a grainy mix and a model with poorer detail

63. Heavy and light body impression materials are used with

   (A) silicone

   (B) alginate
   (C) compound
   (D) plaster

64. A perforated tray is used to carry

   (A) plaster
   (B) mercaptan
   (C) irreversible hydrocolloid
   (D) reversible hydrocolloid

65. Which material is carried in a custom tray?

   (A) high fusing compound
   (B) reversible hydrocolloid
   (C) metallic oxide paste
   (D) irreversible hydrocolloid

66. Which material should be tempered before using?

   (A) alginate
   (B) reversible hydrocolloid
   (C) impression plaster
   (D) metallic oxide paste

67. Compound is a thermoplastic material used to make

   (A) study models
   (B) custom trays
   (C) final impressions
   (D) working models

68. Water-cooled trays are used to carry which impression material?

   (A) reversible hydrocolloid
   (B) silicone
   (C) impression plaster
   (D) irreversible hydrocolloid

69. Copper bands carry which impression material?

   (A) impression plaster
   (B) metallic oxide paste
   (C) silicone
   (D) stick compound

70. When using rubber impression material, it is necessary to coat the tray with

   (A) a separating medium
   (B) petroleum jelly
   (C) a rubber adhesive
   (D) no coating is necessary

71. Vulcanization refers to the setting of

   (A) reversible hydrocolloid
   (B) mercaptan impression material
   (C) zinc phosphate cement
   (D) zinc oxide-eugenol

72. The setting time for mercaptan impression materials is affected by

    (A) the shape of the impression tray
    (B) the bulk of material used
    (C) the amount of accelerator used
    (D) an exothermic reaction

73. The removal of hydrocolloid impressions from the mouth is accomplished with

    (A) a rocking motion
    (B) a jiggling motion
    (C) lateral pressure
    (D) a quick snapout motion

74. When loading a tray with irreversible hydrocolloid

    (A) more material is placed posteriorly
    (B) more material is placed anteriorly
    (C) more material is placed in the palatal area
    (D) the material is placed evenly in the entire tray

75. The setting time of irreversible hydrocolloid can be altered easily by

    (A) using a metal spatula
    (B) using a perforated tray
    (C) varying the water temperature
    (D) adding hard water

76. Placing a reversible hydrocolloid impression in 2% potassium sulfate solution for several minutes results in

    (A) a hard, smooth model surface
    (B) an increase in the gypsum setting time
    (C) a decrease in tear strength
    (D) dies with finer detail

77. After moving an irreversible hydrocolloid impression from the mouth, the operator should

    (A) immerse the impression in a warm bath
    (B) tap the impression to remove saliva
    (C) wash impression to remove saliva, blood, and debris
    (D) let the impression stand in the air for 1 hour

78. Calcination of gypsum determines

    (A) debubblizing techniques
    (B) how impressions are poured
    (C) the physical characteristics of the resulting gypsum products
    (D) the type of impression material that should be used

79. When mixing gypsum products

    (A) add the powder and water to the mixing bowl at the same time
    (B) add the powder to water in the mixing bowl
    (C) add water to the powder in the mixing bowl
    (D) allow powder to be completely absorbed in water, then begin mixing

80. Metallic oxide impression paste is used to make

    (A) final edentulous impressions
    (B) impressions of inlay preparations
    (C) impressions of crown preparations
    (D) impressions for study models

81. Hygroscopic setting expansion occurs in

    (A) noble metals
    (B) waxes
    (C) acrylics after exothermic reactions
    (D) all gypsum products immersed in water after the initial setting

82. To prevent air bubbles in the final model, use

    (A) high water/powder ratio
    (B) boxing techniques
    (C) a mechanical vibrator
    (D) additional catalysts

83. When pouring a model from a full upper impression, add stone

    (A) to the anterior teeth first
    (B) to the same place on the palate
    (C) to the posterior teeth first
    (D) any place desired

84. When pouring a model from a full lower impression, add stone

    (A) when the exothermic reaction begins
    (B) to either heel and continue to add to the same place
    (C) of a watery consistency
    (D) anywhere in the impression

85. A reason for boxing impression is

    (A) to decrease the time necessary to finish the base of the model
    (B) easy storage
    (C) identification
    (D) to increase the hardness of the model

86. Plaster models

    (A) have no dimensional change on setting
    (B) contract on setting
    (C) expand on setting
    (D) have greater crushing strength than do stone models

87. The amount of water needed to mix various gypsum products is related to the

    (A) water temperature
    (B) irregularity of the gypsum particles
    (C) impression material used
    (D) type of mixing bowl used

88. Dental stone is used

    (A) to pour all irreversible hydrocolloid impressions
    (B) for occlusal registration
    (C) to construct casts used in denture construction
    (D) when plaster is not available

89. Increasing the water/powder ratio of stone will result in

    (A) a less porous model
    (B) dies that can be used in constructing crowns
    (C) a weaker model
    (D) a thermoplastic model

90. The working time of a mix of dental stone ends when the

    (A) exothermic reaction is complete
    (B) stone no longer flows
    (C) model can be separated from the impression
    (D) material is the consistency of sour cream

91. Improved stone is used

    (A) to make dies
    (B) to make study models
    (C) for bite registrations
    (D) to invest wax crowns

92. Dowel pins are used to

    (A) articulate impressions
    (B) reinforce stone models
    (C) reinsert individual dies in a model
    (D) calcine gypsum products

93. Casting wax is used

    (A) to replace inlay wax
    (B) to retain asbestos in the casting ring
    (C) as a pattern for metal partial frameworks
    (D) to hold gold casting together

94. Sticky wax is used to

    (A) rebuild cusps on models
    (B) take single tooth impressions
    (C) take bite registrations
    (D) hold fractured denture parts in a fixed position temporarily

95. Utility wax is used

    (A) to wax inlays on models
    (B) as a tray to hold compound
    (C) as periphery wax around trays
    (D) to construct bite rims

96. Impression waxes are used

    (A) for bite registrations
    (B) for study models
    (C) to cast restorations
    (D) to hold dies in position

97. Baseplate wax is used to

    (A) construct wax patterns for crowns
    (B) hold broken parts of dentures together
    (C) contour the edges of impression trays
    (D) determine occlusal relationships in full dentures

98. Gutta percha is used

    (A) as a dental wax
    (B) as a root canal filling material
    (C) as an impression material for gold posts
    (D) only in occlusal restorations of molars

99. The wax used to make a rim around an impression to contain the poured gypsum material is called

    (A) boxing wax
    (B) utility wax
    (C) periphery wax
    (D) blue wax

100. Inlay wax is used to

    (A) temporarily cement inlays
    (B) make inlay wax patterns
    (C) invest inlay patterns
    (D) box models

101. An important property of inlay wax is

    (A) it is brittle at mouth temperature
    (B) it contracts when it is being invested
    (C) its complete burnout
    (D) it is interchangeable with utility wax

102. It is best to invest the inlay wax pattern

    (A) as soon as possible
    (B) after 1 hour
    (C) after 1 day
    (D) any time

103. At mouth temperature, inlay wax should

    (A) produce galvanic stimulation
    (B) constantly flow
    (C) imbibe slightly
    (D) have no flow

104. Which wax is not used intraorally?

    (A) baseplate wax
    (B) sticky wax
    (C) utility wax
    (D) inlay wax

105. When attaching a baseplate rim to a shellac tray, care must be taken

    (A) to avoid burning the patient
    (B) not to warp the shellac tray when heating the wax
    (C) to coat the ridge area with sticky wax
    (D) to use adhesive on the tray first

DIRECTIONS (Questions 106 through 110): Match the term in Column A with the appropriate definition in Column B.

COLUMN A	COLUMN B
106. Exothermic	A. dimensional change of a material under a given load
107. Flow	B. material that speeds up a chemical reaction
108. Galvanism	
109. Catalyst	C. the ability of a material to return to its original shape after stress is released
110. Elasticity	D. release of energy in the form of heat
	E. small electrical currents caused by two different metals contacting in a moist oral cavity

DIRECTIONS (Questions 111 through 130): For each of the items in this section, ONE or MORE of the numbered options is correct. Choose answer

    A if only 1, 2, and 3 are correct
    B if only 1 and 3 are correct
    C if only 2 and 4 are correct
    D if only 4 is correct
    E if all are correct

111. Study models are used

    (1) as references in orthodontic cases
    (2) to show shape, size, and position of teeth
    (3) as an aid in treatment planning
    (4) to fabricate night guards

112. To make a gypsum product set faster

    (1) increase spatulation
    (2) lower the water/powder ratio
    (3) add an accelerator
    (4) increase the water/powder ratio

113. Quicksetting plaster is used

    (1) in transfer registrations when constructing crowns
    (2) as a wash in edentulous impressions
    (3) to record jaw registrations in full denture work
    (4) never

114. When mixing mercaptan and silicone impression materials

    (1) they should be tempered before use
    (2) use a wiping, pressing motion
    (3) mix on a cool glass slab
    (4) use a flexible stainless steel spatula

115. Investment material is used to

    (1) pour final fixed bridge impressions
    (2) prepare molds in which crowns will be cast
    (3) make bite registrations
    (4) help solder fixed bridge units

116. Dental cements are used

    (1) as temporary restorations
    (2) as thermal insulators
    (3) as a luting agent
    (4) to hold denture teeth in place

117. Dies of crown preparations can be made of

    (1) gold
    (2) acrylic
    (3) porcelain
    (4) improved stone

118. Which factors will accelerate the setting time of zinc oxide-eugenol cement?

    (1) increased powder/liquid ratio
    (2) water
    (3) increased temperature
    (4) decreased powder/liquid ratio

119. Acrylic resins are used for

    (1) anterior restorations
    (2) temporary bridges
    (3) denture bases
    (4) temporary trays

120. Which of the following materials are used to polish amalgam restorations in the mouth?

    (1) pumice
    (2) rouge
    (3) tin oxide
    (4) zinc oxide

121. Which factors would decrease the dental team's exposure to mercury vapors?

(1) use of premeasured capsules
(2) smooth tile floors
(3) careful handling of amalgam scraps
(4) use of an automatic plugger

122. Advantages of calcium hydroxide are

(1) ease of manipulation
(2) low solubility in oral fluids
(3) ability to stimulate the production of secondary dentin
(4) high compressive strength

123. When polishing acrylic on a lathe

(1) use low speed to avoid heat buildup
(2) use copious amounts of water with the pumice
(3) keep moving the prosthesis
(4) always use safety (goggles) glasses

124. Bonding resin materials may be used

(1) to repair fractured teeth
(2) to fabricate a temporary crown
(3) for esthetics
(4) only in orthodontic cases

125. Characteristics of pit and fissure sealants may include

(1) self-curing polymerization
(2) acid etching
(3) light-cured polymerization
(4) metallic matrix strips

126. Advantages of glass ionomer cements include

(1) may be used for permanent restorations
(2) high adhesion properties
(3) low abrasion properties
(4) reduced caries due to fluoride-releasing properties

127. Which factors retard the setting time of zinc phosphate?

(1) adding small portions of powder
(2) mixing on a glass slab
(3) decreasing initial acidity
(4) adding a drop of water

128. Synthetic resins are used for

(1) relining dentures
(2) fabricating custom trays
(3) fabricating artificial teeth
(4) sedative fillings

129. To prevent distortion of an inlay wax pattern

(1) manipulate it as little as possible
(2) store it in a dark area
(3) avoid temperature changes
(4) keep it moist

130. When trimming study model casts with a model trimmer, it is best to

(1) wear protective glasses or face shield
(2) begin with the mandibular cast
(3) allow sufficient water to flow through the model trimmer
(4) periodically check casts in occluded position

Answers and Explanations

1. **(A)** The American Dental Association is responsible for establishing criteria and sponsoring research that sets the standards for the accepted specifications for dental materials. The specifications ascertain the highest quality and usefulness of the dental materials for the doctor. Standards affecting the physical and chemical properties of the material are tested, approved, and rated by the American Dental Association for Certification. If a dental material meets the requirements, it becomes Certified. Before purchasing and ordering dental materials, the dental auxiliary must check to see if the dental material is Certified.

2. **(C)** The material used in approximately 75% of all restorations is amalgam.

3. **(C)** To prevent irritating chemicals from reaching the pulp, the dentinal tubules are sealed with varnish. Varnish is placed under zinc phosphate cements and amalgam restorations and other materials that would have deleterious effects on the pulp. Varnish is not placed under materials that have a beneficial effect on the pulp, such as zinc oxide-eugenol and calcium hydroxide.

4. **(D)** Calcium hydroxide is a base placed beneath deep restorations to promote irritation of the pulp and thereby promote the formation of secondary dentin.

5. **(C)** Zinc oxide-eugenol cement sedates pulpal tissue and is, therefore, used when cavity preparations are near the pulp. Zinc oxide-eugenol cement is used also as a temporary restoration and in periodontal dressings.

6. **(D)** Zinc acetate is added to zinc oxide-eugenol cement to accelerate the setting time. Rosin is added to provide strength.

7. **(B)** The desired consistency of zinc oxide-eugenol cement when used as a temporary restoration is puttylike.

8. **(D)** Glass ionomer cements are used as luting agents and exhibit high compressive strength. The powder is composed primarily of an aluminosilicate glass, and the liquid is derived from a polyacrylic acid and water base. The glass ionomers may be mixed on a cool glass slab or a nonabsorbent paper pad. The powder is incorporated into the liquid in two or three large increments and spatulated rapidly over a large surface area. Approximate mixing time range is 45 seconds. The final mix will appear shiny and should be used during this period for maximum adhesion properties to occur. Moisture control is imperative when working with the glass ionomers. The glass ionomers also are used for insulating bases or permanent restorations.

9. **(A)** Excess zinc phosphate cement powder left on the glass slab should be discarded because it may be contaminated. Placing contaminated powder with uncontaminated powder will contaminate all the powder and can change the cement's characteristics.

10. **(A)** Preventive sealant resins are placed in pits and fissures on the occlusal surfaces of the teeth. Pits and fissures are inaccessible for cleaning. Therefore, they are susceptible to decay. The use of sealants has shown a reduction of decay in these areas.

11. **(C)** Fifty percent solution of phosphoric acid is used to etch enamel. Enamel treated in this manner has increased mechanical retention for resin materials.

12. **(D)** The main component of composite (sometimes known as filled acrylic resin) is the inorganic filler. The inorganic filler consists of glass particles, fused silica, and quartz crystals. The organic portion of composites is composed of polymers.

13. **(A)** A plastic spatula is used to mix composite. The filler is so abrasive that abraded metal particles will be incorporated into the material if a metal spatula is used.

14. **(C)** Polymerization is the formation of large molecules (polymers) from smaller units (monomers). When acrylics polymerize, they give off heat and shrink.

15. **(B)** The main component of the acrylic monomer is methyl methacrylate. The powder is composed mostly of polymethyl methacrylate.

16. **(A)** Acrylic may be added to a cavity preparation by small increments, brush or Nealon technique, or by bulk amounts. In the brush technique, two dappen dishes are used, one with monomer and one with polymer. A sable hair brush is wet in the monomer and then placed in the polymer to pick up some powder. The wet powder is then placed in the cavity preparation and allowed to polymerize. This process is repeated until the preparation is overfilled. In the bulk technique, monomer and polymer are mixed on a glass slab or in a dappen dish to a puttylike consistency. The acrylic is then placed in the cavity preparation in bulk until the preparation is overfilled.

17. **(D)** Denture base acrylic needs heat for polymerization. Acrylics used for anterior restorations, temporary crowns, and bridges are self-curing and polymerize by the chemical reaction of their components.

18. **(C)** Placing self-curing acrylics in warm water will speed up polymerization by driving off excess monomer.

19. **(B)** When constructing a custom acrylic tray, excess acrylic is best removed with a knife after adapting the acrylic to the model. The excess can then be used to make a handle for the tray.

20. **(D)** The most esthetic material for anterior bridgework is porcelain fused to metal.

21. **(B)** Noble metals are metals that will not tarnish or corrode in the oral cavity. Gold and platinum are examples of such metals.

22. **(C)** The main component of dental porcelain is feldspar. Silica, also known as quartz, is the second most abundant component of porcelain.

23. **(A)** The primary reason for a porcelain jacket restoration is the excellent esthetic result. Other favorable features of porcelain restorations are that they do not irritate tissues and resist wear.

24. **(D)** Chromium-cobalt alloys are used as frameworks for partial dentures, dental implants, and some fixed bridgework.

25. **(B)** Stainless steel is used for orthodontic wires and bands and preformed crowns.

26. **(C)** Pure gold is used in dentistry to fabricate gold restorations directly in the mouth. Gold alloys are used for cast gold restorations.

27. **(A)** The components of amalgam alloy are, as stated by the ADA, silver (65% minimum), tin (29% maximum), copper (6% maximum), and zinc (2% maximum). The high silver content gives amalgam a high luster.

28. **(D)** Zinc causes water to break down into hydrogen and oxygen gases. This will result in delayed expansion if moisture is present while the amalgam is setting and will weaken the restoration.

29. **(C)** Premeasured amalgam capsules ensure correct proportioning of mercury and alloy and excellent results.

30. **(B)** Insufficient mercury will not wet each alloy particle and will result in an amalgam that is weak, granular, and crumbly and that might have some voids.

31. **(C)** The crushing or compressive strength of amalgam is at least 45,000 psi when it is fully hardened (about 24 hours).

32. **(A)** Amalgamation is the combining, chemically and physically, of mercury with amalgam alloy.

33. **(D)** The purpose of trituration is to remove the protective oxide coat of the amalgam alloy particles. This will allow mercury to react with the individual particles so that they can bond together.

34. **(A)** Undertrituration of amalgam results in expansion of the restoration, reduction in strength of the final restoration, rapid setting of the restoration, and excessive mercury in the final restoration. Overtrituration causes the alloy particles to be crushed. This increases the mercury content of the restoration and results in a weakened restoration. Overtrituration also produces a soft, soupy material that is difficult to manipulate.

35. **(B)** As a result of condensation, amalgam is placed in intimate contact with the cavity preparation, and a dense restoration is achieved by bringing excess mercury to the surface of the restoration. This excess is then removed when carving.

36. **(B)** If amalgam is carved after it has begun to set, it will chip, flake, and possibly fracture.

37. **(C)** The most frequent patient complaint after an amalgam restoration is placed is cold sensitivity in the newly restored tooth. Cement bases, such as zinc phosphate, at least 0.5 mm thick, act as a thermal insulator when placed under amalgam restorations.

38. **(A)** Tarnishing, a surface phenomenon, and corrosion, a chemical deterioration of amalgam restorations, can be reduced substantially by polishing the restorations. Polishing should not take place until 24 hours after placement.

39. **(C)** Overheating the amalgam restoration when polishing may result in damaging the pulp or vaporization of surface mercury, which may pose an occupational hazard to dental staff. During polishing procedures, use a high-speed vacuum system and waterspray.

40. **(D)** Pins are used in restorative dentistry to increase retention of filling materials. Pins are placed in the dentin and are retained by threads, cement, or friction.

41. **(B)** Annealing gold foil removes gaseous impurities from the surface of the gold and makes the gold cohesive. It is accomplished by heating the gold. Underannealing will not remove all the impurities and will result in gold that is not as cohesive as it should be. Overannealing will make the gold brittle and unworkable.

42. **(C)** Casting gold is used for cast restorations (eg, crowns, inlays, posts), wrought wire clasps (for partial dentures), and solder (to join metals together by fusion).

43. **(A)** Flux is used when heating the gold for casting. It removes oxides that form on the gold.

44. **(C)** Pickling removes surface oxides from gold castings. This process is accomplished by placing the gold casting in a strong acid solution.

45. **(D)** When viewing radiographs of teeth with radiolucent filling materials, it is difficult to distinguish between the restoration and recurrent decay. If the materials used are radiopaque, they are easily distinguished from decay.

46. **(B)** Composites have compressive strength of 30,000 psi, which approaches the compressive strength of amalgam (45,000 psi).

47. **(B)** The main component of zinc polyacrylate cement powder is zinc oxide. The liquid is a 40% solution of polyacrylic acid in water.

48. **(C)** The liquid portion of zinc phosphate cement consists of phosphoric acid, water, and dissolved salts. The acid/water ratio is critical, and alterations will affect the setting time of the cement. Evaporation causes a lengthened (slower) setting time, and the addition of water will cause a shorter (faster) setting time.

49. **(B)** Increasing the powder/liquid ratio will decrease the solubility of zinc phosphate cement. Decreased solubility is desirable, and, therefore, as much powder as possible should be mixed into the available liquid until the optimum consistency is reached.

50. **(C)** Zinc phosphate cement remains acidic several hours after it is set and irritating to the pulp. To avoid its irritating effects, cavity varnish often is used to seal the dental tubules before this cement is applied.

51. **(A)** Zinc phosphate cement has the highest crushing strength of dental cements. Zinc phosphate has a crushing strength of 14,500 psi, zinc oxide-eugenol 200 psi, and calcium hydroxide 150 psi.

52. **(D)** Dew point is the temperature at which water vapor condenses. If a glass slab is cooled below the dew point, moisture will collect on the slab and will speed the setting time of zinc phosphate and silicate cements.

53. **(B)** Cleaning dentures in excessively hot water will cause the denture base to warp and distort because processing stresses will be released. Immersion techniques of cleansing dentures are best and may be done with commercial products. A denture brush is recommended for removing soft deposits from the denture.

54. **(A)** To repair a fractured temporary bridge, the bridge is seated in the patient's mouth and dried, small amounts of acrylic are added to the fractured ends of the bridge, the acrylic is allowed to set, and the bridge is then removed from the patient's mouth and polished.

55. **(C)** To repair a fractured denture, the denture is removed from the patient's mouth. The pieces of the denture are luted together with sticky wax on the polished surface, and plaster is poured into the denture to obtain a model of the patient's mouth. After the plaster has set, the sticky wax is removed from the fractured ends, the pieces of the denture are placed back on the model, denture repair acrylic is added to the fractured ends, the acrylic is allowed to set, and the repaired denture is polished and returned to the patient.

56. **(A)** To replace an intact tooth in a denture, the area on the denture where the tooth has popped out is roughened, denture repair acrylic is placed on the area, the tooth is reset, and the acrylic is allowed to set.

57. **(A)** Impressions are used to fabricate restorations outside the mouth. If a restoration is to fit a tooth (eg, a crown) and oral tissues (eg, a denture), the impression must be accurate. An impression is a detailed, accurate negative reproduction of oral tissues. A positive reproduction, or model, which is an exact duplication of the impressed tissues, is obtained by allowing a gypsum product to set in the impression.

58. **(B)** The classification of impression materials is made on the basis of the nature of the material when it is being removed from the mouth. Rigid materials are impression plaster, metallic oxide paste, and impression compound. Elastic materials are reversible and irreversible hydrocolloids, mercaptan or polysulfide, silicone, and polyether impression material.

59. **(C)** Reversible hydrocolloid can change from gel to sol and back to gel by heating and cooling. This material can be reused up to four times.

60. **(D)** Imbibition, the uptake of water by hydrocolloid impressions, causes an expansion of the impression. The resulting model will be inaccurate.

61. **(C)** Syneresis is the exuding of water from hydrocolloid impressions. This loss of water causes shrinkage of the impression, which results in an inaccurate model.

62. **(D)** Undermixing irreversible hydrocolloid impression material will yield a grainy mix that will result in an impression—and subsequently a model—with poor detail. The proper consistency of the material should be smooth and creamy within the mixing time of 1 minute.

63. **(A)** Mercaptan and silicone impression materials use heavy and light body materials to make fine detailed impressions. The light body, or syringe material, has low viscosity and is placed around the prepared teeth. The heavy body, or tray material, has high viscosity and is placed in the impression tray.

64. **(C)** A perforated tray is used to carry irreversible hydrocolloid.

65. **(C)** Materials carried in a custom tray are metallic oxide paste, impression plaster, and rubber impression materials. The custom tray can be constructed of acrylic, shellac, or compound.

66. **(B)** To avoid burning the oral tissues, reversible hydrocolloid should be tempered in a water bath at 110°F to 115°F for 5 to 10 minutes before using.

67. **(B)** Impression compound is used to prepare custom-made trays for edentulous mouths, to make impressions of crown preparations, to border mold custom trays, and to check occlusion for mounting casts. Compound is a thermoplastic material. A material is thermoplastic if it becomes softer when heated and harder when cooled.

68. **(A)** Reversible hydrocolloid is carried to the mouth in water-cooled trays. After the tray is properly positioned in the patient's mouth, cool water is circulated through the tray.

69. **(D)** Copper bands carry low fusing compound used to make impressions of crowns or inlays. The copper band is closely adapted to the prepared tooth before the compound is placed in it.

70. **(C)** When rubber impression materials are used, the tray is coated with a rubber adhesive. Failure to coat the tray can result in the impression separating from the tray.

71. **(B)** The setting or curing of mercaptan impression materials is known as vulcanization.

72. **(C)** The setting time for a mercaptan impression material is dependent on the amount of accelerator, temperature, and humidity.

73. **(D)** Hydrocolloid impressions are removed from the mouth with one firm movement. Rocking or slow removal causes increased deformation of the impression.

74. **(B)** Irreversible hydrocolloid is loaded in a perforated tray with most of the material placed anteriorly. This reduces the amount of material flowing posteriorly and thereby decreases the possibility of the patient gagging.

75. **(C)** The most effective way to adjust the setting time of hydrocolloid is to vary the water temperature. Warmer water will accelerate the set; cooler water will retard the set. Changing the water/powder ratio also will affect the setting time, but it is a poor method because it will weaken the material physically and can alter some of its properties.

76. **(A)** Reversible hydrocolloid impressions immediately on removal from the mouth are placed in a 2% potassium sulfate solution for several minutes. The purpose is to accelerate the setting of the stone model and to give it a hard, smooth surface.

77. (C) After removing a hydrocolloid impression from the mouth, the impression should be washed to remove debris. After washing the impression, excess water must be removed from the impression before pouring a gypsum model.

78. (C) Gypsum products include plaster, dental stone, improved stone, and investment. The calcination of gypsum is the process of heating gypsum to drive off water. This process determines the physical characteristics of the resulting powder and, subsequently, the physical characteristics of gypsum products.

79. (B) When mixing gypsum products, the powder should be added to the water in the mixing bowl. This technique minimizes the amount of air trapped in the mix.

80. (A) Metallic oxide impression material is used to make final impressions of edentulous areas and bite registrations. Metallic oxide paste is mixed on an oil-resistant paper pad to avoid the cleaning problem of using a glass slab. The setting time of metallic oxide paste is decreased by adding a few drops of water and increasing the temperature, the mixing time, and/or amount of accelerator.

81. (D) Hygroscopic setting expansion occurs in all gypsum products immersed in water after the initial set. This increase in volume of the gypsum product will decrease the strength of the model. Hygroscopic expansion is part of the controlled expansion of dental investment.

82. (C) To prevent bubbles from forming in the final model, a mechanical vibrator or vacuum mixer or both are used. The debubblizer is placed in the impression to reduce the surface tension.

83. (B) When pouring a model from a full upper impression, continuously add stone to the same place on the palate. This will allow the stone to flow slowly into the areas where the teeth have been impressed and will move the air out of these areas.

84. (B) When pouring a model from a full lower impression, continuously add stone to either heel of the impression.

85. (A) Impressions are boxed to confine the model material and thereby decrease the time necessary to finish the base of the model.

86. (C) All gypsum products expand on setting. Plaster expands more than stone, which expands more than improved stone. Increased expansion may be caused by increased spatulation, increased water/powder ratio, hygroscopic expansion, and the addition of certain chemicals.

87. (B) The more porous, rough, and irregular the gypsum particles, the higher the water/powder ratio needed to mix the material. With plaster, it is 1:2, with stone, 3:10.

88. (C) Dental stone is used to construct models used in constructing dentures, bite plates, and bite guards. It is also used to make orthodontic study cases.

89. (C) Increasing the water/powder ratio of any gypsum product will result in a porous and, therefore, weaker model.

90. (B) The working time, also known as the initial setting time, begins with the mixing of the gypsum powder and water. It ends when the stone no longer flows, due to the increasing crystallization and viscosity. The final setting time ends when the model can be separated from the impression.

91. (A) Improved stone is the densest gypsum product and is used to make dies from which crowns, inlays, and onlays can be constructed.

92. (C) Dowel pins are used in the construction of individual dies. They permit the accurate replacement of individual dies back in a model. The pin acts as a male attachment and is inserted in a female attachment, which is produced when the model is poured.

93. (C) Casting wax is used as a pattern for the metal framework (gold or chrome cobalt) of partial dentures.

94. (D) Sticky wax is used to hold metallic, acrylic, or gypsum parts in a fixed position temporarily. This wax is sticky only when melted. It is brittle when hard.

95. (C) Utility wax is a soft, tacky wax that often is placed around the periphery of perforated metal trays to improve the contour of the tray.

96. (A) Impression waxes are used to record bite registrations and as impression material for nonundercut areas.

97. (D) Baseplate wax is used to construct bite rims to record occlusal relationships, to set up artificial teeth, and to record bite registrations.

98. (B) Gutta percha is used to seal root canals, as a temporary filling material, and to test teeth for vitality by their sensitivity to heat.

99. (A) Strips of boxing wax are used to form a rim around an impression. This will contain the poured gypsum material and facilitate finishing the model.

100. **(B)** Inlay wax is primarily used to make wax patterns for inlays, individual crowns, and fixed bridges. The main ingredient of inlay wax is paraffin wax (40–60%).

101. **(C)** Some important properties of inlay wax are complete burnout, close adaptation to the prepared tooth, minimal distortion, carvability, maintenance of detail, and flow just above mouth temperature.

102. **(A)** It is best to invest the wax pattern as soon as possible. Stresses introduced into the pattern during fabrication are released after the pattern is removed from the tooth or die. The relaxation of these stresses causes the wax pattern to distort. The longer the wax pattern is stored before investment the greater the possibility of distortion of the pattern.

103. **(D)** At mouth temperature, inlay wax should have no flow, or the pattern will distort before it is removed from the mouth. The flow of inlay wax should take place at temperatures slightly above mouth temperature. If the flow temperature is much higher than the mouth temperature, oral tissues might be injured when using the wax intraorally.

104. **(B)** Sticky wax is not used intraorally because its high melting range will severely burn any oral tissue it contacts.

105. **(B)** Care must be taken when attaching wax rims to a shellac tray to avoid warping the tray. Shellac trays, as waxes, are thermoplastic materials and are easily altered by heat.

106. **(D)**

107. **(A)**

108. **(E)**

109. **(B)**

110. **(C)**

111. **(E)** Study models are used as references to show progress in orthodontic cases, to help in treatment planning in all phases of dentistry, to show arch shape and arch relationship, to help fabricate restorations, such as temporary bridges and mouth guards, to show occlusal relationships, and to help construct custom trays for final impressions. Study models may be entered as evidence in a court of law in conjunction with a malpractice suit.

112. **(A)** To accelerate the setting time of gypsum products, lower the water/powder ratio, increase spat-

ulation, add an accelerator, and use warm water or terra alba.

113. **(A)** Impression plaster, also known as quicksetting plaster, is used to make final impressions of edentulous mouths, to make bite registrations, and to transfer registrations so that dies of crown preparations can be positioned properly.

114. **(C)** In order to mix mercaptan and silicone impression materials, the materials should be proportioned on a paper pad and mixed with a flexible stainless steel spatula using a wiping and pressing motion. The resultant mix should be homogeneous and should be completed in about 1 minute.

115. **(C)** Dental investment is used to prepare molds for cast restorations, such as crowns, inlays, onlays, and partial frameworks, and to hold fixed bridge units in place when soldering.

116. **(A)** Some uses of dental cements are as temporary restoration, thermal insulator, luting material, sedative base, root canal sealer, and pulp capping material.

117. **(D)** Dies of crown preparations can be made of amalgam, electroplated copper, electroplated silver, or improved stone.

118. **(A)** The setting time of zinc oxide-eugenol is accelerated by increasing the powder/liquid ratio or increasing temperature, water, and zinc acetate.

119. **(A)** Some uses of acrylic resins are anterior restorations, bases of full or partial dentures, temporary crowns, and bridges, facings on crowns, prosthetic plastic teeth, bite plates, retainers, custom-made trays, and splints. Advantages of acrylic restorations are that they are insoluble in oral fluids, can be finished in one sitting, are easy to repair and add to the existing restoration, act as a thermal insulator, and are easily manipulated.

120. **(B)** Pumice, emery discs, quartz discs, garnet discs, and tin oxide are included in the materials used to polish amalgam restorations intraorally. Rouge and tripoli are polishing agents but cannot be used in the mouth.

121. **(A)** The toxic effects of mercury can occur through the skin or by inhalation of mercury vapors. Prevention by limited and careful handling, such as the use of premeasured capsules and quick efficient cleanup if any spills occur, is the best way to avoid mercury-related health problems.

122. (B) Calcium hydroxide is easy to manipulate, stimulates the production of secondary dentin, and protects the pulp from irritation from caustic filling materials. It is, however, soluble in oral fluids and does not have a high compressive strength when compared with other restorative materials.

123. (E) Polishing acrylic on a lathe requires the use of low speed, copious amounts of water with the pumice, and continuous movement of the acrylic. These factors will prevent the buildup of heat and deterioration of the acrylic.

124. (B) Bonding resin materials may be used to repair fractured teeth and for esthetics. Severe diastemas may be corrected with the bonding resin material, and badly stained teeth may be covered with the bonding resin. The bonding resins require acid etching procedures before placement and may be light cured.

125. (A) Characteristics of pit and fissure sealants include self-cured or light-cured polymerization and acid etching. A 35% to 50% solution of phosphoric acid is used to etch the enamel surface. The etching solution cleanses the enamel surface and increases the adherence of the sealant material by creating microscopic openings (pores) on the enamel surface. The resin material then penetrates into the pores and creates a resin bond or tag interlocking the sealant material to the tooth and increasing mechanical retention.

126. (E) Glass ionomer cements are very versatile materials that may be used for permanent restorations, luting agents, and thermal base insulators. The glass ionomers exhibit high adhesion properties and low abrasion properties. As a restorative material, the ionomers have the ability to release fluoride ions into the tooth to prevent redecay.

127. (A) Advantages of zinc phosphate cement include its high compressive strength, ease of manipulation, and ability to control the setting time by changing the powder to liquid ratio. ZOP is acidic and, consequently, irritating to the pulp. The setting time of zinc phosphate cement can be retarded by using a cool glass slab, decreasing initial acidity by mixing a very small portion of powder with the liquid, mixing cement over a large area to dissipate the heat, and lengthening spatulation time.

128. (A) Synthetic resins are used to reline dentures and to fabricate custom trays and artificial teeth. A composite type of resin contains fillers, such as crystalline quartz or finely ground glass particles, and is used for permanent restorations of the anterior teeth. Unfilled resin materials or acrylic resins are used to fabricate temporary crowns during fixed prosthetic procedures.

129. (B) To avoid distortion of a wax pattern, it should be invested as soon as possible, manipulated as little as possible, and protected from temperature changes. If it is necessary to store a wax pattern, it should be refrigerated to decrease possible distortion.

130. (E) When trimming study models with a model trimmer, it is necessary to wear protective eyewear to prevent injury to the eyes. A sufficient water flow must be circulating through the model trimmer unit before use to facilitate the trimming of the plaster/stone models. When actual trimming begins, do not allow fingers to come in close contact with the trimming lathe. Begin by occluding models together and trim the mandibular cast first. After trimming procedures, allow the cast to dry for 24 hours before final polishing and labeling.

BIBLIOGRAPHY

Benson HJ, Kipp KE. *Dental Science Laboratory Guide*, 4th ed. Dubuque, Iowa: William Brown Co, 1968.

Buonocore MG. *The Use of Adhesives in Dentistry*. Springfield, Ill: Charles C Thomas Publishers, 1975.

Christensen GJ. Glass ionomer as a luting material. *J Am Dent Assoc*. 1990; 120: 55–57.

Craig RG, O'Brien WJ, Powers JM. *Dental Materials: Properties and Manipulation*, 4th ed. St. Louis: CV Mosby Co, 1987.

Gilmore HW, et al. *Operative Dentistry*, 4th ed. St. Louis: CV Mosby Co, 1982.

Philips RN. *Elements of Dental Materials for Dental Hygienists and Assistants*, 4th ed. Philadelphia: WB Saunders Co, 1984.

Skinner EW, Philips RW. *Skinner's Science of Dental Materials*, 8th ed. Philadelphia: WB Saunders Co, 1982.

Smith DC. Dental cements. *Adv Dent Res*. 1988; 2: 134–141.

Suzuki M, Jordan R. Glass ionomer-composite sandwich technique. *J Am Dent Assoc*. 1990; 120: 55–57.

Torres H, Ehrlich A. *Modern Dental Assisting*, 4th ed. Philadelphia: WB Saunders Co, 1990.

Williams DF, Cunningham J. *Materials in Clinical Dentistry*. New York: Oxford University Press, 1979.

CHAPTER 8

Medical Emergencies

INTRODUCTION

Dental auxiliaries must be properly trained to provide support to the dentist during treatment of an office medical emergency. Medical emergencies may present life-threatening situations, and the auxiliary must be ready to carry out his or her delegated role during an office emergency in a swift and efficient manner. Early recognition of impending medical emergencies and prevention of potential medical complications are the responsibility of each staff member. This chapter provides a synopsis of several specific medical emergencies, including clinical patient signs and symptoms. An overview of related medical emergency procedures and office protocol is given, including medical emergency equipment, supplies, medications, and patient vital signs.

MEDICAL HISTORY

The best way to treat an emergency is to prevent its occurrence. This can be done by collecting information about patients' medical and dental histories that will inform the office personnel of patients' needs and potential emergency situations. These histories must be updated continuously to provide current information.

Each medical history questionnaire must be reviewed before administering direct patient clinical care. Of special concern to the dental team is patient information about drug allergies, prophylactic antibiotic coverage, history of infectious disease, diseases with related oral manifestations, physiologic changes, such as pregnancy, psychologic disorders, and illnesses currently under treatment by the patient's physician that may contraindicate certain dental procedures. The name and telephone number of the patient's personal physician are vitally important and must be documented clearly on the patient's dental chart.

VITAL SIGNS

In addition to reviewing the patient's medical history, critical, life-saving information may be obtained by taking and recording the patient's vital signs. Vital signs include blood pressure, pulse rate, respiration rate, and body temperature. This information often is gathered by the dental auxiliary and documented in the patient's dental record for reference by the dentist before dental treatment.

Blood Pressure

Blood pressure may be defined as the force or pressure exerted on the walls of the blood vessels from the flow of blood during the contraction and relaxation phase of the heart muscle. Blood pressure is measured during systole, the contraction phase of the heart, and measured as the systolic or highest pressure value. During the resting or relaxation phase diastole, the diastolic or lowest blood pressure value is measured.

Blood pressure is measured with special equipment that may include a small portable unit known as a mercury manometer or an aneroid sphygmomanometer. The sphygmomanometer consists of an inflatable cuff, pressure gauge or dial, and hand-controlled pressure bulb. The stethoscope is used to listen to the sounds produced by the brachial artery as the blood flow is altered by the pressure exerted from the sphygmomanometer cuff. These sounds are referred to as Korotkoff sounds. The first sound heard through the stethoscope is the systolic blood pressure, and the last sound heard is the diastolic pressure (Fig. 8–1).

The actual measurement of blood pressure is expressed as a fraction, with the systolic pressure over the diastolic pressure (eg, 120/80). The 120 measurement indicates the systolic reading, and the measurement of 80 represents the diastolic pressure reading.

Average systolic values for adults may vary depending on age, height, weight, and health-related complications. An average range may fall between 100 and 140 for systolic pressure and between 60 and 89 for diastolic pressure.

Unusually high systolic blood pressure values, or hypotension (low diastolic blood pressure values), should alert the auxiliary to possible medical or drug-related problems. Extremely high diastolic blood pressure values, known as hypertension, are also of concern because of increased risk of heart attack and stroke and should be recognized by the dental staff. Appropriate precautions and adjustments to the designated dental treatment procedure should be conducted immediately.

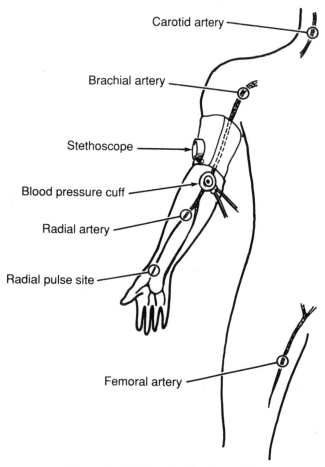

Carotid artery

Brachial artery

Stethoscope

Blood pressure cuff

Radial artery

Radial pulse site

Femoral artery

Figure 8–1. Major arterial pulse points.

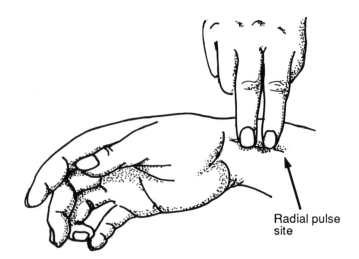

Radial pulse site

Figure 8–2. Position of fingers to monitor pulse.

Pulse Rate

The average pulse rate for adult males is approximately 60 to 100 heartbeats per minute. Women and children generally tend to have slightly higher pulse rates than adult males. Several factors may contribute to slightly higher pulse rates for all patients, including increased activity or exercise, anxiety over impending dental treatment, and certain prescription drugs. The most frequent site for feeling the pulse is at the radial artery, located on the lateral aspect (thumb side) of the wrist (Fig. 8–2). Weak or irregular pulse rates should be recognized and recorded in the patient's dental record. The carotid artery located on the side of the neck often is used to obtain a pulse rate during cardiopulmonary resuscitation procedures.

Respiration Rate

The average respiration rate for adults is approximately 16 to 20 breaths per minute. Respiration rate may range from 12 to 20 breaths per minute, depending on the patient's age and amount of physical activity or inactivity. Respiration is measured as one complete inspiration and exhalation of air by the body. Observations should be made regarding any variations in the rhythm of the respi-

rations or difficulty and labored breathing. Unusual sounds, such as wheezing, should be noted.

No movement of the chest or abdomen indicates respiratory failure, and emergency steps to administer cardiopulmonary resuscitation (CPR) should begin immediately.

Body Temperature

Body temperature is taken orally with a thermometer. The average measurement of body temperature is 98.6°F or 37.0°C. Elevated temperatures may indicate other serious complications or signs of infection and should be treated accordingly.

OFFICE PREPARATION FOR AN EMERGENCY

In order to prevent tragic results in an emergency situation, the office must follow certain procedures. All auxiliaries should be trained to participate in emergency situations and to simulate such situations so that each role is clearly understood.

Emergency support telephone numbers should be prepared in advance and posted in convenient locations near each office telephone. Listings should include local fire departments and emergency room extensions. Telephone numbers of the nearest pharmacy, physician, or medical office if located in the same building as the dental practice may be included.

EMERGENCY KIT AND EQUIPMENT

It is particularly important for all personnel to remain calm and to prevent panic. Procedures should be routine, and materials should be readily available and uncomplicated. An emergency kit should be assembled, and each staff member should be familiar with its use. Basic components of this kit should be emergency equipment, noninjectable drugs, and injectable drugs.

The basic emergency equipment includes an oxygen delivery system, a suction system with tips, syringes, tourniquets, and airways.

Noninjectable drugs should include oxygen, a respiratory stimulant (aromatic ammonia), a vasodilator (nitroglycerin), a bronchodilator (epinephrine), and an antihypoglycemic (sugar).

Injectable drugs that can be used include epinephrine for severe allergic reactions, diazepam as an anticonvulsant, Benadryl as an antihistamine for mild allergic reactions, hydrocortisone succinate as a corticosteroid, and 50% dextrose glucogen as an antihypoglycemic. However, these injectable drugs are administered only by specially trained medical or dental personnel.

RESPIRATORY EMERGENCIES

In a respiratory emergency, a patient's breathing stops or is reduced to a level at which the body cannot support its oxygen needs. Since nerve tissue can easily be injured from loss of oxygen, an interruption of breathing of 4 to 6 minutes can result in permanent damage. Respiratory failure can occur from obstruction of the airway, hyperventilation, bronchial asthma, heart failure, or acute pulmonary edema.

Hyperventilation
Dental patients are most likely to experience respiratory difficulties from hyperventilation as a result of anxiety. Symptoms include impaired consciousness (loss of consciousness is very rare), lightheadedness, and a feeling of faintness. Breathing may be prolonged, rapid, or deep. The usual treatment is to discontinue dental treatment, make the patient comfortable, and have the patient breathe into a paper bag to correct respiratory alkalosis by increasing the blood level of CO_2.

Bronchial Asthma
Bronchial asthma also may cause respiratory difficulty. These attacks may be precipitated by inhalation of materials that produce an allergic reaction or may be caused by irritating inhalants, infections, or emotional upset. Dental treatment should be stopped, and a bronchial dilator or oxygen or both may be administered. Symptoms include difficult breathing and wheezing and possible cyanosis in severe cases.

Heart Failure
Heart failure and acute pulmonary edema also can lead to respiratory problems as a result of the body's inability to transport oxygen adequately. Left-sided heart failure leads to pulmonary congestion, and right-sided failure results in vascular congestion, leading to peripheral edema. Patients suffering from these diseases should not be treated in a supine position. If a problem occurs, seat the patient in an upright position and give oxygen while medical assistance is summoned.

ARTIFICIAL RESPIRATION

In cases of respiratory difficulty, when the heart has stopped beating, artificial respiration and CPR should be instituted. CPR requires special training and should be attempted only by individuals possessing these skills. Outside emergency medical assistance should be sought as quickly as possible.

The objective of artificial respiration is to maintain an open airway and mechanically breathe for the victim. The following steps should be used in an emergency situation.

Steps in Administering Artificial Respiration (Given That the Patient Has a Pulse)
Mouth-to-mouth and mouth-to-mask

1. Place victim on his or her back on the ground.
2. Kneel perpendicular to the victim's body next to the head.
3. Wipe any foreign matter from the victim's mouth with two fingers.
4. Open the airway by tipping the victim's head back until the chin is pointing upward (Fig. 8–3).
5. Place your left ear very close to the victim's mouth and look at the chest and check for breathing; feel for pulse.

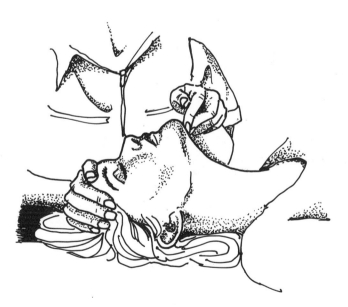

Figure 8–3. Open airway by head tilt and chin lift.

6. If the victim is not breathing, pinch the nostrils with the fingers of the hand on the forehead, and place your mouth over the victim's mouth and deliver two quick full breaths. Do not allow time for the lungs to deflate between breaths.

7. Add a breath every 5 seconds until help has arrived, the victim begins to breathe, or exhaustion overtakes you.

8. Look, listen, and feel for breathing and check the pulse. If the victim begins breathing on his own, discontinue artificial respiration. *If the victim is not breathing and has no pulse, begin to administer CPR.*

Steps in Administering Artificial Respiration (If Severe Injury to the Mouth)
Mouth-to-nose

1. Tip the victim's head as for mouth-to-mouth resuscitation.

2. Keep the victim's mouth closed by covering with your hand.

3. Place your mouth over the victim's nose and blow air until the chest rises one breath every 5 seconds.

4. Place left ear close to the victim's mouth (after removing your hand to allow patient to exhale air) and observe the chest to determine if the patient is breathing. Look, listen, and feel.

5. Add a breath every 5 seconds until help has arrived, the victim begins to breathe, or exhaustion overtakes you.

6. Look, listen, and feel for breathing and check the pulse. If the victim begins breathing on his own, discontinue artificial respiration. *If the victim is not breathing and has no pulse, begin to administer CPR.*

CARDIOVASCULAR EMERGENCY

Congestive heart failure (CHF) is a broad classification of heart problems that result from an inability of the heart to handle the blood supply. CHF results from several cardiovascular problems. Patients suffering from this disability usually have trouble lying in a supine position because of fluid retention in the lungs.

Congestive heart failure is usually the outcome of other cardiovascular diseases, most importantly coronary heart disease (CHD), which includes three major categories: arteriosclerotic heart disease (ASHD), myocardial infarction (MI), and angina pectoris.

Myocardial infarction is caused by a sudden deficiency of oxygenated blood to the heart muscle. Symptoms include shortness of breath, perspiration, severe chest pain, and cyanosis. When dental treatment is given to patients who have previously suffered an MI, fear and anxiety must be diminished. Steps that can be taken include administering nitrous oxide sedation, decreasing the length of appointments (no more than 60 minutes),

and with permission of the patient's physician, administering intravenous sedation. In general, systemically released epinephrine, which is produced by the body as a reaction to anxiety, is more dangerous than a properly given anesthetic with 1:100,000 concentration of epinephrine. The dentist treating a patient who has suffered an MI should consult with the attending physician about choice of anesthesia.

Angina pectoris is a painful condition resulting from a transient deficiency of oxygenated blood supply to the heart. Symptoms include severe constricting chest pain, anxiety, perspiration, and increased blood pressure. The pain can be caused by exertion or excitement. Treatment includes administering oxygen to assist labored breathing and changing the patient to an upright chair position. Nitroglycerin, a fast-acting vasodilator, is given for relief. Consultation with the patient's physician is suggested before dental treatment, and each patient should have nitroglycerin emergency medication readily available and accessible before the dental procedure begins.

Chest pain that may or may not be caused by a cardiac emergency is managed by stopping dental treatment, shifting the patient to a comfortable position, and administering oxygen if necessary. If the pain does not subside, the patient might be suffering from a serious cardiac disorder. Medical assistance should be summoned immediately. If a patient loses consciousness, basic life support techniques should be started. This includes placing the patient in a supine position, maintaining the airway, checking the pulse, and administering artificial respiration or oxygen if necessary. If the pulse disappears, CPR should be started immediately. CPR is a technique that supplements artificial respiration with manual artificial circulation. Special training is required before attempting CPR. An individual who lacks the required CPR skills may actually cause injury to the patient.

SHOCK

Shock occurs when the body's vital functions reach a depressed state. It can be caused by trauma, infection, heart attack, smoke, burns, poisoning, lack of oxygen, or obstruction or injury to the air passage. Shock can be exacerbated by abnormal changes in the body temperature, pain, rough handling, and delay in treatment. In some cases, it can be life threatening.

There are two stages of shock. In the early stage, either the skin is pale and cold or the individual is weak and exhibits a rapid pulse. Breathing may be shallow or deep and irregular, and nausea, vomiting, or anxiety may occur. In the late stage, shock symptoms become more acute. The person becomes unresponsive, and the eyes appear vacant, with dilated pupils. Blood pressure falls and temperature decreases. Loss of consciousness or even death can occur.

Treating shock in a dental office requires that those rendering first aid be skilled in the use of a sphygmomanometer, stethoscope, and oxygen delivery system and knowledgeable about the principles of cardiac and respiratory resuscitation. If it is suspected that a patient is in shock, the following steps should be taken: stop dental treatment, record vital signs, place the patient in a supine position, keep the patient comfortable at room temperature, maintain airway, provide oxygen, and immediately summon medical assistance.

Some causes of shock in patients during dental treatment are cardiogenic shock from acute heart failure, hematogenic shock from hemorrhage, and neurogenic shock from neurologic or psychologic disorders.

Anaphylactic Shock

Anaphylaxis is a sudden allergic reaction to exposure to an allergen in the body. The allergen may be a certain type of food or particular medication that causes an immediate, potentially life-threatening emergency. The rapid release of histamines by the body may cause severe swelling and edema. Of particular concern is the swelling of the bronchi and trachea. If the airway is blocked, the patient may begin to show signs of cyanosis, a bluish skin tone due to lack of oxygen. Management of the emergency requires administration of epinephrine in the arm or thigh and oxygen if possible to assist labored breathing. Vital signs should be closely monitored, and the patient's physician should be consulted if necessary.

Insulin Shock

Diabetes is a metabolic disorder of the body. Hypoglycemia, or insulin shock, may occur when there is too much insulin in the body and the blood sugar level is low. This disorder can occur if the patient forgets to eat on time after taking the insulin medication or from overexertion. Symptoms include headache, feelings of dizziness (vertigo), general weakness, clammy skin, and confusion. Management of this condition includes administering something sweet to eat, such as sugar, candy, or orange juice. If necessary, the patient's physician should be consulted for follow-up treatment.

SYNCOPE

Fainting is a transient loss of consciousness that can occur during any phase of dental treatment. Symptoms include pallor, discomfort, weakness, perspiration, cold clammy skin, and temporary loss of consciousness. It is usually a harmless situation, but all loss of consciousness must be regarded as potentially life threatening. Contributing factors include anxiety, fear, emotional stress, exhaustion, and poor physical condition. The patient should be placed in a Trendelenburg position, where the feet are slightly elevated in relation to the head. The airway should be established, and tight clothing should be loosened. Spirits of ammonia and oxygen may be administered.

POSTURAL HYPOTENSION

Postural hypotension, also known as orthostatic hypotension, occurs when the body's autonomic nervous system is unable to compensate for the changes in blood pressure resulting from rapid changes in body position. Patients who remain in a supine position for a long period of time and suddenly are placed in an upright position may experience postural hypotension. Symptoms include a sudden drop in blood pressure and lightheadedness. Treatment includes placing the patient in a supine position, maintaining the airway, administering oxygen if necessary, and slowly changing the patient's position before dismissal.

CEREBROVASCULAR ACCIDENT

A cerebrovascular accident (CVA or stroke) is a neurologic disorder in the brain caused by a vascular insufficiency resulting from hemorrhage or formation of blood clots that interfere with or stop oxygenated blood flow. Transient ischemia attacks (TIA) are minor strokes that last for minutes or hours and may include symptoms of headache, confusion, difficulty in speech, dizziness, ringing in the ears, weakness in arms and legs, and personality changes. TIAs may be warning for major CVAs.

If a patient undergoing dental treatment suffers a TIA, the procedure should be stopped, and medical attention should be suggested to the patient as soon as possible. Signs and symptoms of major strokes may include unconsciousness, paralysis or weakness of upper or lower extremities, difficulty in breathing, and a problem with speech. If a patient suffers a major stroke, signs and symptoms should be managed, and medical assistance should be summoned immediately. It might be necessary to supply life support, including CPR.

CONVULSIVE DISORDERS

Epilepsy is a chronic disease characterized by convulsion-like seizures. These episodes may be mild seizures (petit mal), symptomized by twitching muscles and momentary disorientation, or more severe seizures (grand mal), including symptoms of muscle spasms, thrashing, foaming or drooling at the mouth, rolling eyes, and a loss of consciousness. Management of grand mal seizures includes placing the patient in a supine position with the head tilted to the side so that saliva and vomitus can exit, thus decreasing the chance of aspiration into the lungs. Loosening tight clothing, maintaining an open airway, and removing objects that might injure a thrashing patient are other recommended procedures. Do not attempt to force any object into the patient's mouth during a seizure. Medical assistance may be necessary. The oral health care delivery team should be supportive of the patient's emotional needs.

CHOKING

Choking may occur from certain dental materials or dental prostheses. The patient should be placed in a comfort-

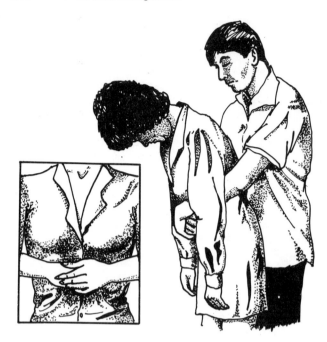

Figure 8–4. Position of hands for Heimlich maneuver.

able position and encouraged to cough in order to remove the obstruction. If a conscious patient is in severe distress, stand behind the patient and deliver abdominal thrusts until the obstruction is cleared. This is known as the Heimlich maneuver (Fig. 8–4). If the choking is not relieved by these measures, medical emergency assistance should be sought as soon as possible. If breathing stops, basic life support measures must be started immediately.

METABOLIC DISORDERS

Diabetes mellitus is a chronic disease associated with carbohydrate, fat, and protein metabolism. The diabetic patient in the dental office can present several types of emergencies, including those related to the vascular consequences of the disease (MI, angina, and stroke). Most emergencies, however, will be caused by insulin therapy, resulting in a blood sugar level that is either too high or too low.

If a patient suffers from hyperglycemia as a result of above-normal levels of blood sugar, he or she may suffer abdominal pain, nausea or vomiting, and intense thirst. The breath might have an acetone odor, and the skin may appear dry and flushed. Medical assistance should be summoned immediately.

Avoidance of an emergency associated with diabetes mellitus can be enhanced by following general rules. Diabetic patients should be treated in the morning and questioned to determine whether diet and insulin therapy are properly coordinated.

Hyperthyroidism is a disease caused by excessive pro-

duction of thyroid hormones. In general, patients with this problem have an increased basal metabolic rate that might be manifested in rapid heart rate, sweating, headache, increased blood pressure, and anxiety. In addition, there might be an increase in cardiac problems. If these symptoms appear, dental treatment should be stopped, and a medical consultation should be suggested. Additionally, local anesthesia containing epinephrine should never be given to such patients, since it may intensify the condition.

BLEEDING DISORDERS

Simple bleeding can occur as a result of certain dental procedures. Careful medical histories should be elicited so the doctor can be aware of any conditions that might predispose a patient to prolonged bleeding. There are three sources of bleeding: arterial bleeding, when the blood is bright red and spurting, venous bleeding, when the blood is darker and flows continuously, and capillary bleeding, when the blood is bright red and flows slowly and steadily. Most bleeding can be controlled by isolating the area and applying pressure as directly as possible. The patient should be watched carefully for signs of shock. If bleeding does not subside with pressure, the area should be anesthetized in preparation for further treatment. If the bleeding is of capillary origin, sponges impregnated with epinephrine hydrochloride (1:1000) or adsorbable gelatin sponges can be packed in the bleeding site. Closing the wound tightly with sutures also can stop the bleeding.

TABLE 8–1. DOSAGE GUIDELINES FOR LOCAL ANESTHETIC AGENTS

Drug	Class	Maximum Safe Dosage
Lidocaine (Xylocaine) 2% without epinephrine	Amide	4.4 mg/kg up to 300 mg (8.3 carpules)
Lidocaine (Xylocaine) 2% with epinephrine	Amide	6.6 mg/kg up to 500 mg (13.8 carpules)
Mepivicaine (Carbocaine) 3% without vasoconstrictor	Amide	270 mg (5 carpules)
Mepivicaine (Carbocaine) 2% with 1:20,000 Neocobefrin	Amide	180 mg (5 carpules)
Prilocaine (Citanest forte) with 1:20,000 epinephrine	Amide	8 mg/kg up to 600 mg (8 carpules)
Propoxycaine (Ravocaine) 0.4% and Procaine (Novocaine) 2% with 1:30,000 levophed	Ester	The manufacturer recommends average dose of 1.8 mL, although this dose may be doubled if necessary

Note: The maximum recommended dosage without significant effect at any one time is 0.2 mg which is approximately equivalent to 10 carpules of 1:100,000. Cardiac patients should always be evaluated closely with regard to the use of epinephrine. Dosage is defined as a body mass-dependent variable. Guidelines based on healthy adult male weighing approximately 70 kg.

DRUG-INDUCED EMERGENCIES

Complications may arise from local anesthesia. Allergic reactions have decreased dramatically with the introduction of amide anesthesia. (The traditional anesthesia is of the ester type.) Some reactions do occur, however, and may range from a simple dermatitis to fatal anaphylactic shock. Often these reactions occur in response to preservatives or other ingredients in the anesthetic solution. The most common reaction from local anesthesia is tachycardia caused by an exogenous release of epinephrine. Dental treatment should be stopped, and the patient should be made comfortable in a supine position until symptoms subside.

An overdose of anesthetic can cause convulsive reactions or even death (Table 8–1). Factors that can affect the dosage are age (younger and older patients are more sensitive), low body weight, impaired liver and kidney function, or a metabolic disorder. Since an overdose of anesthetic is preventable, it is incumbent on the dentist to evaluate each patient for correct dosage. If the patient has a reaction to the anesthetic, dental treatment should be stopped, basic life support steps should be undertaken, and emergency medical assistance should be summoned if needed as quickly as possible.

Questions

DIRECTIONS (Questions 1 through 59): Each of the questions or incomplete statements in this section is followed by four suggested answers or completions. Select the ONE lettered answer or completion that is BEST in each case. Check your answers with the correct answers at the end of the chapter.

1. Medical emergencies can be prevented by

   (A) thoroughly charting all existing oral conditions
   (B) presetting instrument trays
   (C) keeping the operatory as sterile as possible
   (D) being alert to signs and symptoms of impending emergencies

2. Acute symptoms are

   (A) severe, with quick onset
   (B) dull and steady
   (C) of long duration
   (D) somniferous

3. Chronic symptoms are

   (A) of short duration
   (B) sharp and quick
   (C) of long duration
   (D) extremely painful

4. Health history questionnaires must be completed

   (A) at every dental appointment
   (B) before rendering clinical dental care
   (C) in ink at the end of the dental treatment
   (D) only if a surgical procedure is indicated

5. The primary responsibility for treating a patient who is experiencing a medical emergency lies with the

   (A) laboratory assistant
   (B) dentist
   (C) dental hygienist
   (D) certified dental assistant

6. The office emergency kit should be checked weekly by the

   (A) dentist
   (B) dental hygienist
   (C) dental auxiliary
   (D) laboratory assistant

7. Preparation and training for medical emergencies are necessary for the

   (A) dentist only
   (B) dental hygienist
   (C) dental assistant
   (D) all dental team members

8. The definition of first aid is

   (A) the immediate and temporary care given the victims of an accident until the services of a physician can be obtained
   (B) the temporary care given the victim of an accident or sudden illness
   (C) the immediate care given to a person who has been injured or has been suddenly taken ill
   (D) the care and treatment given to a victim of an accident or sudden illness

9. A reason for first aid training is to

   (A) prevent accidents
   (B) eliminate the need for a physician in emergency situations
   (C) avoid contagious diseases
   (D) practice office emergency drills

10. The instruments for measuring blood pressure are

   (A) a barometer and stethoscope
   (B) stereoscope and sphygmomanometer
   (C) sphygmomanometer and stethoscope
   (D) sphygmomonoscope and stethoscope

11. When taking a blood pressure reading, the first sound heard is the

  (A) diastolic pressure
  (B) systolic pressure
  (C) carotid pressure
  (D) pulse pressure

12. Which of the following would be a normal systolic pressure reading for an adult male?

  (A) 60 mm Hg
  (B) 80 mm Hg
  (C) 100 mm Hg
  (D) 120 mm Hg

13. In the blood pressure reading 148/60, the number 60 represents

  (A) systolic pressure
  (B) diastolic pressure
  (C) hypertension
  (D) radial artery pressure

14. The color of the oxygen cylinder tank is always

  (A) green
  (B) blue
  (C) red
  (D) white

15. The lower edge of the sphygmomanometer cuff is positioned

  (A) 2 inches above the crease of the elbow
  (B) 4 inches above the crease of the elbow
  (C) 1 inch above the crease of the elbow
  (D) 1 inch below the crease of the elbow

16. During blood pressure measurement, the exhaust valve is released at a rate of

  (A) 2–3 mm Hg/second
  (B) 4–6 mm Hg/second
  (C) 3–5 mm Hg/second
  (D) 5 mm Hg/second

17. The antecubital fossa is located at

  (A) the wrist
  (B) the elbow
  (C) the knee
  (D) the temporomandibular joint

18. Pulse readings are taken most frequently at the

  (A) carotid artery
  (B) brachial artery
  (C) temporal artery
  (D) radial artery

19. To obtain a pulse reading on a patient

  (A) gloves must be worn
  (B) the patient must be supine
  (C) use the first two fingers of your hand to palpate the radial artery
  (D) a stethoscope is used

20. The average resting pulse rate for an adult is

  (A) 40–50 beats per minute
  (B) 60–100 beats per minute
  (C) 120–140 beats per minute
  (D) 150 beats per minute

21. The oral thermometer should be left in the mouth

  (A) 2 minutes
  (B) 3 minutes
  (C) 4 minutes
  (D) 5 minutes

22. A normal oral temperature reading for a healthy adult is

  (A) 98.6°F
  (B) 96.8°F
  (C) 100°F
  (D) 101°F

23. The best time to record the patient's respiration rate is

  (A) after the patient has coughed and cleared the throat
  (B) during administration of local anesthesia
  (C) when the patient is completely unaware of what the auxiliary is doing
  (D) at the end of the dental procedure

24. Normal respiratory rate per minute for an adult is

  (A) 10–12 breaths per minute
  (B) 12–14 breaths per minute
  (C) 14–16 breaths per minute
  (D) 16–20 breaths per minute

25. The amount of air that cannot be expired from the lungs is called the

  (A) tidal air
  (B) residual air
  (C) vital capacity
  (D) alveolar air

26. Short appointments are given to patients with a history of

   (A) allergies
   (B) cardiac problems
   (C) aphthous ulcers
   (D) rampant caries

27. The depressed state of many body functions is called

   (A) shock
   (B) depression
   (C) psychosis
   (D) mental retardation

28. When treating for shock, the body position is

   (A) head lower than the rest of the body
   (B) based on the injury
   (C) head and shoulders raised 8–12 inches
   (D) flat, with head turned to the side

29. Syncope refers to

   (A) a sudden state of excitement
   (B) loss of consciousness
   (C) dizziness after an injection
   (D) hypertension

30. Inhalation of spirits of ammonia is used to treat

   (A) insulin shock
   (B) respiratory collapse
   (C) circulatory collapse
   (D) syncope

31. If a patient faints, the assistant should

   (A) seat the patient upright
   (B) place the head lower than the rest of the body
   (C) hold the patient's head in his or her lap
   (D) sharply slap the patient's face

32. Chronic respiratory problems affect the

   (A) type of prosthesis a patient can wear
   (B) prognosis of root canal therapy
   (C) positioning of the patient in the dental chair
   (D) type of x-rays taken

33. The proper sequence in an emergency situation is

   (A) treat for shock, control severe bleeding, restore breathing
   (B) restore breathing, treat for shock, control severe bleeding
   (C) restore breathing, control severe bleeding, treat for shock
   (D) control severe bleeding, restore breathing, treat for shock

34. The administration of an excess amount of a drug is known as

   (A) an overdose
   (B) an overkill
   (C) hyperactivation
   (D) hypokinesis

35. If circulatory collapse occurs, the patient should be

   (A) given a drink of warm water
   (B) left alone
   (C) given external cardiac massage
   (D) seated upright

36. Proper preparation of a victim for artificial respiration is

   (A) wipe foreign matter from mouth and tilt head backward with chin pointing downward
   (B) wipe foreign matter from mouth and tilt head backward with chin pointing upward. Put one hand on the victim's forehead and tilt the head back. With the other hand bring the chin forward and lift jaw to maintain an open airway. Pinch nostrils shut and seal your mouth tight around the victim's mouth
   (C) tilt head backward with chin pointing upward, put one hand under victim's neck and lift. Place heel of other hand on forehead and rotate backward, pinch nostrils shut, and seal your mouth tightly around the victim's mouth
   (D) wipe foreign matter from mouth and tilt head forward with chin pointing downward. Put one hand under victim's neck and lift. Place heel of other hand on forehead and rotate backward. Pinch nostrils shut and seal your mouth tightly around victim's mouth

37. A method used for removing swallowed objects on which a victim is choking is the

   (A) Silvester method
   (B) Herman maneuver
   (C) Albin method
   (D) Heimlich maneuver

38. Breathing air containing insufficient oxygen, carbon monoxide, or other toxic gases may cause

   (A) acute asthma
   (B) asphyxia
   (C) circulatory collapse
   (D) inhalation collapse

39. A partial denture becomes lodged in a patient's throat. The proper first aid measure is to

   (A) give the patient a glass of water

(B) allow the patient to cough out the object
(C) attempt to quiet the patient
(D) have the patient sit up and bend over

40. Anaphylactic shock is

(A) a chronic allergic condition
(B) the result of aspirating a foreign object
(C) a sudden violent allergic reaction
(D) a reaction to mental depression

41. The drug that best counteracts analphylactic shock is

(A) Novocaine
(B) Xylocaine
(C) epinephrine
(D) a barbiturate

42. When treating a patient with a history of rheumatic heart disease, the patient should

(A) be treated without any special precautions
(B) never be placed in a supine position
(C) be referred to a specialist
(D) be treated with a prophylactic antibiotic before the scheduled dental appointment

43. A patient taking anticoagulation medication could pose a problem related to

(A) the length of the appointment
(B) hemorrhage control
(C) stress and anxiety of the dental situation
(D) muscular coordination and trismus

44. Sharp cuts bleeding freely are

(A) incisions
(B) abrasions
(C) lacerations
(D) punctures

45. Wounds that are jagged, irregular and associated with considerable tissue damage are

(A) abrasions
(B) incisions
(C) lacerations
(D) punctures

46. Angina pectoris is

(A) an embolism in the brain
(B) a painful condition of the heart
(C) cancer of the chest
(D) a spasm of chest muscle

47. Symptoms of postural hypotension include

(A) profuse sweating
(B) elevated (high) blood pressure
(C) low blood pressure
(D) a sudden state of excitement

48. To reduce the possibility of injury during an epileptic seizure, the operator or assistant should

(A) remove anything nearby that might get in the way, such as furniture or equipment and not interfere with the patient during seizure
(B) place padded tongue depressors between the patient's teeth
(C) attempt to hold the patient absolutely still
(D) seat the patient in a straight back chair

49. If a patient begins to have convulsions in the waiting room, the operator or assistant should

(A) administer oxygen
(B) cover patient with a blanket
(C) administer stimulants orally
(D) protect the patient from injury by moving objects out of reach

50. A patient walking to the operatory suddenly keels over. There is no pulse or breathing. What should be done?

(A) cover the patient with a blanket
(B) do not treat until help arrives
(C) keep the patient's head below his or her feet
(D) summon help and begin artificial respiration and external cardiac massage

51. Your patient is leaving the office and begins to feel severe pain in the chest and left arm, along with nausea and lightheadedness. The appropriate medical emergency treatment includes

(A) allow patient to rest quietly and summon medical support as quickly as possible
(B) administer oxygen
(C) have patient lie in supine position with feet elevated
(D) apply hot compress to painful area of arm

52. When performing chest compressions, the heel of the hand should be placed

(A) near the xiphoid process
(B) at the center of the chest just below the heart
(C) two or three fingerwidths above the lower end of the sternum
(D) just above the heart

53. To prevent foreign objects, such as amalgam, from flying in the eyes, the dentist and assistant should

    (A) blink frequently if wearing contact lenses
    (B) wear a face mask
    (C) wear safety glasses
    (D) work standing up

54. If a foreign object becomes embedded in a patient's eye

    (A) irrigate the eye with tap water
    (B) rub the patient's eye
    (C) attempt to remove the object with a sterile instrument
    (D) cover the eye and seek medical attention quickly

55. If a permanent central incisor is accidently avulsed, what is the treatment?

    (A) throw the tooth away—it cannot be saved
    (B) promptly reinsert tooth and see the dentist immediately
    (C) keep tooth moist in tap water until medical help can be summoned
    (D) reinsert tooth and keep teeth as clean as possible

56. To avoid injuries to teeth while playing contact sports, athletes should

    (A) have regular dental checkups
    (B) ask the dentist to fabricate a protective mouth guard
    (C) wear orthodontic braces
    (D) have fluoride treatments daily to strengthen teeth

57. An antidote

    (A) counteracts the effects of a poison
    (B) is a form of artificial respiration
    (C) is a central nervous system stimulant
    (D) is a central nervous system depressant

58. Insulin shock is due to

    (A) too much blood sugar
    (B) too much insulin in the blood
    (C) too little insulin in the blood
    (D) overeating

59. Medical emergency procedures for a patient going into insulin shock include

    (A) have patient ingest sugar cubes or a sweet drink
    (B) give an injection of insulin immediately
    (C) place a nitroglycerin tablet sublingually
    (D) send the patient home, then call his or her physician

DIRECTIONS (Questions 60 through 76): For each of the items in this section, ONE or MORE of the numbered options is correct. Choose answer

    A if only 1, 2, and 3 are correct
    B if only 1 and 3 are correct
    C if only 2 and 4 are correct
    D if only 4 is correct
    E if all are correct

60. Knowledge of the patient's medical and dental history might affect

    (1) the treatment plan
    (2) the drugs prescribed
    (3) the length of the scheduled appointments
    (4) the method of payment

61. The condition of the skin when a patient is in shock is

    (1) pale
    (2) cold and clammy
    (3) moist
    (4) palms feel sweaty

62. Some symptoms of an allergic reaction are

    (1) swelling and rash
    (2) pain in the extremities
    (3) inability to breathe or swallow
    (4) a craving for sweets

63. Placing a nitroglycerin tablet under the tongue is the suggested emergency treatment for a patient suffering from

    (1) syncope
    (2) epilepsy
    (3) anaphylactic shock
    (4) angina pectoris

64. Emergencies in the operating environment can be prevented by

    (1) being alert to signs of impending emergency in your patients
    (2) being careful of comments that may upset or frighten the patient
    (3) keeping the operating site free of debris and bloody gauze
    (4) playing music in the office

65. Lawsuits can be avoided by

    (1) keeping accurate and complete records
    (2) understanding the state Dental Practice Act and its limitations
    (3) knowing your patient's health history and contraindications
    (4) obtaining appropriate patient consent before treatment

66. The first aid measures for a person in shock in the dental office are

    (1) administer stimulants
    (2) maintain a comfortable temperature
    (3) keep the patient moving
    (4) keep the patient lying down

67. Some causes of syncope in the dental office are

    (1) fear
    (2) spirits of ammonia
    (3) seeing blood
    (4) smoking

68. Due to lack of oxygen, brain cells begin to die after

    (1) 30 seconds
    (2) 1 minute
    (3) 2–3 minutes
    (4) 4–6 minutes

69. For an operative dental appointment, which vital signs must be taken?

    (1) blood pressure
    (2) pulse
    (3) respiration
    (4) height and weight

70. Acetone breath, dry mouth, thirst, and weak pulse are possible symptoms of

    (1) hypertension
    (2) epilepsy
    (3) kidney disease
    (4) diabetic coma

71. Medical emergency treatment for the patient who is hyperventilating includes

    (1) have patient take deep, slow breaths
    (2) administer oxygen quickly
    (3) place paper bag over nose and mouth
    (4) have patient lie down in supine position

72. Symptoms of a (CVA) stroke may include

    (1) irregular, thready pulse
    (2) slurred speech
    (3) cyanosis
    (4) generalized body rash

73. During dental treatment, the patient begins to feel severe chest pain. What basic emergency procedures should be implemented?

    (1) elevate feet of patient
    (2) sit patient upright
    (3) allow patient to rest for 5 minutes, then continue treatment
    (4) call for medical assistance immediately

74. A basic office emergency armamentarium includes

    (1) portable oxygen tanks
    (2) intravenous armamentarium and related drugs
    (3) sponges and tourniquets
    (4) sugar packs

75. If performing CPR on a patient with a history of an infectious disease, the rescuer should always

    (1) wear disposable latex gloves
    (2) not perform CPR until medical assistance arrives
    (3) use protective devices or a microshield
    (4) obtain a thorough health history first before beginning CPR

76. The patient with a history of liver disease (hepatitis) should be given which drug in limited quantities?

    (1) oxygen
    (2) dilantin
    (3) nitrous oxide
    (4) local anesthetics

Answers and Explanations

1. **(D)** The best way to treat an emergency is to prevent the occurrence of one. The dental auxiliary must always be alert to any signs or symptoms of impending emergencies that may be exhibited by the dental patient.

2. **(A)** Acute symptoms are those that are severe and occur with a quick onset.

3. **(C)** Chronic symptoms are characterized by their long duration.

4. **(B)** Health history questionnaires must be completed before rendering clinical dental care. A patient's medical history can affect all phases of a patient's treatment, including prescriptions, preoperative and postoperative instructions, and length of appointments.

5. **(B)** The primary responsibility for treating a patient who is experiencing a medical emergency lies with the dentist. The dental auxiliary and dental hygienist may serve as a support team with preassigned designated emergency responsibilities.

6. **(C)** The office emergency kit should be checked weekly by the dental auxiliary.

7. **(D)** All dental team members must be trained properly to administer emergency medical treatment if necessary. CPR training is recommended for all members of the dental team.

8. **(C)** First aid is the immediate care given to a person who has been injured or has been suddenly taken ill.

9. **(A)** Some reasons for first aid training are to promote prevention of accidents, provide emergency care, and prevent additional injury due to improper care.

10. **(C)** The instruments used to measure blood pressure include the sphygmomanometer and stethoscope. The stethoscope is used to listen and magnify the sounds of the blood pressure flow. The sphyg-momanometer consists of an inflatable cuff and rubber tubing attached to a hand-controlled bulb. The cuff may have a pressure gauge dial (aneroid type manometer) attached directly to it, or a portable mercury-gravity manometer with a mercury column gauge may be used to record the blood pressure measurement. When using the mercury type manometer, the mercury column should be at the operator's eye level for an accurate reading.

11. **(B)** When taking a blood pressure reading, the first sound heard is recorded as the systolic pressure measurement. Systolic blood pressure is the pressure exerted on the walls of arteries when the heart contracts.

12. **(D)** In healthy young adults, the average blood pressure is 120/80. The number 120 is recorded as the systolic blood pressure measurement.

13. **(B)** The number 60 represents the diastolic blood pressure measurement. Diastolic blood pressure is the pressure exerted by blood on the walls of arteries when the heart is at rest.

14. **(A)** The color of the oxygen cylinder tank is always green. Oxygen tanks should be checked periodically to ensure that they are full and functioning properly.

15. **(C)** The lower edge of the sphygmomanometer cuff should be placed approximately 1 inch above the (antecubital fossa) elbow crease. The cuff should be deflated before placement and wrapped evenly and firmly around the arm.

16. **(A)** During blood pressure measurement, the sphyg-momanometer cuff is deflated by releasing the exhaust valve at a rate of 2 to 3 mm Hg per second.

17. **(B)** The antecubital fossa or space is located at the elbow.

18. **(D)** Pulse readings are taken most frequently at the radial artery. The radial artery is located at the lateral aspect of the wrist (thumb side of the hand).

19. **(C)** The most common site to obtain a pulse reading on a patient is at the radial artery located on the wrist. The first two fingers of your hand are used to palpate and record the pulse. Other pulse sites are the temporal artery located on the side of the head in front of the ear and the carotid artery on the side of the neck.

20. **(B)** The average resting pulse rate for an adult is 60 to 100 heart beats per minute. A normal pulse rate should have a relatively regular rhythm. The pulse rate can increase with exercise and decrease with sleep.

21. **(A)** The oral thermometer should remain in the closed mouth for approximately 2 minutes.

22. **(A)** The average or normal oral temperature reading for an adult is 98.6°F. Fever is an increase in oral temperature in excess of 101°F.

23. **(C)** The best time to record the patient's respiration rate is when the patient is completely unaware of what the auxiliary is doing. Patients who are aware that they are being observed tend to begin breathing abnormally (either faster or slower), causing an inaccurate reading. A respiration is measured as one breath taken in and let out.

24. **(D)** The average respiratory rate for an adult is 16 to 20 breaths per minute.

25. **(B)** The residual air is the amount of air remaining in the lungs after the deepest exhalation that cannot be expired from the lungs through a voluntary effort. Tidal air is the amount of air that can be handled in a normal inhalation and a normal exhalation.

26. **(B)** Short appointments are recommended for patients who have either a physical or mental problem and can be easily stressed by long dental appointments. Patients who have a history of cardiac problems are normally scheduled for shorter dental appointments to avoid undue stress on an already weakened heart.

27. **(A)** The depressed state of many body functions is called shock. The severity of shock depends on the cause. Some forms of shock are neurogenic, insulin, and anaphylactic.

28. **(A)** When treating a patient for shock, the victim's feet should be raised 8 to 12 inches above the rest of the body to increase blood circulation in the head.

29. **(B)** Syncope refers to the lack of blood to the brain for a short period. This is caused by dilation of blood vessels in the body and results in loss of consciousness.

30. **(D)** Inhalation of spirits of ammonia is used as a reflex stimulant that causes a patient to regain consciousness after fainting. It is stored in individual vials that are broken at the time of use.

31. **(B)** The treatment for syncope is to place the head lower than the rest of the body, administer aromatic ammonia inhalant, loosen tight clothing, administer oxygen, and give reassurance.

32. **(C)** Patients with chronic respiratory problems must be positioned in such a manner that may facilitate the breathing process and comfort. In many cases, these patients cannot be placed in a supine position.

33. **(D)** The proper sequence in an emergency situation is to control severe bleeding, restore breathing, and treat for shock. Only severe bleeding—bleeding that is spurting from a wound as the heart beats—must be controlled immediately. If bleeding is not severe, the immediate priority is to establish an airway.

34. **(A)** An overdose is the term used to identify administering an excess amount of a drug.

35. **(C)** If circulatory collapse occurs, the patient should be given external cardiac massage. This procedure artificially continues the circulation until the patient's heartbeat has been restored or until medical help arrives.

36. **(B)** Clear foreign matter from the mouth, tilt the head backward with chin pointing up, put one hand on the victim's forehead, and apply firm backward pressure with the palm of the hand to tilt the head back. Place the fingers of the other hand under the bony part of the victim's lower jaw to bring the chin forward, lift the jaw to bring the teeth close together, but do not close the victim's mouth in order to maintain an open airway. Pinch the nostrils shut and form a seal over the victim's mouth with your mouth.

37. **(D)** The Heimlich maneuver includes placing the victim in a forward-bending position, standing behind him or her, and placing arms around the victim's waist. A fist is made and placed one hand's length above the patient's navel. The rescuer makes quick inward and upward thrusts, forcing air through the trachea to dislodge trapped particles.

38. **(B)** Asphyxia, or suffocation, may occur when the air does not contain sufficient oxygen to support the respiratory process.

39. **(B)** If a foreign object, such as a denture, becomes lodged in a patient's throat, allow the patient to cough the object out first. If this is not successful, use the Heimlich maneuver and begin artificial respiration. If there is complete obstruction, attempt to re-

move the object physically. If the patient loses consciousness and cannot breath, a tracheotomy is the last resort.

40. **(C)** Anaphylactic shock is a sudden violent allergic reaction. Two drugs used in dentistry that may cause this reaction are local anesthesia and penicillin. A detailed accurate medical history of past adverse drug reactions could indicate whether a drug could cause this reaction.

41. **(C)** The drug that best counteracts anaphylactic shock is epinephrine; 0.5 mL of 1:1000 epinephrine is injected subcutaneously for this purpose.

42. **(D)** Patients who have a history of rheumatic heart disease must be protected against bacterial endocarditis, a microbial infection of the endocardium or heart valves. Prophylactic antibiotic coverage is required before the scheduled dental appointment. A review of the patient's medical history is required for the appropriate premedication regimen. Consult the patient's physician if necessary. Recommended antibiotic coverage for dental procedures and guidelines are available through the American Heart Association.

43. **(B)** Patients taking anticoagulation medication must be watched for bleeding problems because this medication diminishes the ability of the blood to clot.

44. **(A)** Incised wounds are caused by sharp objects. The amount of bleeding depends on their depths and the tissues that are cut.

45. **(C)** Lacerated wounds are jagged and irregular. They are associated with considerable tissue damage and with free bleeding if blood vessels are severed.

46. **(B)** Angina pectoris is a painful condition of the heart caused by lack of blood to the heart muscles. Patients who have this condition should be treated with techniques that decrease anxiety, pain, and other stressful situations that may promote an attack.

47. **(C)** Postural hypotension is most likely to occur when the patient's chair position is changed too quickly. Symptoms include lightheadedness, possible loss of consciousness, and low blood pressure. Predisposing factors include patients taking antihypertensive medications, antidepressants, narcotics, and drugs for Parkinson's disease. To avoid postural hypotension raise the patient in the dental chair slowly from a supine position to an upright position.

48. **(A)** The first aid measures that should be rendered to a patient during an epileptic seizure are moving objects away from the patient, loosening the patient's clothing, supporting the patient's breathing if

necessary, allowing the patient to rest, and reassuring the patient.

49. **(D)** If a patient begins to have convulsions in the waiting room, the operator or assistant should protect the patient from injury by moving objects out of his or her reach. Summon professional medical support if necessary.

50. **(D)** If a patient suddenly keels over with no pulse or breathing, summon help immediately, support respiration by mouth-to-mouth resuscitation, and support circulation with external cardiac massage.

51. **(A)** The appropriate medical emergency treatment for the patient who suddenly feels acute severe pain in their chest and left arm, along with nausea and lightheadedness, would be to allow the patient to rest quietly and summon professional medical emergency support as quickly as possible. The symptoms described may be indicative of a serious cardiac problem requiring immediate medical attention.

52. **(C)** During CPR, chest compressions must be given with the victim lying on a firm flat surface. The victim's head should be at the same level as the heart. Begin by locating the lower edge of the victim's ribcage. Gently slide your hand so that the index and middle fingers are placed up the edge of the ribcage to the notch where the ribs meet the (sternum) in the center of the lower part of the chest. The heel of the other hand is placed on the sternum right next to and above the two fingers of the hand resting on the notch.

53. **(C)** To prevent foreign objects from flying into a person's eye, the best precaution is to wear safety glasses.

54. **(D)** If a foreign object is embedded in a person's eye, an eye patch should be placed over both eyes and medical attention should be sought. Attempting to remove an embedded foreign body may result in further irritation and damage.

55. **(B)** The treatment for an accidently avulsed central incisor is to rinse the tooth in lukewarm water, reinsert it as soon as possible, and stabilize the reinserted tooth until professional help arrives.

56. **(B)** To avoid injuries to teeth while participating in contact sports, athletes should wear mouth guards. Mouth guards are usually made of flexible materials that will absorb some of the impact of a traumatic blow.

57. **(A)** An antidote counteracts the effect of a toxic drug.

58. **(B)** Insulin shock results from excess insulin in the blood and can be counteracted by eating a food with high sugar content.

59. **(A)** Patients with a medical history of diabetes complications should be monitored closely during dental treatment. Medical emergency procedures for a conscious patient undergoing insulin shock include the administration of orange juice, candy, sugar water, soft drinks, or other oral carbohydrates that easily can be made available in the dental office. Office emergency kits should contain packets of sugar if a refrigerator is unavailable to stock other perishable items. The treatment of an unconscious patient in insulin shock requires immediate basic life support procedures and immediate medical attention. Intravenous administration of dextrose usually is required.

60. **(A)** A patient's medical and dental history can affect all phases of a patient's treatment, including appointment and prescriptions.

61. **(E)** Signs and symptoms of a patient in shock include a change in skin color. The skin may appear pale and feel moist and cold and clammy. Other symptoms of shock include rapid or shallow breathing, weakness and nausea, low blood pressure, and confusion.

62. **(B)** Signs and symptoms of an allergic reaction include skin rash, itching, and swelling. Mucous membranes, such as the lips and larynx, may become swollen, leading to more serious complications and distressed respiration. Pulse rate is usually thready and weakened, and medical support should be sought immediately.

63. **(D)** Patients with a medical history of angina pectoris may be treated with nitroglycerin. Nitroglycerin is a vasodilator and should be administered sublingually for quick onset of the drug. The patient can be made more comfortable by seating in an upright position and administering oxygen if necessary.

64. **(A)** Emergencies in the operating environment can be prevented by being alert to signs of impending emergency in all patients and by keeping the operating site free of bloody debris. Avoidance of phrases or words that might upset or frighten the patient also is recommended.

65. **(E)** Lawsuits can be avoided by keeping accurate records and completely documenting all dental procedures rendered. Entries must be made in ink, and medical health histories must be updated periodically. Appropriate patient treatment consent forms must be signed and on file in case of a potential lawsuit. Each state sets certain standards and limitations regarding dental auxiliary procedures that must be adhered to strictly in order to remain within the defined legal boundaries of the state Dental Practice Act.

66. **(C)** First aid measures for a person in shock in a dental office are to maintain a comfortable temperature, keep the patient lying down, be encouraging to the patient, loosen any tight clothing, and call the patient's physician.

67. **(B)** Some causes of syncope in the dental office are fear, visual disturbances (such as seeing blood or a needle), pain, and the injection of local anesthetic directly into a blood vessel.

68. **(D)** The human brain requires oxygen to function. Without oxygen, a state of unconsciousness will occur rapidly. In emergency situations where airway obstruction exists, permanent brain damage (brain cell death) will occur within 4 to 6 minutes.

69. **(A)** The vital signs taken before an operative dental appointment include blood pressure, pulse, and respiration. A patient's height and weight are recorded at the first visit on a medical history questionnaire and do not need to be monitored before each operative dental visit.

70. **(D)** Symptoms of diabetic coma (ketoacidosis) include weak pulse, low blood pressure, dry mouth and thirst, flushed skin tone, confusion, general weakness or drowsiness, and acetone breath odor. Diabetic coma may occur from an insufficient amount of insulin or failure to take insulin medication when indicated.

71. **(B)** Medical emergency treatment for the patient who is experiencing hyperventilation includes reassuring and calming the patient and having the patient take several deep slow breaths. A paper bag may be held gently over the patient's mouth and nose to correct the hyperventilation syndrome by having the patient breathe in his or her own exhaled air, which contains carbon dioxide.

72. **(A)** Cerebrovascular accident (CVA) is known also as a stroke. A CVA is caused by a sudden loss of brain function due to an interruption of the blood supply to the brain. Symptoms of CVA may include an irregular or thready pulse, slurred speech, dilated pupils, slow labored breathing, and cyanosis (bluish discoloration of the skin).

73. **(C)** Basic emergency procedures for the patient who begins to feel severe chest pain during dental treatment include discontinue dental treatment immediately and seat patient in an upright position to

help ease the chest pain. Medical support assistance should be summoned as quickly as possible, and if indicated, an oxygen mask should be applied to assist the patient in breathing more easily.

74. **(E)** A basic office emergency armamentarium includes intravenous armamentarium and related drugs, sponges, tourniquets, syringes, mouth props, and sugar packs. A portable oxygen tank also is considered a basic necessity of the medical emergency kit.

75. **(B)** If performing CPR on a patient with a history of an infectious disease, the rescuer should wear disposable latex gloves and use a protective microshield over the victim's mouth and face.

76. **(D)** The patient with a history of liver disease (hepatitis) should be given limited quantities of local anesthetic. Liver damage may indicate difficulty in metabolizing the injected anesthetic drug, causing an elevated anesthetic level in the patient's blood.

BIBLIOGRAPHY

American Red Cross. *Advanced First Aid and Emergency Care*, 2nd ed. New York: Doubleday and Co, Inc, 1980.

American Red Cross. *Standard First Aid and Personal Safety*, 2nd ed. New York: Doubleday and Co, Inc, 1979.

American National Red Cross. *American Red Cross Community CPR Wookbook*. 1988.

American National Red Cross. *American Red Cross Standard First Aid Workbook*. 1988.

Malamed SF. *Handbook of Medical Emergencies in the Dental Office*, 3rd ed. St. Louis: CV Mosby Co, 1987.

McCarthy FM. *Emergencies in Dental Practice; Prevention and Treatment*, 3rd ed. Philadelphia: WB Saunders Co, 1979.

Rose LF, Kaye D. *Internal Medicine For Dentistry*, 2nd ed. St. Louis: CV Mosby Co, 1990.

Sande MA, Volberding PA. *The Medical Management of AIDS*, 2nd ed. Philadelphia: WB Saunders Co, 1990.

Soltero DJ, Whitacre RJ. *Vital Signs*. Seattle: Instructional Services, 1978.

Veterans Administration Medical Center. *Periodontal Resident Manual*. West Los Angeles: VA Medical Center, 1990.

Wilkins EM. *Clinical Practice of the Dental Hygienist*, 6th ed. Philadelphia: Lea & Febiger, 1989.

CHAPTER 9

Behavioral Sciences

INTRODUCTION

Dental assisting is a profession that involves working with people. As a member of the treatment team, the dental assistant functions as an important extension of the dentist. The dental assistant who is able to function as a successful professional in health care delivery has knowledge of the psychology of individuals and groups and understands the skills necessary for effective patient motivation and interoffice communication. This chapter focuses on several key behavioral science concepts and techniques for effective patient management and interpersonal office skills.

COMMUNICATION

Communication is the development of shared meaning. Communication is a process, not an event. Many individuals believe that they are engaged in an act of communication when they speak to another person, but often they are wrong. It is not enough just to send a message. The message must be perceived and understood. The receiver, rather than the sender of the message, finally defines both the quality and meaning of the message. Almost all interaction taking place in the dental office is based on communication. To be effective, the assistant must exchange clear and accurate messages with the dentist, patients, and other staff members. The auxiliary must be able to fully understand the nature of the communication process.

In the busy office, patients often depend on the auxiliaries to convey their needs, concerns, messages, and questions to the dentist. In turn, the dentist may depend on the staff to be the liaison for important communication with patients. The auxiliary must convey information to the patient in the form of instructions and explanations. Besides telling the patient when to come to the office, how to pay for treatment, where to sit, and so on, the assistant also may provide oral health care instruction and answer patient's questions about office policy, dental insurance, and office records. The auxiliary must elicit and clarify information presented by the patient. Often the auxiliary requests basic personal information from the patient before or during an initial appointment.

TABLE 9–1. METHODS OF COMMUNICATION

1. Build redundancy into messages
2. Focus the attention of the receiver
3. Request feedback
4. Use active listening
5. Provide clear instruction
6. Be specific when giving instruction
7. Do not overload the recipient

Communication also may be intended to influence or modify behavior. The auxiliary through proper selection of words and tone of voice can praise a patient, punish a patient, or encourage a desired behavior.

The dental assistant will want to support the patient by sharing feelings. The right gesture or words often provide the patient with the support necessary to survive an anxious moment. The ability to express empathy is a key factor in the assistant's attempts to be helpful.

Finally, communication is a part of creating and modifying personal relationships. The very act of communication bonds people together, and most relationships are defined by the quality of their communications.

METHODS OF COMMUNICATION

It is possible for the dental assistant to increase the probability that accurate communication occurs. Some of the obvious methods are knowing the subject being discussed, using words the other person understands, and listening carefully (Table 9–1).

Build Reinforcement into Messages

The same message can be given in different forms. For example, the auxiliary not only should tell the patient how to brush but also could demonstrate the techniques. Often, providing the patient with written as well as verbal information will help ensure that the message is received.

Focus the Attention of the Receiver

Before providing information, tell the receiver what you

plan to present. Help your listener to decide on what to focus his or her attention.

Request Feedback

After the message has been sent, ask the listener to tell you what you have said. At times, you might want the patient to demonstrate a skill you have just presented.

Use Active Listening

Active listening is a method used to help the message sender increase the ability to be understood. As a dental assistant, you will want to ensure that you accurately understand the patient's message and that the patient feels he or she is being heard and receiving attention. There are three types of receiver activity involved: restatement, reflection, and clarification.

Restatement. The receiver tells the message sender what he or she has just heard. The receiver does not add information but merely, in his or her own words and those of the sender, repeats the message received.

Reflection. The receiver tells the sender the feelings are being received. In other words, the receiver provides his or her own interpretation of the emotional meaning of the message.

Clarification. The receiver asks the sender to add information in areas that were unclear in the original message. Thus, the sender is given the opportunity to expand and explain those elements of the message that were originally unclear.

Provide Clear Instruction

The dental assistant often is called on to provide patients with home care instruction. There are specific guidelines for providing clear, usable instructions.

Begin by giving the patient a clear overview of the task. The patient should be told what the task is supposed to accomplish and what the patient is to learn.

The second step is to determine the receiver's perception, expectations, and knowledge of the required task. The instructor should determine the receiver's readiness and willingness to undertake the task. The instruction should be tailored to the needs of the receiver.

Allow time for questions, feedback, and correcting misconceptions. Build in redundancy. The best instruction should be not only verbal but also visual.

The instructor should be open to the receiver's ideas and perceptions. If the instructor listens to the receiver, he or she is more likely to be clear and helpful.

Be Specific When Giving Instruction

Use the correct name for objects and avoid vagueness in terms and instruction. When steps are involved, they should be numbered and given in order.

Do Not Overload the Recipient

A person can learn only so much in one sitting. At the same time, evaluate the receiver's knowledge. Where possible, allow the receiver to demonstrate his or her knowledge and understanding. Finally, give reinforcement, praise, and encouragement.

PERSONAL PERCEPTIONS

An important aspect of the dental assistant's job is providing the emotional support and information necessary to the patient for accepting and cooperating with dental treatment. It is not required that the auxiliary be a psychotherapist, but it is important that he or she be able to understand and relate to the patient's behavior. The behavior of others can be modified by changing one's own behavior and perceptions. Although the assistant cannot control the patient directly, he or she can help change the patient's perceptions of the situation. Self-knowledge and social skills are the tools the dental assistant applies when working with others. Dental care often makes people anxious, frightened, and confused. In these states, people might behave in ways that can cause problems during treatment. The assistant must respond to this behavior in ways that are helpful to the patient. Several areas of personal functioning are important in this activity.

Effective Presentation of Self Is Crucial to Professional Functioning

People learn something about each other when they first meet. They use the clues that are given to determine who others are and how they should behave. The assistant can control the messages he or she provides by paying attention to dress, posture and movement, eye contact, and personal tempo.

The clothes people wear and how they wear them reveal information about themselves. For example, a white uniform informs the patient that the auxiliary is a part of the treatment team and is engaged in an efficient, no-nonsense activity.

Upright posture and purposeful, directed activity convey to the patient that the auxiliary is engaged in important work, is conscientious, and knows what he or she is doing.

Direct eye contact conveys interest, alertness, and attention. Through appropriate eye contact with the patient, the auxiliary begins to establish or continue the relationship with the patient.

The Dental Assistant Should Be Centered When Interacting with Patients

Since the dental patient often is anxious, feeling a little out of control, and not thinking clearly, it becomes the auxiliary's responsibility to preserve the stability of the situation. The auxiliary must avoid being thrown off balance by the patient's misperceptions, upset, or inappropriate behavior. Ceramicists speak of centering their clay on the potting wheel so that the clay will respond only to the pressure of their fingers and will not wobble because it is unbalanced. In much the same way, the auxiliary must center himself or herself within the treatment situation and create an internal calmness and receptiveness so that the only response given is to the actual behavior of the patient. The auxiliary's response is not to be distorted by outside concerns brought from home or from previous patient behavior. Instead, the auxiliary should react to the actual treatment situation.

Establishing A Clear and Acceptable Interpersonal Contract Is an Important Key to Patient Management

A contract is the expectation for certain behavior or behaviors that one person develops concerning the other. These contracts are not legal or written—they are psychologic. Often, the expectations are not even shared with the other. Whether the contract is explicit (shared) or implicit (not discussed), it is helpful to negotiate clear, explicit contracts. The patient should be told exactly what is expected of him or her in the office. In the same way, the auxiliary should try to discover the patient's expectations of the staff and office and clarify them if they are unreasonable or unrealistic.

WORKING IN THE DENTAL TEAM

The interactions and communication among team members also influence the way the dental patient perceives the practice. An important responsibility of the dental assistant is functioning as a productive and cooperative member of the dental team. Understanding behaviors that lead to successful group interactions should be demonstrated by all dental team members on a regular basis.

Conflict

Interpersonal conflict is an issue in any work group. Conflict often is attributed to personality differences, but it is seldom this simple. In a work group, conflict is not likely to arise out of the structure of the working situation itself. There are two types of conflict. The first is called zero-sum conflict. This type of conflict often arises when two or more people are competing for the same object. The object could be desk space, the right to provide patient education, or priority on vacation time. What is important is that the individuals are in conflict because they want the same thing—not because of feelings about each other. This type of conflict is best resolved by negotiation, compromise, and the addition of new resources. Clarifying the conflict is not helpful, since it only serves to make the competition more open and intense. A helpful method of breaking the impasse and developing interdependence and trust is for one party to give to the other something the other values but that does not cost the giver. This is known as the Osgood solution and is a commonly used strategy even between nations.

The second type of conflict is more personal and usually involves feelings of betrayal. This conflict arises when one individual fails to meet the expectations of the other. The results of contract violation lead to a desire to punish.

In this situation, the parties involved must sit down, clarify their perceptions and feelings, and work out their differences.

The number of individuals in the work group is important. Groups of fewer than five have special properties because of the possibilities of becoming imbalanced. Groups of three and five tend to be unstable because of the probability of uneven numbers in each subgroup.

Power

Power is the ability to control or influence the behavior of others. In most groups, an informal pecking order is established that determines who influences whom. In the dental office, four sources of power exist. *Expert power* is derived from having the knowledge and skills necessary for accomplishing a task. In the office, every member at one time or another will assume leadership because of the possession of some special knowledge. However, the people who have been in the office longest and know most about the way things are done tend to control office activity. *Reward power* is derived from being able to control the rewards available. For example, the person who holds the pursestrings of the office or who is in charge of hiring and firing often is quite powerful in day-to-day activity. The receptionist who controls the patient's access to the dentist has this power over the patient. *Position power* is based on each individual's formal job title. For example, the office manager, by virtue of the job title, is able to control the office. Finally, *referent power* is a form of social power that stems from one person's identification with another. In terms of optimum functioning, expert power, because it supports the organizational structure, is the most legitimate source of power.

PATIENT MANAGEMENT STRATEGIES

Dental patients can be separated into four age groups: children, adolescents, adults, and the elderly. Each age group faces social, emotional, and intellectual challenges and opportunities as a result of their level of physical, psychologic, and societal maturation. Each group presents different concerns in the office and requires different management strategies.

The Child

Children are focused on their actual experience. A child's thinking and understanding are concrete. The word and the experience are perceived as being the same; that is, a child takes what is said literally instead of symbolically. For example, when a child hears that the dentist is going to use a hatchet, he or she pictures teeth being chopped. It is, therefore, important that the dental assistant select words carefully to convey nonthreatening, familiar images to the child. Thus, the injection, or shot, might be referred to as "sleepy water," which will be squirted near the tooth or gums to "put the tooth to sleep." In addition, young children often make a direct causal connection between discomfort experienced as the dentist works and punishment. It is very important for the dentist and auxiliary to clarify for the patient that the dental treatment is not punishment and that the child has not done something bad or wrong in taking care of his or her teeth. Parents should not be allowed to use the dental visit as a threat or punishment to force a child to adopt desired oral care habits.

A related issue for children is body integrity. A child believes that each part of the body is crucial to personal identity. Loss of a body part or a change in appearance (such as the loss of a tooth) can be upsetting. Fear of mutilation, such as having a tooth drilled, is more threatening than the possibility of pain. Providing a child with a mirror so that he or she can see that the dentist is not causing damage is an effective strategy for calming the child's anxiety. If a tooth must be extracted, it is a good idea to allow the child to take it home and to control its disposal.

A third crucial issue for a child is competence. Children judge their own worth in terms of what they can do. Actions are concrete demonstrations of one's value. Because a child has acquired the cognitive and physical capacity to perform tasks by the end of nursery school, teachers and peers expect the child to demonstrate a level of competence. Children feel they must earn the approval of peers and adults. The auxiliary, in giving instruction and correcting behavior, should concentrate on what a child does well rather than on what is done wrong. Success leads to success. Children's behavior is best controlled by telling them exactly what is expected. A child should be guided step by step through the visit. The desire to do things correctly is a powerful motivator. This developmental period is an excellent time in which to instill positive oral habits.

Related to children's concern with competence is their concern with self-control. Children often panic when they feel out of control, so it is important to avoid restraining or immobilizing a child unless it is necessary for treatment or to prevent the child from acting out. By carefully explaining what is going to happen, the auxiliary can help the child retain a sense of control. A good technique is the method of *Tell-Show-Do*.

Tell the child what is going to be done.

Show the child the setting and demonstrate how the equipment works.

Do the procedure, explaining to the patient what is happening.

A final note regarding children is in order. Research shows that the negative dental habits and feelings about dentists expressed by adults often are the result of negative childhood dental experiences. Positive dental experiences as a child can be the key to positive dental health in adulthood.

The Adolescent

Adolescents tend to be focused on themselves. In psychologic terms, the adolescent is considered egocentric. That is, an adolescent perceives and judges the world in terms of his or her own needs and philosophy. Because he or she has developed physically into a mature body and intellectually to the point of being able to think abstractly and for the long term (like an adult), the adolescent starts to assume adult status. Thus, the adolescent is beginning the process of establishing himself or herself as an independent entity separate from parents. Two psychologic patient management issues become critical. First, although adolescents desire independence, parents are very much concerned with both the economic and dental–medical aspects of treatment. Involving parents in the dental treatment is a tricky problem. On the one hand, the parents are paying the bill, and they are legally responsible for their child's welfare. Often, problems of living (eg, sexually transmitted diseases, signs of stress, changes in health status) are revealed in the dental examination. On the other hand, the adolescent wishes to preserve autonomy and privacy. Developing an alliance with the parents can place the treatment team in the center of a family power struggle. As a general rule, it is better to work directly with an adolescent patient. Rather than ask parents to reinforce appointment keeping or home care compliance, it is more effective to form a therapeutic alliance with the patient. To do this, it may be necessary to consider very carefully an adolescent's need for privacy before involving parents in the resolution of social and medical problems discovered in the course of treatment.

A second psychologic patient management issue is related to the adolescent's search for an autonomous identity. Since adolescents are questioning their parents' standards and values, they must look elsewhere for new criteria, often to the judgments of peers and other nonfamily adults. Other people's judgment determines an adolescent's standard of personal value. Appearance becomes very important, and the approval of others is crucial. A primary issue for adolescents is whether teeth are straight and pretty and whether speech is clear. An adolescent is less concerned with how well he or she does than with whether people judge him or her as intelligent, nice, or special. When giving health instruction or responding to an adolescent's questions and requests concerning treatment, it is important that the adolescent not feel patronized or negatively perceived. It is helpful to tell the patient what he or she is doing correctly and incorrectly. It is important to convey the impression that whether the action or request is correct or not, you respect the person. Negative statements should be avoided.

Adolescents can be extremely provocative as they test to see whether others will reject them or become involved with them. Some patients will become hostile and very touchy. Others will become seductive or intrusive or both. The auxiliary's patience and tolerance will be challenged. The appropriate stance with an adolescent is to maintain an accepting, warm, but nonpersonal manner. It is important to maintain a nonjudgmental, professional attitude and to avoid becoming involved in the adolescent's very intense life struggles. One can listen, offer support, and accept the person without becoming a major actor in the drama. It is important to create the type of atmosphere that will allow the patient to cooperate and benefit from the dental treatment.

The Adult

Adults tend to be focused on time, convenience, and function. The primary pressure faced by an adult patient is getting done all the things for which he or she is responsible. Job pressures, family responsibilities, and social relations tend to take precedence over dental care. Patients usually are more concerned with how long the treatment will take, how much their daily functioning will be impaired, and how much treatment will cost them than they are with esthetics, the dental staff's opinion, or treatment discomfort. To meet the dental patient's need and to elicit cooperation, the auxiliary must enter into a clear exchange with the patient regarding expectations. The office hours and office policies regarding punctuality and payment must be discussed clearly. After the treatment plan is presented by the dentist, the schedule of office visits and payment should be discussed by the auxiliary with the patient. Treatment is likely to fail and the relationship with the patient to sour if the expectations of both the dental office and the patient are not defined clearly. Appointments should be arranged that will fit within the patient's work and family obligations. Financial arrangements must be consistent with the patient's ability to pay. Adults will require information about their insurance benefits and accurate documentation of their treatment and its cost.

In providing patient education, the auxiliary should focus on the immediate and long-term effects of oral functioning. Adults can plan ahead and will be concerned with their long-term health and the economic consequences of noncompliance. They recognize that they will suffer for their mistakes and benefit from their diligence. They will be able to accept short-term inconvenience in the hope of long-term benefit. For adults, dental health care is an investment. The auxiliary must convince an adult that the investment is worthwhile.

The Elderly

The elderly patient is concerned with loss of function and loss of social identity and importance. Old age is more a function of social expectations (social age) and current physical state (physical age) than it is of the passage of years (chronologic age). Socially, retirement, reduced financial ability, and family status changes (children marrying and leaving home, birth of grandchildren, and death of family members and close friends) define a person as getting on in years. Physically, decline in fitness or flexibility of cognitive functioning is an indicator of aging. As the individual enters old age, his or her ability to do things for himself or herself decreases. For example, the loss of teeth and the necessity of wearing dentures will affect the patient's ability to talk and eat, as well as appearance and self-concept. The loss will have an impact on all aspects of the individual's functioning. Chronic illness is both the cause and the result of a gradual physical deterioration of the body. Once body functioning is disrupted by chronic disease often related to aging, it is not unusual for the entire social and physical functioning of the individual to decline. The result of these changes is an increased dependence on others.

Two problems faced by the auxiliary who works with the elderly patient are hypochondriasis and depression. Hypochondriasis is an excess anxious concern with the functioning of body parts. For instance, patients will become very concerned with small lesions, the way their various dental prostheses fit and look, and their general oral health. They will experience a greater need for sympathetic attention and concern.

Depression is a morbid sadness and feeling of loss. In an elderly person, it is usually the result of the loss of self-esteem that occurs when the individual is unable to contribute to personal welfare and the welfare of others. The aging person feels useless and a burden to those around and may experience a loss of purpose that was provided by a defined job and family roles.

The auxiliary can provide relief of these negative feelings by according the patient special attention. It is helpful to allow the patient to share his or her experiences. Listening respectfully to the patient's opinions and advice is beneficial to the patient and may even be of help to the auxiliary. Reminiscence is therapeutic to elderly persons. It allows them to reinstate social roles and contributions. Finally, the dental visit, because it is a personal process of taking care of one's needs, is often an important event in the elderly person's life. It involves planning and getting ready for the visit and receiving focused concern and attention. It often is an important topic of discussion with friends.

Because of the changes in cognitive and emotional functioning, elderly patients may need special support in the dental setting. Dental treatment can be demanding physically. Patients may become disoriented and confused. It is helpful to suggest that the patient arrange to be accompanied by a friend or member of the family when he or she comes for treatment. It may be necessary, if the patient does come to the office alone, to ensure that the patient gets home safely by arranging transportation.

In addition, elderly patients have some difficulty adapting to new ideas or demands. It is helpful if the auxiliary builds on the patient's past experiences, beliefs, and habits when giving instruction in necessary home care techniques. New procedures and methods, as well as appointment times and directions, should be written out and given to the patient to take home. Providing this support will enable the elderly patient to cooperate satisfactorily with treatment.

SPECIAL PATIENT CIRCUMSTANCES

Some patients will come to the office with physical problems. Other patients may be emotionally disturbed. In each case, it may be necessary to make special provisions for these people.

Patients with physical handicaps might require special modifications of the treatment apparatus. Patients in wheelchairs may have to be treated in their wheelchairs if it is too difficult to transfer them to the dental chair. Many patients with physical handicaps needlessly avoid treatment because of embarrassment or feeling that they are unacceptable for treatment. The dental auxiliary can make it easier for these patients by making the necessary provisions in advance of the patient's arrival or introduction into the treatment room. The auxiliary should review the patient's chart before treatment and make any needed preparations so that the patient will not be forced to be embarrassed.

Patients who experience psychologic or emotional difficulty may require that the office environment be simplified. The staff should decrease the activity level of the treatment room for the disturbed patient. Too much stimulation can confuse the patient and make him or her more anxious or disoriented. Patients who are easily confused or upset should be placed in quiet environments and focused onto the treatment taking place so that they do not become disoriented and panic. The patient should be guided carefully through each step of treatment. The dental assistant must be alert to the signs and symptoms of suspicious or irrational patient behavior that may be related to drug or alcohol abuse. Patient behavior patterns may vary from extreme restlessness to impaired judgment or slurred speech. If the dental assistant remains responsive and alert to the dental patient's concerns and physical behavior, management problems can be prevented, and the dental treatment will be accepted in a calm and cooperative manner by the patient.

PATIENT MOTIVATION

Often the dental assistant is called on by the dentist to help educate or manage a patient. Several approaches for improving patient behavior are discussed in the following sections.

Motivation

If an individual is to perform a task, whether it be as a patient fulfilling home care instruction or as an employee meeting job expectations, the person must understand how he or she is supposed to behave. In addition, the individual must be willing to perform the task. This willingness to act is called motivation. Motivation is the result of personal impulse or desire to obtain a particular object or experience. In other words, motivation may be defined as inducing somebody into action relative to something. The inner forces that drive a person into action are called needs. These needs might be for attention, love, respect, safety, and so on. Abraham Maslow, a psychologist, has described a hierarchy of needs. He states that one must satisfy lower-order needs before being gratified by higher-order needs (Fig. 9–1).

The first level of need is related to survival concerns. The individual ensures that he or she will not starve, die of thirst, suffer terrible pain, or be physically attacked before being able to focus on the next level of concern. For example, if a patient has pain, the pain must be relieved

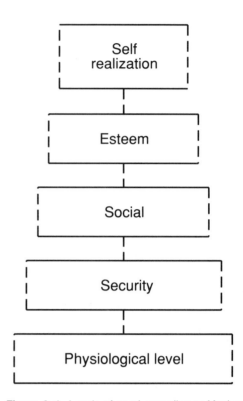

Figure 9–1. Levels of need according to Maslow.

before the patient will listen to discussions of oral hygiene, reliability, or long-term treatment plans. The second level of need is for security, which is the need for protection. This may include protection against physical or economic instability or fear of the unpredictable. The third level of need is for acceptance and approval and includes the social needs. Patients often are concerned about whether the dental staff accepts, respects, and approves of them. The fourth level of needs has to do with esteem, specifically, those needs dealing with personal self-worth, competency, and the esteem of others. The highest order of need may be termed the level of self-realization or actualization. This involves needs that drive the individual to grow and to develop one's potential to the highest order.

The dental assistant can elicit the patient's motivation by creating situations in which the patient's needs can be fulfilled by responding to the dental assistant's requests. Furthermore, if the dental assistant focuses on the patient's sufficiency needs (higher-order needs, such as oral health, reliability, responsibility) rather than on the patient's deficiency needs (lower-order needs, such as fear of pain or loss), the patient is more likely to develop positive dental habits.

There are three steps in eliciting a patient's motivation. The first is helping the patient assume ownership of the particular task or problem. If the patient is to take responsibility, he or she must recognize that a problem or need exists, see what can be done to resolve the problem,

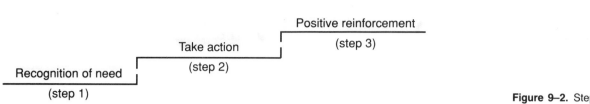

Figure 9–2. Steps to motivation.

and exhibit a readiness to act. The second step is to show the patient that there is a reasonable probability of success following action. Finally, once the patient acts, the behavior should be reinforced (Fig. 9–2).

Behavior Modification

Behavior modification is a technique that developed from observing how all organisms, including people, learn. Behavior modification generally is used to meet one of three objectives: to increase the rate or frequency of a desired behavior, to decrease the rate or frequency of an undesired behavior, or to substitute a new behavior for an existing undesirable one.

When an individual is reinforced (rewarded) for a particular response, he or she is more likely to exhibit the same response to that stimulus in the future. However, when the response is met with punishment, the individual is less likely to exhibit the same behavior. By controlling the outcomes or contingencies to a patient's behavior, the dental assistant can increase the probability that the patient will behave appropriately. All individuals, in part, learn how to behave by observing the consequences of their behavior.

Shaping

Shaping is a technique based on the principles of operant conditioning. It was developed by Dr. B.F. Skinner. It is a useful method of improving patient behavior. Shaping is based on the principle of systematically reinforcing successive approximations up until the final task, at which time a reward is earned, and the task has been mastered by shaping the behavior a step at a time. With shaping, the patient can learn in small incremental steps. The desired behavior is reinforced at each step by feedback or some form of acknowledgment until finally the task is mastered. An example of the application of the shaping theory may be visualized with teaching toothbrush instruction. At first, the toothbrushing technique that the patient demonstrates is not effective in removing plaque, as visually indicated by a disclosing agent. The patient is given instructions and allowed to brush again. At the second visit, the teeth are disclosed again after the patient brushes. Marked improvement can be observed visually by noting less plaque-covered tooth surfaces. The auxiliary should praise and reinforce the correct behavior (technique) demonstrated by the patient after evaluating the brushing. A third and possibly fourth visit may be necessary until the toothbrushing technique is mastered and demonstrates a plaque-free score. By systematically shaping the patient behavior at each visit in small incremental steps, the desired goal of correctly brushing is reached.

Desensitization

Sometimes the patient's primary response to the dental situation is fear, avoidance, and anxiety. This reaction may block the patient's ability to cooperate with treatment. Desensitization is a technique used to decrease the likelihood of this response. This is done by teaching the patient a new response that is incompatible with the frightened or anxious response. For example, the patient can be taught to relax and think pleasant thoughts in response to a signal. Then the patient is gradually introduced to aspects of the dental situation and signalled to relax when he or she perceives each aspect. Gradually, a new response (the relaxation and thinking pleasant thoughts) that is incompatible with the phobic response (getting anxious and frightened) is substituted for the old one.

DENTAL FEAR AND ANXIETY

Dental treatment often elicits an anxiety reaction in patients. Anxiety is different from fear in that fear usually is a focused response to a specific, observable threat, whereas anxiety is a generalized response to a situation. Anxious patients often hyperventilate and may even faint. They may exhibit behavior that creates patient-management problems. In addition, the anxious patient's psychologic and physiologic responses may increase resistance to anesthesia, making it more difficult for the dentist to perform treatment comfortably. The auxiliary often can help the patient cope with or decrease the anxiety response by awareness of behavioral and psychologic issues involved.

An important issue is the patient's need for control. Depending on upbringing and experience, people exhibit characteristic needs to control their social and physical experience. Some people cope with their anxiety in the dental office by demanding to know everything about their treatment and requesting that they be consulted on every decision. Others go to the other extreme, desiring to turn everything over to the dental team and avoiding being given any information. Often, this second group will voice the wish that they could be put to sleep and awakened when everything is over. Of course, most people fall along the continuum between these two extremes. It is important that the auxiliary be aware of the patient's needs and responsive to these concerns.

The overcontrolling patient will be less of a problem if he or she is given complete information and allowed to participate in treatment planning within clearly defined limits. The patient should understand that the dental team must set certain rules if successful treatment is to be accomplished, but the auxiliary should realize that this patient will initiate fewer problems when kept fully informed. The patient who desires to give up all control and avoid knowledge may be even more of a problem. This patient often fails to fulfill home care instructions and, at times, may fail to provide informed consent to treatment. This patient also needs information to decrease anxiety, but, in this case, the patient should be educated slowly and carefully. Where possible, the patient should be encouraged to ask questions and participate in the decision making. Often, the overly compliant patient will secretly resist treatment and express hidden resentment at being controlled by failing to understand directions and becoming helpless in the chair.

A second issue is the way in which the patient perceives the events occurring around him or her and interprets the sensations felt in treatment. Besides the patient who has a firm hold on reality and who perceives accurately the events occurring in treatment, there are other types of patients. Some patients amplify every sensation they experience. Mild pressure or discomfort may be classified as pain. Every experience is magnified out of proportion. In their response to anxiety, these patients increase their vigilance. In contrast, some patients deny they feel or experience anything. They report to the dentist that they are not feeling any pain and that the dentist can proceed even without anesthesia. These patients may be so anxious about their pain and discomfort that they pretend that nothing is really happening. Unfortunately, when pain becomes overwhelming or the anxiety too great, the defense breaks down. The patient can no longer deny his or her experience and may panic. Another type of patient may distort the actual reality of the situation. For example, a very suspicious patient seeing two auxiliaries talking may assume they are talking about him or her.

With each of these types of patient behaviors, the auxiliary and dentist must work to improve the ability to perceive reality clearly. For example, the hypersensitive patient can be helped to distinguish between pressure and pain so that he or she can clearly determine what actually is being experienced. The clearer perception will reduce concern over treatment. The denying patient can be guided to recognize and accept the experience of treatment and to allow the dentist to provide appropriate anesthesia. The distorting patient should be given more information before and during treatment. At each point in treatment, what is occurring should be explained both carefully and slowly.

The third issue is the patient's perception of the dentist and the treatment team. Most people use their past experience to guess how new people will behave and think. They project characteristics about others. In the dental situation, the anxious patient often sees the members of the dental team as authority figures. The patient then irrationally expects them to have special powers, knowledge, or abilities. This psychologic process is called *transference*. Often, the patient will react to the dentist or dental team members positively or negatively in terms of these perceptions. The dental assistant should be alert to these magnified expectations and help the patient develop a more appropriate understanding of the treatment situation.

Questions

DIRECTIONS (Questions 1 through 42): Each of the questions or incomplete statements in this section is followed by four suggested answers or completions. Select the ONE lettered answer or completion that is BEST in each case. Check your answers with the correct answers at the end of the chapter.

1. The most effective method of decreasing a zero-sum conflict is to

   (A) clarify expectations
   (B) develop interdependence
   (C) make people agree to get along
   (D) ask each person to be more tolerant of the other

2. The best way to motivate adolescents toward good oral hygiene habits is by

   (A) social acceptance and appearance
   (B) monetary considerations
   (C) a detailed discussion of dental plaque
   (D) establishing feelings of security

3. An important method of improving the quality of interpersonal contracts is to

   (A) continually enforce the elements of the contract
   (B) make explicit expectations of the other
   (C) make the rewards more attractive
   (D) increase the dimensionality of the contract

4. One of the most important tasks of the auxiliary when attempting to support an anxious patient is to

   (A) be efficient
   (B) be calm and cool
   (C) be centered
   (D) be strong

5. The dental assistant's primary responsibility in patient management and the application of dental psychologic principles is to

   (A) enable the patient to accept and tolerate dental procedures

   (B) help the patient resolve psychologic problems
   (C) keep the patient still and quiet until the treatment is completed
   (D) maintain his or her own sanity

6. A major source of office conflict in a busy office is

   (A) laziness on the part of some of the staff
   (B) intolerance of interpersonal differences
   (C) tension resulting from working with many patients
   (D) unclear job roles and duties

7. Effective communication can take place only when

   (A) the sender (speaker) has presented himself or herself in a clear and concise manner
   (B) the message being sent is clear
   (C) the receiver understands the message being sent
   (D) feedback is present

8. One important aspect of communication is perception of the message being sent. What is one of the major influences affecting message perception?

   (A) the intentions of the sender
   (B) the expectations held by the receiver
   (C) the length of the message
   (D) the complexity of the message

9. A major determinant of how a particular behavior is interpreted is

   (A) the setting in which the behavior takes place
   (B) the level of anxiety of the receiver
   (C) the level of calmness of the sender
   (D) the timing of the behavior

10. An assistant has been providing oral health instruction to a 16-year-old girl who is receiving periodontic treatment. Her mother comes with her at each visit. The assistant notices that despite the amount of education he or she provides, the girl's oral health status does not improve. What might the assistant do?

 (A) inform the mother that she should remind the girl to take care of her mouth
 (B) tell the girl that if she does not begin to develop oral hygiene habits, she will lose her teeth
 (C) yell at the girl for being so uncooperative
 (D) teach the girl how to assess the health of her oral cavity

11. The major purpose of giving feedback to another person is

 (A) to induce the other to change behavior
 (B) to let the other know that he or she is being heard
 (C) to correct behavior that has gotten out of hand
 (D) to provide information for decision making

12. In managing the hostile or aggressive patient, the auxiliary is most likely to be successful if he or she

 (A) directly challenges the patient and threatens to dismiss him or her
 (B) gives up, backs down, and lets the patient have his or her way
 (C) establishes clear but limited options for the patient
 (D) refuses to see the patient until the patient agrees to behave

13. If applying Maslow's hierarchy of needs to plaque control instruction

 (A) feelings of self-actualization must be present before learning can begin
 (B) the basic need of the patient is to relate well to the auxiliary
 (C) if the patient has not satisfied his basic needs, he will be more receptive to changes in oral hygiene
 (D) certain needs of the patient must be satisfied before practicing oral hygiene

14. When treating a pedodontic patient, the dentist's first concern should be

 (A) to establish a rapport with the parents
 (B) to obtain a thorough dental–medical history
 (C) to establish a rapport with the child
 (D) to ensure that both parents and child know the dentist is the boss while the child is at the dental office

15. A patient always does exactly what she is told. She never asks questions or makes any requests. How can an assistant help her to increase the likelihood that her treatment will really meet her needs?

 (A) give her very clear instructions and always be firm in expectations
 (B) encourage her to ask questions and to express her doubts
 (C) request the dentist to take very special care of her
 (D) ask her to bring in someone else with her to be present when you give her information or education

16. In a dental office, a characteristic of the work group that is very likely to be noticed by the patient but not by the people working in the office is

 (A) a special language that has developed among the staff
 (B) a set of norms and rules that has developed among the working staff
 (C) a set of power hierarchies that have developed
 (D) the efficiency and interest of the working class

17. The first step in eliciting a patient's compliance with a home care regimen is

 (A) telling the patient that he or she must take better care of the oral tissue
 (B) educating the patient how to care for his or her teeth and other oral tissues
 (C) helping the patient recognize that home care is necessary for healthy teeth
 (D) warning the patient that if the oral tissues are not taken care of, he or she will lose the teeth

18. Most defensive behavior represents

 (A) basic personality structure
 (B) learned behavior
 (C) difficulty in accepting treatment
 (D) an inability to relate to authority

19. A patient has come into the office with a troubled look on his face and a complaint. He starts his conversation with an insult and then begins to criticize everything about the office and the dentist. The assistant's most appropriate response at this point would be to

 (A) ask the patient to leave
 (B) provide an explanation or apology for each complaint
 (C) engage in active listening
 (D) become occupied in some paper work or other work until the patient calms down and behaves more appropriately

20. Active listening involves

(A) being alert and attentive
(B) checking perceptions
(C) leaning forward and showing interest
(D) being a concerned listener

21. The primary requirement of reinforcement when used to modify behavior is that it is

(A) visible and tangible
(B) simple for the auxiliary to administer
(C) inexpensive and easily obtained
(D) adequate to elicit the behavior

22. One reason that the use of restatement will help stop an argument is

(A) the persons involved are forced to listen to one another
(B) the persons involved can distinguish between understanding and agreement
(C) it slows down the pace and forces the participants to think
(D) it forces each party to more closely examine the other's ideas

23. An 80-year-old man who has been a patient of the same dentist for a long time is having problems with his dentures, which were constructed 2 years ago. They just do not feel right to him. The doctor has told the patient that there is nothing really wrong with the dentures and suggested that the patient likes the attention and expects special treatment, since he has been a patient for many years. The patient has just called for a long appointment because he feels that his dentures need a lot of adjustment. The assistant checks the doctor's schedule and discovers that the next available appointment is 2 weeks away and informs the patient, who becomes very angry, refuses the appointment, and demands to speak to the dentist. What probably went wrong?

(A) the patient is just a general problem, and the assistant should not have had to deal with him
(B) the patient is getting senile and does not understand that the doctor is very busy
(C) the patient expects that he will be taken immediately and cannot stand the frustration of being put off for so long
(D) the patient does not feel that the assistant is giving him the attention and concern he deserves

24. A very effective method of lowering patient anxiety is to

(A) sing to him or her
(B) use a quiet voice and show a calm manner

(C) give clear explanations
(D) ignore the upset and work slowly giving the patient time to calm down

25. It is very important that the dentist elicit the patient's most mature level of coping with the anxiety raised by the dental visit. One form of coping that can create real problems with treatment is

(A) denial
(B) aggression
(C) countertransference
(D) transference

26. A patient in the office is a very intense 7-year-old girl. She asks the assistant many questions about her teeth and seems to be very interested when the assistant teaches her how to brush her teeth. In fact, the dentist had to fill cavities in four different teeth and would like to get her to brush more often. How might the assistant encourage her to become more involved in her home care?

(A) tell her that she will have more cavities if she does not brush
(B) promise her a prize if she has no cavities on her next visit
(C) give her a new toothbrush
(D) provide her with disclosing tablets and teach her how to use them

27. A major fear that many handicapped patients feel when coming to the dental office is

(A) that they will not be able to tolerate treatment
(B) that the dentist will not want to treat them
(C) that they will be further mutilated
(D) pain

28. A 35-year-old woman is having trouble disciplining herself to comply with appropriate oral care activities. The assistant and patient have decided to develop a behavior modification protocol to help her establish new habits. After establishing that she desires to change her present behavior, the first step for the assistant is to

(A) specify the behavior she wants to change
(B) develop a very special rapport with the patient
(C) give the patient encouragement
(D) tell the patient how great her mouth is going to feel when she develops new oral habits

29. Two auxiliaries in the office have managed to get locked into a competitive struggle over who is going to do patient education and work chairside. It seems that one person—the one who works with patients—gets all the interesting jobs, and the other always ends up doing paper work and answering phones. The conflict is beginning to interfere with performance. A good approach toward ending the conflict would be for each auxiliary to

(A) sit down with the other and talk it out
(B) go to the dentist and tell him or her to choose between them
(C) ignore the other
(D) accommodate the other without inconveniencing himself or herself

30. A dental assistant is charged with the responsibility of providing support to anxious patients. The auxiliary must always remember that

(A) fatigue causes depression and feelings of helplessness
(B) if fears and anxieties are not focused on, they will go away
(C) feelings are real
(D) everyone is motivated by their unconscious

31. A mother has brought her 5-year-old son to the office because one of his primary teeth was slow to fall out. The dentist had to remove the tooth. It would be helpful to allow the child to take his tooth home because having the tooth will allow him to

(A) make money from the tooth fairy
(B) relieve his sense of body harm or loss
(C) bring a gift to his mother
(D) remember what went on in the office

32. A 59-year-old man has been told that because of periodontal problems and resultant bone loss, he is going to lose several teeth. His primary concern is likely to be

(A) that he is going to look bad
(B) that he is losing health and vitality
(C) that his body is going to suffer harm
(D) that the dentist disapproves of him for allowing this to occur

33. The most difficult type of behavior to change is

(A) approach behavior
(B) habitual behavior
(C) escape behavior
(D) aggressive behavior

34. A dental assistant has been talking to a quiet, withdrawn woman about 24 years old concerning oral health self-care and is concerned about her responses. Since the patient does not talk much, the assistant is uncertain as to whether she is really listening. How might the assistant discover whether the patient is involved?

(A) observe how the patient positions her body relative to the assistant
(B) check to see whether the patient maintains eye contact
(C) ask the patient whether she understands
(D) watch to see how often the patient says, "I understand," "Okay," "Yes," and other such comments

35. A patient is always 15 minutes to a half-hour late for her dental appointments. At each appointment, the assistant reminds her to come on time, but she continues to be late. What might the assistant do to reduce the probability that the patient will continue to arrive late?

(A) inform them later of an extra charge
(B) threaten to not give the patient an appointment if she comes late again
(C) cancel the patient's appointment if she is more than 5 minutes late
(D) schedule their appointment in your appointment book 15 minutes after the time you listed on their appointment card

36. When meeting the patient for the first time, the auxiliary should be aware of his or her tendency to

(A) want to take care of the patient
(B) stereotype the patient
(C) like the patient
(D) accept what the patient says

37. Sometimes a patient will elicit strong anger in an assistant. At those times, the assistant will probably be most effective if he or she

(A) swallows the anger and gets on with the job
(B) punishes the patient and gets it over with
(C) recognizes the anger and tries to understand what it is that leads to the reaction
(D) recognizes that since he or she gets along with most patients, there is probably something wrong with the patient

38. In the office, feedback to other auxiliaries or to patients is most likely to be helpful when it is

(A) given gently
(B) given nonjudgmentally
(C) given firmly
(D) very tactful

39. A patient persists in exhibiting inappropriate behavior in the office each time he comes. He makes wisecracks at the auxiliaries and goes into the office, where he does not belong. The dental auxiliary can help this patient by

(A) reminding him firmly of office rules
(B) asking the doctor to offer him premedication (sedation)
(C) yelling at him and threatening to throw him out of the office
(D) calling his wife and requesting that she deal with him

40. A 15-year-old orthodontic patient is not properly or consistently cleaning his teeth and oral tissues under his appliance. Despite reminders from the dentist and continual pressure from his parents, he continues to neglect his care instructions. To increase compliance, the dentist should

(A) check to see whether the patient has friends who are telling him it is unnecessary to be so worried about his teeth. If so, provide him with better instruction and education
(B) check to see whether the parents are using correct terminology when speaking with their son and to see whether they fully understand what is to be done
(C) attempt to establish an agreement with the adolescent concerning the self-care needed and the probable outcome of neglect
(D) threaten to discontinue treatment if the adolescent does not shape up

41. One of the best cues for discovering how receptive one person is to another is to observe

(A) the number of statements of interest
(B) the tone of voice
(C) the amount of eye contact that occurs
(D) body posture and body language

42. People who do not face the person to whom they are speaking are often

(A) being rude
(B) avoiding intimacy
(C) not involved in the discussion
(D) in a hurry

DIRECTIONS (Questions 43 through 46): For each of the items in this section, ONE or MORE of the numbered options is correct. Choose answer

A   if only 1, 2, and 3 are correct
B   if only 1 and 3 are correct
C   if only 2 and 4 are correct
D   if only 4 is correct
E   if all are correct

43. Children and adolescents are similar in some ways but very different in others. Which patient management strategies tend to be different for adolescents and children?

(1) the use of praise
(2) enlisting the parents' support and cooperation
(3) avoiding particular words
(4) showing interest and concern regarding the problem

44. Letting a child hold a mirror and watch what the dentist is doing in his or her mouth is based on the notion that

(1) children will be distracted from their concerns by playing with the mirror
(2) children fear mutilation and are calmed by seeing that they are not being extensively damaged
(3) children need something to do while they are being treated
(4) children have a need to participate actively in their treatment

45. A very experienced dental assistant has gained a position of power and influence in an office after being there for only a short period of time. What has likely led to her position of influence and power?

(1) she takes the time to find out what is going on in the office
(2) she keeps quiet and waits to be asked to participate in office activities; she is not pushy
(3) she is very experienced and lets everyone know
(4) she offers to help out wherever she can

46. Being able to provide appropriate and helpful feedback is an important skill for the dental assistant to possess. Feedback is likely to be most effective when it is

(1) used to describe a particular behavior just exhibited by the patient
(2) used to alert or reassure the patient that the assistant is paying attention
(3) used to inform the patient about a problem that was the result of his or her behavior
(4) used tactfully to tell a patient that he or she has stepped out of line

Answers and Explanations

1. **(B)** Zero-sum conflicts are the result of competition. The individuals are in conflict because they want the same thing or object, such as vacation time or desk space. This type of conflict is best resolved by negotiation, compromise, and the addition of new resources.

2. **(A)** The best way to motivate adolescents toward good oral hygiene habits is by emphasizing the relationship between good daily oral hygiene and social appearance. This will encourage social acceptance among their particular age group.

3. **(B)** The quality of the interpersonal contract is based on the clarity and mutual understanding and acceptance of its provisions.

4. **(C)** The anxious patient needs to test reality. The auxiliary must give the patient his or her complete attention and not become distracted by other events occurring in the office. In addition, the auxiliary must be careful not to bring problems from home into the office. The reaction to the patient's behavior should be to that behavior and not the result of a delayed reaction to a problem at home.

5. **(A)** The goal of the dental assistant is to decrease patient problems during treatment. Just keeping the patient quiet is not enough, as it is important for the patient to participate in his or her treatment. It is not the dental assistant's job (or training) to resolve psychologic problems that arise in the office.

6. **(D)** A sense of resentment and betrayal is often a result of a confusion over who is to do what. Most office conflicts are not a result of personality clashes or personal problems but rather are a result of a lack of cooperation among staff in getting work done.

7. **(C)** Communications success is determined ultimately by the receiver's ability to understand the message sent, not by the sender's skill in sending the message. Communication is, by definition, the development of a shared meaning, not simply sending a message.

8. **(B)** The receiver interprets what he or she hears, feels, and sees. The human organism is an information-processing organism, and all information is interpreted in the light of its meaning for the receiver. Therefore, expectations (eg, suspicions, hopes, fears) will determine the importance and meaning of the information received.

9. **(A)** Behavior always occurs within a social context. The context determines, in large part, the appropriateness and meaning of a behavior.

10. **(D)** An adolescent needs to feel respected by adults. By enlisting the patient in her treatment, the auxiliary signals the feeling that the patient is capable and dependable. Attacking the patient will further alienate the patient. Since adolescents are trying to develop independence from their parents, enlisting the parents is likely to cause more problems than it solves.

11. **(B)** Feedback is, by definition, a process of mirroring an individual's behavior. Feedback is information about the outcomes of one's behavior.

12. **(C)** Establishing clear but limited options is a method of guiding the patient in a nonhostile or nondefensive way. Attacking the patient or giving in to the patient is not likely to produce a productive outcome for the office or the patient.

13. **(D)** According to Maslow, lower order needs must be satisfied before the patient will be receptive to learning and accepting new dental procedures, such as oral hygiene instruction. If a patient is hungry or very apprehensive, he or she will not respond well to the dental auxiliary's instructions, since lower-order needs must be satisfied first before learning.

14. **(C)** Children are very self-centered. The dentist must begin by establishing a positive relationship with the patient so that the patient will want to please him or her.

15. (B) Often, anxious or highly dependent patients give up all decision making and control to the dentist. This can be a problem both legally and in terms of self-care. One way to elicit ownership of a patient's dental problems and his or her care is to support the patient in questioning and raising issues about his or her state of oral health.

16. (A) In all groups, norms, rules, and power relationships are developed and explicitly supported by their members. The office members introduce patients and new members of the office to these characteristics. However, as people work together, their working vocabulary changes. They adopt special words and phrases that speed up communication. These code words become commonplace to the group members and go unnoticed by them, but the patient will be aware of these words because of their unfamiliarity in general discussion.

17. (C) All efforts to elicit a patient's motivation begin with having the patient recognize that a problem exists and that the patient's activity will make a difference. Just telling a patient that he or she should be concerned or threatening the patient with long-term punishment is not likely to be effective. Education in method should occur after the patient's interest is elicited.

18. (B) Most situational behavior as defensive behavior is a result of past experience.

19. (C) Some people react to feelings of anxiety with aggression or hostility. Active listening will enable the dental assistant to identify and respond helpfully to the anxiety or concern presented by the patient. Hostility or defensiveness tends to provoke more hostility. Ignoring the patient is a form of aggression.

20. (B) Active listening is by definition a process in which the listener works with the speaker to create meaning. In the process of checking perceptions, the listener clarifies and corrects his or her perceptions. Signaling or pretending that one is paying attention is not active listening.

21. (D) Unless the reinforcement is attractive enough to elicit the behavior desired of the patient, it will not be adequate for use in a behavior modification protocol.

22. (A) In order to restate another's comments, an individual must be able to understand and formulate what he or she said. In addition, this process makes clear to the other that the disagreement is not due to lack of understanding but a different perception of the situation.

23. (D) The patient believes that he has developed a special relationship with the office and the dentist. In his mind, the contract calls for special attention. He, therefore, feels the assistant is violating this contract and treating him unfairly. If he felt that the assistant was aware and respectful of his special status, he would probably accept the appointment offered.

24. (C) Anxiety is a fear of something fantasized or unknown. The explanation will serve to focus the patient's concerns and enable him or her to apply specific skills.

25. (A) Denial is a way of fending off anxiety. However, when pain or discomfort becomes too intense to deny, the patient is likely to feel out of control and panic. Countertransference is not a form of coping. Aggression can be controlled easily by clear limits and firmness. Transference is a valuable support for therapeutic alliance as long as distortions are clarified.

26. (D) Since the child is 7, she is likely to be concerned with her ability to do things and very concrete in her thinking. Disclosing tablets will enable her to actually see the problem of plaque and recognize when she has been successful in cleaning her teeth. Threatening her and promising a prize are external motivators and less likely to be effective on a daily basis.

27. (B) Handicapped patients often pose special problems of logistics in delivery of treatment. These problems might previously have led health providers to reject the patient.

28. (A) All behavior modification protocols begin with a specification and measurement of the actual target behavior. Behavior is the focus of the effort rather than an attempt to change attitudes or feelings.

29. (D) Since the conflict is not related to a violated expectation or a betrayal but is related to a competition for scarce resources, it is more effective to engage in tradeoffs and bargaining. The Osgood solution is an effective strategy for zero-sum conflicts.

30. (C) For the patient, the feelings he or she experiences are current reality. To deny the feelings is to deny the patient's experience. It is the auxiliary's job to help the patient to clarify his or her perceptions of the dental office experience.

31. (B) A primary concern of the young child is body integrity. The child sees the alteration or loss of any body part as an assault on the body's integrity. The lost tooth is an important (psychologic) part of the child's body.

32. **(B)** In middle age, the individual becomes aware of his or her own mortality. The loss of teeth is seen by the patient as a signal of loss of vitality or health. It is important to reassure the patient that the progress of disease can be halted, and the loss of teeth is not a sign of a general body deterioration or aging.

33. **(C)** Escape behavior is self-reinforcing and, therefore, beyond the control of the auxiliary. The outcomes of approach behavior and aggressive behavior usually are accessible to the auxiliary, and habits can be intercepted or modified by presenting alternative behavioral possibilities.

34. **(A)** Body language is less amenable to conscious control than verbal reactions. Eye contact often is not a good indicator because many people are taught to make eye contact when speaking to an authority and do so in the absence of real attention.

35. **(D)** It may be best to make the appointment entry 15 minutes after the time listed on the patient's appointment card to ensure that a habitually late patient will arrive on time.

36. **(B)** In an effort to predict the patient, the auxiliary is likely to project personal characteristics on the patient that he or she has observed in similar patients in the past. Everyone uses experiences to prepare for new situations. Wanting to take care of the patient, liking the patient, and accepting what the patient says are actions resulting from the auxiliary's stereotyped impressions of the patient.

37. **(C)** The anger is the result of a reaction to the behavior of another. The behavior is not the cause of the anger. If the auxiliary understands the source of the anger, he or she will be better able to adapt suitably to the patient's behavior.

38. **(B)** Feedback is intended to be informational. Its goal is to provide information that can be used in self-change. If the feedback is judgmental, regardless of how tactfully or gently it is given, it will evoke the patient's need to defend himself or herself.

39. **(A)** The patient's inappropriate behavior is probably due to his anxiety concerning dental treatment. The dental assistant can help him control his anxiety by more clearly structuring the situation for him. Punishing him is only going to increase his anxiety; sedating him will only increase his sense of helplessness and confusion.

40. **(C)** The most effective method of working with an adolescent is to establish a therapeutic alliance in which the adolescent's need to be appropriate and responsible is elicited. Adolescents are concerned about the quality of their relationships with impor-

tant others. By building a positive relationship, the dentist can increase the patient's need to comply with treatment.

41. **(D)** Body posture is a form of body language. Body orientation and the way the body is held (eg, tense, alert, slumped) provide important clues to the person's emotions, concerns, and interests.

42. **(B)** Body orientation is an indicator of psychologic attention. Often when an emotional reaction to the interaction is too intense for the participant, he or she will turn away to decrease the sense of contact.

43. **(A)** Since children are very concerned with competence, the dental assistant should avoid criticism. Adolescents, being more concerned with how the dental assistant feels about them, are more likely to benefit from a balance of praise and criticism. Parents will play a strong part in the child's treatment but the treatment will probably be more effective if the parent is not included in the adolescent's treatment. Including the parents may elicit the normal power struggles of adolescence. Children are more sensitive to loaded words than are adolescents.

44. **(C)** Children are very concrete in their thinking. Their fantasies are more frightening than reality. Being able to see exactly the limits of what is occurring will allow them to cope appropriately with their fears. Children feel more comfortable if they are actively participating rather than being passive. It is important to tell the child what to do rather than what not to do.

45. **(B)** Knowledge is a primary source of power. People tend to listen to the individual who appears to have the knowledge necessary to complete the current task. The auxiliary who either enters with technical knowledge or has acquired information about the office is most likely to be able to influence the outcomes of others.

46. **(B)** Feedback should be presented nonjudgmentally and serve the function of providing factual information a patient can use to modify his or her behavior.

BIBLIOGRAPHY

Berni R, Fordyce W. *Behavior Modification and the Nursing Process*, 2nd ed. St. Louis: CV Mosby Co, 1977.

Craig CJ. *Human Development*, 5th ed. Englewood Cliffs, NJ: Prentice-Hall, 1989.

Dworkins SF, Ference TP, Giddon DB. *Behavioral Science and Dental Practice*. St. Louis: CV Mosby Co, 1978.

Froelich RE, Bishop FM, Dworkins SF. *Communication in*

the Dental Office: A Programmed Manual for the Dental Professional. St. Louis: CV Mosby Co, 1976.

Goffman E. *The Presentation of Self in Everyday Life.* New York: Doubleday and Co, Inc, 1959.

Havinghurst R. *Developmental Tasks and Education*, 3rd ed. New York: McKay Publishers, 1972.

Hirsch S, Hittelman E. Effective communication. *General Dentistry*, 1978; **26**:38–43.

Ingersoll B. *Behavioral Aspects in Dentistry.* New York: Appleton-Century-Crofts, 1982.

Malamed B, Siegel S. *Behavioral Medicine: Practical Application in Health Care.* New York: Springer Publishing Co, Inc, 1980.

Mayerson E. *Putting the Ill at Ease.* New York: Harper & Row, 1976.

Morton J, et al. *Dental Teamwork Strategies*, 6th ed. St. Louis: CV Mosby Co, 1987.

Morton JC, Rickey CA. *Building Assertive Skills.* St. Louis: CV Mosby Co, 1980.

Smith F. Management of the child patient and the handicapped patient. *Clinical Dentistry* Vol. 1, Chapter 33.

Weinstein P, Getz T. *Changing Human Behavior: Strategies for Preventive Dentistry.* St. Louis: CV Mosby Co, 1979.

CHAPTER 10

Dental Practice Management

INTRODUCTION

Dentistry is both a profession and a business. Practice administration, as it is perceived in the world of modern dentistry, is crucial to establishing an efficient, effective practice. A dental practice cannot be effective unless it is efficient, and both can be accomplished only when the entire dental team uses basic operational business skills. The responsibilities of the business office assistant may include basic accounting and bookkeeping skills, appointment control, collections and financial payment arrangements, maintenance of the office inventory system, corresponding and processing dental insurance forms, and implementing supervisory skills when indicated. This chapter provides an overview of the business aspect of the dental practice and the role of the business office auxiliary.

THE OFFICE MANUAL

An office manual is a reference guide that contains detailed descriptions of all office policies and procedures. Information about the following aspects of the practice should be included.

1. The doctor's philosophy of practice (ie, goals and objectives)
2. Job descriptions for all members of the dental team
3. Employment policies (eg, working hours, vacation, sick leave, overtime, holidays)
4. Office policies for the staff (eg, dress code, conduct, staff meetings)
5. Guidelines for appropriate office communication (eg, telephone technique, reception policies, written correspondence, patient education)
6. Policies for management of office records (eg, clinical and financial patient records, payment and collection procedures, accounts receivable, accounts payable, insurance coverage, recalls, inventory)
7. Guidelines for clinical procedures (eg, preparation of tray setups, sterilization techniques, prescriptions, laboratory interactions)
8. Medical emergency office protocol and procedures

The guidelines set forth in the manual summarize office policies, reflect the characteristics of the practice, and enable the office to run smoothly from both a clinical and a management perspective. In addition, when a new employee joins the practice, the manual facilitates his or her integration into the practice. The office manual, which should be updated regularly, is an invaluable resource that promotes sound management and allows the office to run more efficiently.

The business assistant clearly performs an integral role in office administration. Tasks may vary as a function of the managerial style of the dentist, but the application of well-organized management techniques results in a successful office that provides fulfillment to the doctor, staff, and patients. It is the business assistant's responsibility to understand the principles of office administration and to employ them daily.

TELEPHONE COMMUNICATION

Every assistant should be aware that the telephone is an essential piece of equipment in the dental office. Without it, and more importantly, without using it properly, a dentist cannot practice effectively. More than 95% of a dentist's business results from telephone calls, and the majority of new patients make the initial contact by telephone. Therefore, it is imperative that the telephone image conveyed by the auxiliary encourage a friendly, trusting attitude in the caller.

The production of dental services is the main function of the dentist. To maximize the delivery of services, it is necessary to keep delaying factors at a minimum level. Delaying factors include most telephone calls from patients, unexpected salespeople, family, and friends. All calls should be screened so that the doctor speaks only to patients who cannot be helped by the assistant.

When a caller questions fees, his or her concern should be addressed by an explanation that fees are contingent on procedures involved. Since a diagnosis cannot be determined over the telephone, a patient inquiring about fees should be scheduled for an examination and told that the dentist will discuss all fees before rendering any treatment.

If a telephone answering machine is used when the

office is closed, the recorded message should be clear and understandable. The speaker should request pertinent information (eg, name, telephone number, including the area code, and purpose of the call, that is, chief dental problem) and provide the caller with a clear understanding of what will happen as a result of the call (eg, the call will be returned, the caller should contact the doctor at another number, or the caller should contact another doctor who will see patients in emergency situations).

In all telephone communication, the assistant's courtesy, diplomacy, and poise can make the difference between a steady stream of loyal, cooperative patients and a steady stream of frustration and problems.

PATIENT RECEPTION

The business assistant is the key public relations member of the office team because he or she makes the first contact with patients, both on the telephone and in the reception area. During the initial interaction with new patients, first impressions often form lasting impressions, and consequently the assistant should make an effort to be courteous and pleasant at all times. The first meeting is a time for exchanging information and familiarizing the patient with office procedures. A warm friendly greeting by auxiliaries can engender the same feelings toward the doctor even before the patient and doctor meet. Apprehensive patients are extended a feeling of reassurance and calmness by the office assistant.

The reception area must be clean, and patients should be greeted promptly on arrival. Patient arrivals should be made known to the doctor as quickly as possible via a signal system. If the dentist is delayed, patients who are waiting should be notified and told approximately how long it will be before they will be seen by the doctor. This information will clarify to all patients that the office has respect for both their time and the doctor's, and this consideration is always appreciated.

PATIENTS' RECORDS

A series of records should be maintained for each patient. A case history form that includes the patient's past and present medical and dental health histories should be updated periodically to avoid potential medical emergencies and legal problems. Diagnostic materials include x-ray films, information noted at the clinical examination, and study models. A patient information sheet contains the record of existing conditions and a prioritized treatment plan designed for each patient on the basis of the doctor's diagnosis. The plan enables the dentist to systematically meet the dental needs of the patient and enables the business assistant to facilitate the course of treatment by knowing the procedures required, the order of procedures, the person who will perform each procedure (ie, the dentist, an assistant, or a hygienist), the time required for each procedure, and the total fee for services to be rendered. Permanent record cards are maintained for each

patient and contain specific notations of all treatment performed, the date on which it was performed, materials used, the prognosis, and other relevant information.

Individually and collectively, these records protect both the patient and the dentist should treatment discrepancies arise. Patient records are confidential histories of financial and treatment experiences that cannot be released or made public without the patient's permission. Before any records leave the office (eg, for insurance purposes or consultation with a specialist), duplicate copies should be made for legal protection.

RECORD AND BOOKKEEPING SYSTEMS

A record and bookkeeping system encompasses all paperwork pertaining to the dental practice, ranging from the appointment book, which is usually the first place that the patient's name appears, to collection control, which is often the last. The system must be completely standardized and organized, since accurate and adequate records provide a comprehensive history of past and present patient treatment, production records that enable the dentist to assess expenses periodically through cost accounting, and precise tax information. These records also can prevent or resolve malpractice involvement. All records must be complete and accurately documented in ink for legal purposes. Keep in mind that the dental record is permissible as evidence in a court of law and usually the single most valuable piece of evidence in a malpractice case.

APPOINTMENT BOOK AND DAY SHEET

The appointment book is the control center of office activity. A mismanaged appointment book can destroy a potentially fine practice by wasting the doctor's productive time or by creating a schedule that results in a reception room becoming a waiting room filled with unhappy patients. For optimum control, the appointment book should be the responsibility of the business assistant, who has an overview of all doctor–patient activity, knowledge of patient availability in relation to office availability, and an understanding of the amount of time necessary for treatment planned.

Time and motion studies have shown that one of the most efficient formats of an appointment book is the week-at-a-glance style. The format enables the assistant to balance the workload appropriately by noting available time during the week. The patient's name, phone number, and procedure scheduled for that time slot should be printed in pencil to provide easy reading and to allow any changes to be entered neatly.

In advance, certain periods of time should be matrixed or blocked out (eg, lunch and dinner hours, holidays, when the office will be closed, vacation time, and professional meetings when the doctor will not be in the office).

Time should be prioritized to reflect the periods of the

day that are valued most highly and the type of patients who will be appointed during that time. The preferences of the doctor and working schedules of business people should be reflected in this determination. Elderly patients and young children should be scheduled early in the day, a time when they will be most cooperative. Patients with special needs, such as medical problems or handicaps, also should be considered when scheduling dental appointments. In addition, a philosophy for emergency patients should be developed. Some offices reserve buffer periods for unexpected emergencies, whereas others work them into existing schedules.

Broken appointments and cancellations may disrupt the most organized office. Patients who repeatedly break appointments or cancel them with insufficient notice should be made aware that this is unacceptable behavior. Time created, however, should be used efficiently, and a call list that contains patients' names, telephone numbers, and times they are available on short notice should be created for maximum use of office resources.

Most efficient offices schedule patients in time units. The most frequent unit selected is a period of 15 minutes. Therefore, a patient being appointed for a procedure requiring 45 minutes would be scheduled for three units of time in the appointment book. Unit scheduling provides a realistic mechanism for controlling the workload and allows the dental team to adhere to the schedule throughout the day. Scheduling a patient for a 15-minute appointment when the actual time needed is a half-hour is one of the reasons that some offices consistently work overtime. To alleviate improper scheduling and to ensure that each patient will be appointed appropriately for the next visit before he or she is dismissed, the doctor or the chairside assistant must provide the person controlling the appointment book with information about the procedure planned in units of time required for the patient's next appointment.

Adequate time should be allotted between appointments if indicated to complete necessary dental laboratory work for the scheduled dental patients of the day.

The day sheet is a replica of the appointment book for the day and should be placed in each treatment room. This schedule provides the dentist and auxiliaries in the operatories with the information necessary to eliminate checking the appointment book to determine who is expected, when he or she is expected, and the treatment planned. The day sheet also enables the staff to plan ahead and minimize delaying factors by preparing the next patient in the treatment room with necessary instruments and materials.

THE RECALL SYSTEM

A responsive recall system is essential to every dental office. It reflects a supportive attitude that encourages patients to maintain proper oral health for a lifetime. At the end of each series of treatments, the dentist or the assistant should remind the patient that they should return for an examination after a given interval of time. The atmosphere created should be motivating and reflect concern for the patient's health, but it should be clear that maintenance and recall are a dual responsibility, and patients who fail to respond may compromise their oral health.

Recall methods vary. Some offices telephone patients, others send written reminders, and others use a combination of telephone and mail notices. Once the method. of recall is chosen, a recall file that can be used and updated easily should be established. A patient's recall card should be separated from his or her clinical chart, and each family member should have an individual recall card, since the length of time between examinations may vary.

A standard recall method of record keeping includes the two-card system for each patient: one card is designated by the month during which the recall visit should occur, and the other is alphabetical by patient name. For reference, the monthly card should be filed in a box divided in the same manner. Each card should include the patient's name, complete home and business address, telephone number, and preferred type of reminder (written or phone). The recall card can be used also to keep a record of the patient's recall pattern.

Alphabetical cards can be filed on a revolving desk file and should include the patient's name, type of reminder preferred, and date of the last appointment. This file also serves as a tickler file and is easily accessible if a patient should call to inquire about the recall or to request treatment earlier than the scheduled time. Some newer record-keeping systems employ the computer to update monthly patient recalls and send out reminders for the patients who have not made an appointment.

FINANCIAL RECORD KEEPING, PAYMENT ARRANGEMENTS, AND COLLECTION

Accurate financial records must be maintained for both efficiency and legal protection, and the actual bookkeeping is only as valuable as the detail and accuracy with which it is maintained. The simplest system is single-entry bookkeeping, which records only payments. The double-entry system records both the debit (charges) and credit (payments) for each office transaction. The two entries provide the necessary information to balance the financial records and provide duplicate records in the event that a patient's card is lost or destroyed. Many offices use a pegboard system, a form of double entry that allows two or more office records to be written at one time through the use of carbon paper and pegs that stabilize punched forms in the correct position. Some large dental practices use electronic data-processing systems involving computers to record production and financial data, recall dates, and any other desired information.

Every office has a policy about payments. A dental practice cannot survive if there is an inordinate amount of accounts receivable (money owed to the dentist for treatment completed). Fees charged for services rendered represent the dentist's earnings, but only payments actually received constitute income. For the practice to be profitable, income must exceed overhead, which is the cost of the resources needed to produce dentistry, including rent, salaries, supplies, laboratory procedures, and so forth.

Credit experts indicate that delinquent accounts over 90 days old are the most difficult and often impossible to collect. In order to minimize accounts receivable, all patients should be informed of the exact financial obligation before treatment is begun. Various payment policies and methods should be offered as a means of making the responsibility less burdensome. Payment methods include cash, checks, money orders, credit cards, and bank plans. There are many payment policies, but those shown in Table 10–1 are the most common.

Although proper payment arrangements may be made, some patients fail to fulfill their obligations and honor the method of payment to which they have agreed. The business assistant should monitor payment arrangements continuously. As a patient makes the next appointment, the assistant should check to see whether payment is due. If the patient is defaulting and payment is not forthcoming, the assistant should address the issue. Patients should not be given the option of whether to pay but rather of how to pay. If patients offer excuses rather than payments, they should be informed that they may either mail the payment (a stamped, self-addressed envelope should be provided) or bring it in at the next visit.

If a patient continues to default, the assistant should remind the patient that arrangements were agreed on and

determine whether there is a need to renegotiate the contract and ask the patient to select an alternate method of payment. Although many people tend to pay dental obligations last, most will adhere as agreed after being reminded of their responsibilities.

Statements should be used minimally as a mechanism for reminding patients of balance to date, when a patient has stopped treatment before completion, or when they have finished treatment sooner than expected. Statements are used to remind patients of divided payment agreements, noting the dates and amounts of expected payments.

A small percentage of patients complete treatment with an outstanding balance. These patients should be sent several statements at regular intervals (eg, every 30 days). If the patient does not respond, telephone follow-up should be initiated. If these efforts are unsuccessful, the patient should be informed that if payment is not received on a specified date, the matter will be referred for collection. Most people are concerned with collection referral, since their credit rating can be jeopardized.

THIRD PARTY CARRIERS (INSURANCE PROCEDURES)

An increased number of people have dental insurance coverage, and it is estimated that this population will be enlarged annually. As a result, insurance claim management is an important duty of the business assistant. Managing insurance coverage in a positive manner often results in practice growth because

1. Patients accept comprehensive care, since the cost of treatment is defrayed by coverage
2. People who previously did not seek oral health care are taking advantage of third party coverage
3. Accounts receivable often are reduced substantially due to payments received directly from insurance carriers.

Many forms of insurance coverage exist. Insurance companies may reimburse the doctor or the patient for dental services rendered. The amount of reimbursement may be based on usual, customary, or reasonable fees (UCR)—an amount considered standard for the procedure in a given community—or on a fixed amount determined by the carrier for each procedure. Some plans are organized on a prepayment basis, such as HMOs and PPOs, where the doctor receives a fixed amount of money for each patient for a specified period of time. Under this system, also known as capitation, the dentist receives the same amount of money regardless of the type and amount of care delivered. Patients covered by this type of insurance seek care only from participating dentists, who constitute a closed panel. The business assistant should be familiar with the organization of different types of coverage and understand how they affect the payments between the dentist and the patient.

For maximum efficiency, a patient's insurance forms should not be located with the clinical records. A separate

TABLE 10–1. PAYMENT POLICY METHODS

Method	Definition
Advanced payment	Payment before treatment is the most desirable, since billing, collection problems and accounts receivable are eliminated.
Fixed amount	The total fee is divided by the approximate number of sessions projected for completion of the treatment, and a fixed amount is expected from the patient at each visit, regardless of the actual charge for particular treatment rendered during the visit.
Divided payment	The total fee is divided into three amounts. The initial payment, usually larger than the other two, is collected when treatment commences. The balance, which is divided in half, is due when treatment is half completed and a visit or two before treatment is completed.
Open account	Patients are sent statements (forms indicating the financial status of their accounts) after treatment is rendered. This method often results in high accounts receivable, since most patients are unaware of their obligations until they receive statements, are often unprepared to pay for services rendered, or take a substantial amount of time to complete payment.

insurance file should be maintained and checked periodically to ensure prompt claim processing.

The insured patient should be aware of individual benefits, and the business assistant often can increase or clarify this understanding. This knowledge encourages acceptance of total treatment plans because the patient understands his or her financial responsibilities and those of the insurer. The doctor's treatment planning also may be affected by this type of coverage. When a patient calls for an appointment, he or she should be told that all forms, benefit booklets, and other relevant information should be brought to the office on the first visit. The business assistant then has the opportunity to initiate the payment process and alleviate or diminish any potential problems.

INVENTORY SYSTEMS

For efficiency, every office must maintain a well-organized inventory system. An inventory system can be created simply by using index cards or the pages of a loose leaf binder. Each major disposable item used in the office has its own card or page and contains the following information.

1. The name of the item (eg, anesthetic)
2. The brand name (eg, Carbocaine 2%)
3. The name of the supplier and the supplier's address and telephone number
4. How the item is sold (eg, box, case, package)
5. The quantity to order for the most advantageous price
6. The time at which the item should be reordered (eg, when only three cases of a material are left)
7. Back orders, which are items previously ordered but not shipped by the supplier because of temporary unavailability

When an item is removed from the supply storage area, it should be recorded in the supply log book in order to keep accurate records of the current stock on hand. When new supplies are ordered, the assistant must not change the inventory record until the items are actually delivered in order to keep an accurate accounting of what is on hand and what is back ordered.

Careful planning and periodic evaluation of the office inventory system can result in several advantages for the dental practice. For example, information about the quantity of any given material used in a time period enables the office to take advantage of savings resulting from quantity buying. Awareness of the rise of the price of dental materials enables the dentist to adjust fees using cost accounting methods. An efficient office supply system allows the practice to run smoothly by preventing critical shortages of necessary supplies during patient treatment procedures.

In order to maintain an efficient office supply system, a perpetual inventory should be performed at regular intervals. If at all possible, stocking space should be marked with the proper item name or item number to correspond with the inventory control card. This will assist in accountability of the inventory and ensure control. Appropriate security measures (eg, locked cabinet) and strict inventory control should be conducted for prescription drugs stored in the office.

To assist you in preparing for the Specialty Examination in Dental Practice Management, it is recommended that you review Chapter 4, Biomedical Sciences, Chapter 5, Chairside Assisting, Chapter 6, Dental Radiology, Chapter 8, Medical Emergencies, and Chapter 9, Behavioral Sciences.

Questions

1. Ethics refers to

   (A) accreditation by the ADA
   (B) professional standards of conduct
   (C) jurisprudence
   (D) membership in the ADAA

2. What determines which duties the dental auxiliary can perform?

   (A) state law
   (B) federal law
   (C) common law
   (D) the dentist

3. Who is responsible for duties delegated to auxiliaries?

   (A) the receptionist
   (B) the office manager
   (C) the dentist
   (D) the patient

4. The period of time in which a patient may bring suit against a dentist is known as

   (A) probationary time
   (B) libel
   (C) tort
   (D) statute of limitations

5. A patient suing for malpractice may include in the suit

   (A) the dental auxiliary
   (B) the dentist only
   (C) the hygienist and dentist only
   (D) anyone working in the dental practice

6. Patient records are

   (A) public information
   (B) available only to relatives
   (C) confidential records and private property
   (D) released at the assistant's discretion

7. An appropriate response when answering the phone is

   (A) "This is Dr. Smith's office. Ms. Jones speaking. May I help you?"
   (B) "Who's calling?"
   (C) "With whom would you like to speak?"
   (D) "May I help you?"

8. A patient calls and complains about the treatment given. The receptionist should

   (A) justify the dentist's position
   (B) engage in a verbal duel
   (C) take the patient's side
   (D) allow the dentist to handle the situation

9. A telephone caller asks the price of a full mouth rehabilitation. The receptionist should

   (A) estimate the price
   (B) ask the patient to come in for an examination
   (C) put the dentist on the phone to quote prices
   (D) refer the person elsewhere

10. What is a contract?

   (A) an analysis of assets against liabilities
   (B) an agreement between two or more people
   (C) records of work completed
   (D) an unexpected action

11. A case presentation is

   (A) a treatment conference with the patient
   (B) a case that is sent to the laboratory for construction

(C) a paper or speech presented by the doctor to a dental society

(D) a study model used to diagnose a case

12. Which person traditionally controls the appointment book?

(A) dentist
(B) chairside assistant
(C) receptionist
(D) hygienist

13. An office manual is

(A) a procedural guide for all office activities
(B) detailed information on how the equipment should be serviced
(C) the doctor's instructions for operating equipment most efficiently
(D) the record that the business assistant keeps for the accountant

14. Overhead is

(A) net income
(B) the cost necessary to practice dentistry
(C) assets of the practice
(D) the break even production point

15. The money paid to the dental practice is known as its

(A) gross income
(B) liabilities
(C) net income
(D) expenses

16. A day sheet in each treatment room provides which of the following data?

(A) any serious medical problem that could affect treatment
(B) the patient's occupation
(C) the procedure to be performed and length of the appointment
(D) the number of visits needed to complete treatment

17. Mr. Jones completed his dental treatment in September. For a 6-month recall he should return in

(A) January
(B) March
(C) April
(D) June

18. Change in the office procedure involving auxiliary personnel is best planned

(A) by an appointment
(B) by the patient
(C) at a staff meeting
(D) by a consultant

19. A list of equipment and supplies present in the office is known as

(A) expendables
(B) overhead
(C) the office manual
(D) an inventory

20. An invoice is a

(A) statement of money collected
(B) statement of items shipped
(C) cash receipt
(D) form of vertical filing

21. If the dentist is delayed, patients who are waiting should be

(A) kept busy as a distraction
(B) ignored
(C) notified of the delay
(D) told to leave

22. If a patient does not keep a scheduled appointment, the business assistant should

(A) wait until the patient contacts the office
(B) contact the patient as soon as possible
(C) send the patient a statement with a charge for the broken appointment
(D) close the patient's file

23. An effective method to ensure that the patient will keep an appointment made over the telephone is to

(A) overlap appointments
(B) charge the patient for missed appointments
(C) send a written confirmation
(D) repeat the appointment time before hanging up

24. Factors to be considered in appointment scheduling include all of the following EXCEPT

(A) the emergency patient
(B) management of prime time
(C) young children or elderly patients
(D) the business assistant's lunch time

25. A patient requires several appointments, each a week apart. The best scheduling would be to assign the patient

(A) the same time and day each week
(B) randomly
(C) Monday the first week, Tuesday the second week, Wednesday the next week, and so forth
(D) relative to the payment arrangements

26. Which of the following statements is NOT true about double-entry bookkeeping?

(A) clearly shows both the debit and credit for every office transaction
(B) provides the necessary components to balance books
(C) assists the dentist in determining fees
(D) provides a record if a patient's payment card is lost or misplaced

27. Third party refers to

(A) children of patients
(B) insurance carriers
(C) a group of general dentists and specialists
(D) patients receiving public assistance

28. Insurance forms should always be

(A) accompanied by x-ray films
(B) accompanied by study models
(C) duplicated for office records
(D) mailed first class

29. A truth-in-lending form is

(A) a contract signed by the patient
(B) a contract signed by the doctor
(C) a government requirement to protect all patients who pay for treatment in advance
(D) a government requirement to protect patients from hidden finance charges in installment payments

30. Dental records

(A) are not admissible as evidence
(B) should always be typed
(C) are legally admissible as evidence
(D) minimize a dentist's risk of liability if filled out in ink

31. What records are kept in an inactive file?

(A) records of all patients who have completed treatment
(B) records of patients who will return in 1 year
(C) records of patients no longer seeking treatment at the office
(D) records of patients who receive treatment at a discount

32. Accounts receivable are

(A) money owed to the dentist from insurance carriers
(B) all monies owed to the dentist for completed treatment
(C) all monies that the dentist owes to creditors
(D) all monies owed to the dentist for future treatment

33. As accounts receivable age, they

(A) increase in value
(B) remain the same in value
(C) decrease in value
(D) are placed in an inactive file

34. Duties of the secretary or business assistant include all of the following EXCEPT

(A) expose x-rays
(B) greet patients
(C) handle the telephone
(D) schedule appointments

35. Third party precertification (or prior authorization) will inform the

(A) dentist and patient of the obligation assumed by the third party
(B) dentist of the correct treatment plan
(C) dentist that prepayment is available
(D) patient of the dentist's skills

36. A patient denies payment responsibilities. The next course of action is

(A) to forget about the bill
(B) to contact a collection agency
(C) harassment
(D) to notify the patient's employer

37. Appointments should be placed in the appointment book in

(A) black ink only
(B) red ink
(C) pencil
(D) blue ink

38. In the appointment book, each line or unit is usually for

(A) 1 minute
(B) 5 minutes
(C) 1 hour
(D) 10–15 minutes

39. When you go through the appointment book and block off time, such as staff meetings, this is called

(A) deleting
(B) outlining

(C) scheduling

(D) confirming

40. If a patient is habitually late, the assistant should

(A) not give them another appointment

(B) give them a stern lecture on the importance of being on time

(C) schedule their appointment in your appointment book 15 minutes after the time you listed on their appointment card

(D) inform them later of an extra charge

41. Patients should come in for a recall

(A) whenever they think they need a checkup

(B) whenever they have a toothache

(C) at periodic intervals

(D) whenever the hygienist can fit them into the schedule

42. All insurance carriers use

(A) the same table of benefits

(B) different tables of benefits depending on the type of coverage to which the subscriber is entitled

(C) a percentage of the dentist's usual and customary fees

(D) closed-panel dental care for their subscribers

43. On any given day, a business assistant encounters a good deal of pressure, frustration, and interruption. He or she can cope with this if he or she

(A) takes a personal day off now and then

(B) can delegate tasks to other auxiliaries

(C) takes the phone off the hook during busy periods

(D) remains calm and systematically completes tasks until they are done

44. When a patient calls and insists on speaking to the doctor, the assistant should

(A) call the doctor to the phone as promptly as possible

(B) explain to the patient that it is the responsibility of the assistant to respond to phone calls

(C) explain that the doctor is treating a patient and that he or she will return the call as soon as possible

(D) tell the patient to call back at a specific hour

45. Assignment of benefits means that

(A) the patient is entitled to complete reimbursement for his or her dental care in each given year

(B) the dentist receives direct payment from the insurance carrier in the amount that the patient's insurance plan designates

(C) all members of the immediate family of the insured are entitled to insurance coverage in a given year

(D) if a patient does not use his insurance benefits in a given year, he or she can allot these benefits to an immediate family member

46. A patient cancels an appointment an hour before he is due. A good course of action is to

(A) close the office at the appointment time

(B) allow the dentist to resolve the problem

(C) call a patient who is available on a short notice

(D) announce a coffee break to the dentist and rest of the staff

47. The rights of a patient during the treatment phase do NOT include

(A) the right to be informed about his or her condition

(B) the right to refuse treatment

(C) the right to confidential records

(D) the right to dictate the course of treatment

48. Cross-training means

(A) auxiliaries are knowledgeable about each other's jobs

(B) dental assistants can perform some of the procedures usually delegated to the hygienists

(C) auxiliaries are trained in a school environment

(D) auxiliaries receive on-the-job training

49. If a dental office is managed by sound business principles, the business assistant should make every effort to

(A) arrive promptly every morning

(B) conserve the doctor's time

(C) complete all the bookkeeping promptly

(D) maintain recalls

50. A bank statement will show which of the following?

(A) only deposits made

(B) the customer's credit account

(C) checks paid, deposits, and the balance

(D) customer credit card charges

51. The patient's name should be entered in the appointment book

(A) before the day's treatment is complete

(B) after mailing the recall appointment

(C) when the appointment is made

(D) after the appointment is completed

52. When a patient suffering pain of dental origin calls for an appointment, the assistant should

    (A) have the patient come in immediately for temporary relief
    (B) make an appointment for next week
    (C) make an appointment the following day
    (D) refer to another dentist

53. Net pay refers to

    (A) salary after deductions
    (B) total collections minus office expense
    (C) taxable wages plus tips
    (D) total amount used to figure payroll taxes

54. Gross pay refers to

    (A) total collections of accounts receivable per month
    (B) salary after deductions
    (C) salary before deductions
    (D) total collections minus office expenses

55. Which of the following taxes is NOT a payroll tax?

    (A) State Disability Insurance
    (B) Social Security
    (C) Federal Income Tax
    (D) Federal Excise Tax

56. A recall system based on making advance appointments is called

    (A) standby appointments
    (B) continuing appointments
    (C) chronologic file system
    (D) instant reference system

57. In the filing rule regarding surname, the correct indexing order is

    (A) first name, middle name, surname
    (B) surname, first name, middle name
    (C) middle name, first name, surname
    (D) surname, middle name, first name

58. The most frequently used adult charting system is to

    (A) number the teeth from 1 to 32 beginning with the maxillary right third molar
    (B) number the teeth in each quadrant from 1 through 8 beginning with third molars
    (C) number the teeth in each quadrant from 1 through 8 beginning with central incisors
    (D) letter the teeth beginning with the maxillary right third molar

59. UCR stands for

    (A) unusual, coverage, regular
    (B) usual, carrier, reasonable
    (C) usual, customary, reasonable
    (D) usual, claim, rider

60. When storing supplies, you should

    (A) store frequently used items in an easily accessible area
    (B) store frequently used items out of reach
    (C) store film near a heat source
    (D) store cements in the refrigerator

DIRECTIONS (Questions 61 through 65): Match the items in Column A with the appropriate definition in Column B.

COLUMN A

61. Alphabetizing
62. Copayment
63. Authorization to release information
64. Filing
65. Carrier

COLUMN B

A. the patient's signature giving consent for the release of information relative to his or her claim
B. the act of classifying and arranging records so they will be preserved safely and in such a manner that records can be retrieved easily
C. an arrangement under which the carrier and beneficiary are each responsible for a fixed share of the cost of dental services
D. the arrangement of captions and indexing units in strict alphabetical order
E. the insurance company or dental plan that agrees to pay the benefits

DIRECTIONS (Questions 66 through 79): Each of the questions or incomplete statements in this section is followed by four suggested answers or completions. Select the ONE lettered answer or completion that is BEST in each case. Check your answers with the correct answers at the end of the chapter.

66. Necessary information required for the patient account record includes all of the following EXCEPT

    (A) home telephone number
    (B) home address
    (C) name and address of employer
    (D) hours worked each week

67. A treatment plan is a (an)

    (A) approach to collections
    (B) inventory control system
    (C) peer evaluation system
    (D) systematic approach to meet the dental needs of the patient

68. A running inventory is

    (A) a system of altering the supply list to know which supplies are present in the office
    (B) moving the inventory from place to place
    (C) a billing technique
    (D) an inventory updated once a year

69. The main advantage of purchasing a large quantity of a particular supply at one time is

    (A) it is easy to store
    (B) to save money when buying in bulk
    (C) the billing is easier
    (D) the dental materials have an indefinite shelf life

70. When recalling patients by telephone, the business assistant should

    (A) call early in the day
    (B) leave a message on the answering machine
    (C) insist that the patient commit to a specific time
    (D) have the patient's recall record ready for reference

71. All fees charged and payments received should be entered promptly on the daily journal page and

    (A) patient ledger card
    (B) charge slip
    (C) receipts
    (D) appointment book

72. An office manual is most effective when it is

    (A) purchased from a reputable dental supply company
    (B) organized by a professional management consultant who has evaluated the practice
    (C) organized by the dentist and the staff in keeping with the office's philosophy, goals, and objectives
    (D) a collection of directions that the dentist believes is appropriate for his or her mode of dental care delivery

73. Pegboard accounting materials include all of the following EXCEPT

    (A) receipts and charge slips
    (B) ledgers
    (C) daily journal page
    (D) bank deposit slips

74. Which of the following does NOT describe an active file?

    (A) waiting insurance approval
    (B) patient under treatment
    (C) treatment complete but with balance
    (D) treatment completed and paid

75. Mark Jones received the following dental treatment: an examination and x-rays ($25), five surfaces of amalgam restorations (at $8 per surface), two extractions (at $10 per extraction). The total fee for his dental treatment is

    (A) $85
    (B) $43
    (C) $75
    (D) $77

76. When filling out a deposit slip, the auxiliary must

    (A) not endorse the checks before depositing
    (B) list checks and currency separately
    (C) only list deposits over $100.00
    (D) list all checks in alphabetical order

77. When a check from a patient has been returned, it is best to

    (A) immediately send the patient to collections
    (B) convert the missing money from petty cash
    (C) adjust the balance of the patient's account accordingly
    (D) ask patient to initiate a stop payment order

78. With reference to a stop payment order on checks, all of the following are true EXCEPT

    (A) the stop payment indicates insufficient funds
    (B) the stop payment order may be made by phone
    (C) the stop payment order may be made by filling out proper bank forms at the bank
    (D) payment can be stopped if there is reason to believe the check has been lost

79. To double-check entries on the daily journal record and patient ledger cards to ensure that all entries and calculations are accurate refers to

    (A) proof-of-posting
    (B) monthly summary
    (C) cross-reference
    (D) computer processing

		SHEET NO.	A	B	C	D	

PROFESSIONAL SERVICE	CHARGE		PAID		NEW BALANCE		PREVIOUS BALANCE		NAME
BALANCE FWD.	2								
Ex, X, P, (ck)	30	00	30	00	—		—		Mary Knight
SR.	24	00	—		36	00	12	00	Lisa Daniels
G.T. (cs)	16	00	28	00	—		12	00	Robert Smith
Ex, X, D.S. (ck)	89	00	34	00	55	00	—		Charles Johnson
C & B (ck)	375	00	100	00	275	00	—		Harold Turner

534   192   366   24

PROOF OF POSTING

The bank deposit for this day should total ___192___

The total for column A is _____

The total for column C is _____

The total for column B is _____

The total for column D is _____

Column D total: _____

Plus column A total: _____

Subtotal: _____

Minus column B total: _____

Equals column C balance: _____

Figure 10–1.

+24
534
558

DIRECTIONS: Refer to Figure 10–1 to answer Questions 80 through 85.

80. The bank deposit for this day is

(A) $100.00
(B) $192.00
(C) $275.00
(D) $375.00

81. The total for column A is

(A) $275.00
(B) $375.00
(C) $534.00
(D) $540.00

82. The total for column C is

(A) $275.00
(B) $366.00
(C) $375.00
(D) $396.00

83. The total for column B is

(A) $100.00
(B) $175.00
(C) $192.00
(D) $292.00

84. The total for column D is

(A) $12.00
(B) $21.00
(C) $23.00
(D) $24.00

85. To perform proof-of-posting properly, the subtotal for column D plus column A would be

(A) $534.00
(B) $558.00
(C) $366.00
(D) $24.00

DIRECTIONS (Questions 86 through 100): Each of the questions or incomplete statements in this section is followed by four suggested answers or completions. Select the ONE lettered answer or completion that is BEST in each case. Check your answers with the correct answers at the end of the chapter.

86. The office manual includes all of the following EXCEPT

(A) statement of purpose or objectives
(B) staff policies
(C) medical emergency procedures
(D) payroll records

87. When a patient is injured by a dentist's employee

    (A) the dentist is not liable
    (B) the employee is the only one who can be sued by the patient
    (C) the employee is not liable
    (D) the employee and dentist are liable

88. Things to avoid during an interview include all of the following EXCEPT

    (A) chewing gum
    (B) lacking a neat appearance
    (C) using eye contact
    (D) talking about salary and hours immediately

89. Consent to an operation or to a course of treatment

    (A) must be actual only
    (B) is a professional duty to the public
    (C) is not necessary for the dentist to obtain
    (D) may be expressed or implied

90. Anything done to a person without consent is

    (A) a skill and judgment
    (B) a judgment
    (C) a trespass
    (D) proof of freedom from contributory negligence

91. Written records on patients kept by the dentist

    (A) are of little value in malpractice cases
    (B) should always be filled in erasable ink
    (C) are the single most important factor in the defense of most malpractice cases
    (D) make expert testimony unnecessary

92. Professional liability claims are most likely to be based on

    (A) the charge of a faulty patient medical history
    (B) the charge of faulty patient x-rays
    (C) the charge of faulty or erroneous diagnosis
    (D) the charge of faulty dental equipment

93. Negligence is

    (A) a legal duty to the public
    (B) a general duty to the dental profession
    (C) a general duty to the legal profession
    (D) the failure to exercise reasonable and ordinary care to avoid injury to others

94. Supplies can be divided into all of the following categories EXCEPT

    (A) capital items
    (B) expendable items
    (C) nonexpendable items
    (D) receivables

95. The most acceptable payment arrangements in a dental office include all of following the EXCEPT

    (A) open accounts
    (B) advance payments
    (C) fixed amount each visit
    (D) divided payments

96. Canceled checks

    (A) are never enclosed with a monthly bank statement
    (B) are the same as voided checks
    (C) should be credited to the account
    (D) have been paid and charged to the depositor's account

97. Which of the following is true in reference to petty cash?

    (A) it is money to pay for inexpensive office items
    (B) it is the same as the Christmas fund
    (C) a $50 check is written every 6 months to replenish
    (D) the cash can be used by the doctor for office uniforms

98. A cashier's check

    (A) is also called a certified check
    (B) is a bank's own check drawn on itself
    (C) is the same as a canceled check
    (D) need not be endorsed

99. Which of the following steps is NOT included in the bank reconciliation procedure?

    (A) compare canceled checks to bank statement
    (B) calculate deposits in transit
    (C) list outstanding checks
    (D) subtract bank service charges from the bank statement total

100. Responsibilities of the business assistant may include which of the following?

    (A) exposing x-rays
    (B) assisting in operative procedures
    (C) interviewing and training new employees
    (D) keeping the treatment area updated with supplies

DIRECTIONS (Questions 101 through 105): Match the items in Column A with the appropriate definition in Column B.

COLUMN A

101. Third party plan
102. Cash
103. Credit
104. Divided payment plan
105. Office budget plan

COLUMN B

A. a belief that the individual is willing and able to fulfill his financial obligation
B. extended installment plans arranged by means of an office contract
C. usually two or three installment payments consisting of a downpayment before treatment begins and the balance being paid when treatment is completed
D. payment in full at each visit for all charges incurred at that visit
E. involves the use of an outside insurance carrier to reimburse partial payments

DIRECTIONS (Questions 106 through 112): For each of the items in this section, ONE or MORE of the numbered options is correct. Choose answer

A if only 1, 2, and 3 are correct
B if only 1 and 3 are correct
C if only 2 and 4 are correct
D if only 4 is correct
E if all are correct

106. Facts that should be obtained when interviewing for a job are

(1) working hours
(2) vacation policy
(3) length of probation period
(4) salary and benefits

107. If a patient presents inappropriate behavior while in the patient reception area, the business assistant should

(1) ask the chairside assistant to seat the patient immediately
(2) allow the patient to continue disrupting the other patients
(3) refer the patient to another office
(4) speak directly to the patient in a firm but professional manner

108. Appointment control will

(1) prevent faulty dentistry
(2) organize the doctor's production time
(3) prevent emergency patients
(4) keep hours within desired limits

109. Record keeping

(1) provides production records
(2) provides a history of treatment success or failure
(3) is needed legally to avoid possible malpractice involvement
(4) avoids the need of an accountant

110. During an office medical emergency situation, the business assistant should

(1) assist the doctor and chairside assistant where needed
(2) update the patient's health history form
(3) call for emergency medical support personnel
(4) administer CPR immediately to the patient

111. Identify where to seek employment opportunities

(1) want ads
(2) dental assisting schools
(3) employment agencies
(4) dental assisting associations

112. Postoperative telephone calls

(1) remind patients of postoperative care they should be carrying out
(2) remind patients of their appointment for postoperative treatment
(3) show patients special concern
(4) are only necessary if sutures have been placed

Answers and Explanations

1. **(B)** Ethics is the moral obligation that dictates the standards of conduct expected by the dental profession. The ADAA has a written code of ethics to which the assistant is expected to adhere.

2. **(A)** The various state Dental Practice Acts determine which duties the dental auxiliary can perform. These laws, as all laws, are subject to change, and many have been revised recently to expand the duties of auxiliaries.

3. **(C)** The dentist is responsible for duties delegated to auxiliaries on his or her dental team. He or she must supervise the performance of these duties and ensure the quality of the final product.

4. **(D)** The statute of limitations specifies a period of time in which a patient may bring suit against a dentist. This time varies according to many factors, such as the age of the patient and the reason for the suit.

5. **(D)** A patient suing for malpractice may include in the suit anyone working in the dental practice. Under the principle of respondeat superior, "Let the higher one answer," the dentist (employer) is ultimately responsible for the wrongful acts of the staff (agents) while such acts are performed within the employment setting of the employer. Each individual employee may be named in a lawsuit and should individually carry personal liability insurance.

6. **(C)** Patient records are a confidential written history of financial and treatment experiences. These records should not be released or made public without the permission of the patient. Records include dental treatment plan, x-rays, study models, charting records, insurance records, and financial statements.

7. **(A)** An excellent response when answering the phone is, "This is Dr. Smith's office. Ms. Jones speaking. May I help you?" The most important part of this communication is the identification of the office.

8. **(D)** The receptionist should allow the dentist to resolve patient problems dealing with the patient's dissatisfaction with treatment. Technical explanations often are required, which are the responsibility of the dentist.

9. **(B)** Fees have many contingencies that cannot be determined over the telephone. Therefore, patients seeking fee quotations should be scheduled for an examination.

10. **(B)** A contract is a legal agreement between two or more people. Contracts may be explicit (verbal or written) or implicit (implied, not explicitly expressed). Examples of dental contracts are schedule arrangements, payment arrangements, and job duties.

11. **(A)** The case presentation is the treatment conference where the dentist explains to the patient the findings of the examination and discusses what treatment procedures are necessary in order to restore the patient's mouth to optimum oral health.

12. **(C)** One person should control the appointment book at all times. It is usually the receptionist in an office where several auxiliaries are employed.

13. **(A)** Every office should have a current manual that details all office tasks, policies, and procedures, in addition to goals, objectives, and philosophy of practice.

14. **(B)** Overhead is the cost needed to produce dentistry. It includes rent, supplies, and salary.

15. **(A)** The money paid to the dental practice is its gross income. The gross income minus the overhead results in the net income.

16. **(C)** A day sheet provides the dentist and office staff

with the day's procedures and the length of each appointment.

17. **(B)** A patient who has completed dental treatment in September and is placed on a 6-month recall will be rescheduled in March.

18. **(C)** Changes in a dental office with multiple auxiliary personnel should occur with input from those individuals the change will affect. An excellent technique is to have a staff meeting to resolve potential problems and permit input into decision making.

19. **(D)** A list of equipment and supplies on hand is known as an inventory. One person in the office should be responsible for maintaining the inventory.

20. **(B)** An invoice is an itemized bill of supplies sent to the dentist. Before paying this bill, the invoice should be checked against the supplies received.

21. **(C)** If the dentist is delayed, patients who are waiting should be notified of the delay. The patient's time must be respected if the dental office expects the same in return. If the delay is extensive, the patients should have the right to reschedule their appointments.

22. **(B)** It must be made very clear to all patients that the time scheduled for appointments is specifically reserved for them and that broken appointments are unacceptable behavior.

23. **(C)** To ensure that the patient will keep an appointment made over the telephone, the receptionist should send a written confirmation.

24. **(D)** Although it is necessary for the business assistant to have a lunch break, this is not considered a prime factor in appointment scheduling. The patient always comes first.

25. **(A)** A patient needing a series of visits should be given appointments at the same time and day each week. This pattern helps the patient remember the appointments.

26. **(C)** Fees are determined by a careful analysis of expenses, (eg, office overhead). The purpose of a double-entry bookkeeping system is to record income (both collected and outstanding).

27. **(B)** In a dental office, third party refers to an insurance carrier. All money paid by a particular insurance company is known as third party payment.

28. **(C)** Insurance forms records, x-ray films, study models, and other items that leave the office for any reason should be duplicated in case of loss.

29. **(D)** Any office that makes arrangements for patients to pay for their dentistry via installments is required by law to provide the patient with a truth-in-lending form. This form indicates whether or not a finance charge will be added if there is a default on payment.

30. **(C)** Dental records are often the most important piece of evidence in court and are legally admissible as evidence. Records must always be kept updated, and all entries must be made in ink. Radiographs and models may be included as part of the dental treatment record and should be properly labeled, including patient name and date.

31. **(C)** The two patient records that are filed as active or inactive are treatment and financial records. The treatment record is placed in an inactive file if the patient is no longer seeking care at the office. The financial record is placed in an inactive file if the account has been fully paid.

32. **(B)** All treatment that has been completed and is unpaid is considered an account receivable.

33. **(C)** As accounts receivable age, they decrease in value and become more difficult to collect. Therefore, firm payment arrangements are a necessity for a successful practice.

34. **(A)** Duties of the business assistant do not include exposing dental x-rays. Primary duties of the business assistant may include greeting patients, handling the telephone, and scheduling appointments.

35. **(A)** Third party precertification will inform the dentist and patient of the obligation assumed by the third party. The money allocated by the insurance company is usually partial payment and is given to the patient or dentist after treatment is completed.

36. **(B)** Each office has a policy about payment. If a patient has had dental work completed and then denies payment responsibility, the dentist usually will contact a collection agency to begin appropriate legal action.

37. **(C)** Appointments should be placed in the appointment book in pencil. Erasable entries are best in an appointment book because of the frequency of adjusting the schedule in cases of cancellations and emergencies. All entries should be legible and accurate.

38. **(D)** In the appointment book, each line or unit represents time increments of 10 or 15 minutes. An

appointment that would take 30 minutes to complete would require three units (lines) equivalent to 10 minutes each, or if using the 15-minute time increments, two units (lines) would be necessary to equal a 30-minute block of time.

39. (B) Outlining the appointment book designates what time periods the office is closed, such as days off, lunch time, holidays, and vacation time. Outlining the appointment book also indicates blocks of time per day that have been set aside to handle emergency appointments or staff meetings.

40. (C) A good procedure to follow to ensure that a habitually late patient will arrive on time is to schedule the appointment in the book 15 minutes after the time listed on the patient's appointment card.

41. (C) At the completion of a course of treatment, a patient should be informed of the necessity of returning for a checkup at regular intervals designated by the dentist.

42. (B) It is important that benefits be determined before treatment begins and that the patient be made aware of how much (or little) he or she might receive from the insurance company.

43. (D) The prime personality trait of a good business assistant is being able to remain calm and to complete all tasks of the day systematically.

44. (C) In an effort to conserve the doctor's time and also permit him or her to provide the appropriate attention to the patient in the chair, the business assistant should make every effort to cope with all telephone calls. In those situations wherein it is necessary for the patient to speak to the doctor, the assistant should explain that the doctor will return the call as soon as possible. It is then the assistant's responsibility to see that this promise is kept.

45. (B) The dental office that accepts assignment of benefits must be sure the patient signs that portion of the insurance form that indicates the money should be sent directly to the dentist. This is done before treatment commences.

46. (C) A cancellation close to the appointed time can be handled by calling a patient who is available on short notice, by extending the visit of the patient who is present before the cancellation, or by moving a patient to be seen late in the day into the time slot.

47. (D) Although patients have many rights pertaining to professional care, the right to determine the proper cause of treatment belongs to the dentist.

48. (A) It is important for every dental assistant to be aware of his or her own job description and be capable of fulfilling those specific tasks in the most efficient manner. A dental assistant who is cross-trained also has a working knowledge about the procedures assigned to other assistants and is capable of performing those tasks should it become necessary in time of absence or during a particularly busy period.

49. (B) Although a competent business assistant will arrive promptly, refrain from making personal calls, and complete all assigned tasks, his or her prime responsibility is to conserve the doctor's time. Since the income of the office is in direct proportion to how thoughtfully time is managed by the business assistant, time and productivity are synonymous.

50. (C) A bank statement is issued by the bank and is a record of all transactions, including deposits, withdrawals, canceled checks, and the existing balance. Bank statements usually cover a specific time period and may be calculated on a monthly basis.

51. (C) The patient's complete name, telephone number (home or work), and type of treatment to be rendered must be entered legibly in the appointment book. All appointment book entries should be made in pencil and be erasable in case of a change. In order to minimize appointment errors, it is best to enter this information in the appointment book at the time that the appointment is being made. The appointment card should be completed after the appointment book entry is made. It is best to confirm by phone all appointments made through the mail before entering the name in the appointment book.

52. (A) When a patient suffering from pain of dental origin calls for an appointment, the dental auxiliary should obtain basic information regarding the nature of the pain, such as duration of pain, which tooth or area is involved, or if there has been a traumatic injury to the area. This basic information will assist the doctor and chairside assistant in preparing for the emergency appointment. The patient should be given an immediate appointment for temporary relief.

53. (A) Net pay refers to salary earned after deductions. The net pay plus all deductions will equal the gross pay.

54. (C) Gross pay refers to the total amount earned before deductions, or the gross salary earnings.

55. (D) Federal law requires that Social Security Tax and Income Tax (withholding) be withheld from each employee. Most states also require a withholding state tax, such as State Disability. Federal Excise Tax is not a payroll tax. It is a separate operational fee that must be paid by the business owner to operate the place of business. The Federal Excise Tax is a requirement imposed by the Federal government.

56. **(B)** A recall system based on making advanced appointments is known as a continuing appointment system.

57. **(B)** In the filing rule regarding surname, the correct indexing order is surname (last name), given name (first name), and middle name or middle initial.

58. **(A)** The most frequently used adult charting system is the Universal numbering system, which numbers the teeth from 1 through 32, starting with the maxillary right third molar, which is numbered 1 and continuing across to the maxillary left third molar, which is numbered 16. The mandibular left third molar is numbered 17, and the numbering continues across to the mandibular right third molar, which is numbered 32.

59. **(C)** The abbreviation UCR is associated with the dental insurance fee-for-service concept. A method of calculating fee-for-service benefits is the usual, customary, and reasonable concept. *Usual* refers to the fee that the doctor charges private patients for a specific service. *Customary* fees are established if the fees fall in the same range of fees of several doctors within the same geographic area. *Customary* fees between specialists are grouped together and are considered separately from the general practitioners' fees. *Reasonable* is the concept applied to justify higher fees in cases where treatment rendered required extra time or skill due to the nature of the procedure. In these special circumstances, the doctor will increase the usual fee.

60. **(A)** When storing supplies, frequently used items should be stored where they can be reached easily. The operatory or dental laboratory storage areas are best suited for small consumable items and supplies that are used continuously. Manufacturer's storage recommendations must be considered when storing supplies. X-ray film should not be stored near a light or heat source, and certain types of cements must be stored at room temperature. Less frequently used supplies should be stored in a supply room and need not be as easily accessible.

61. **(D)**

62. **(C)**

63. **(A)**

64. **(B)**

65. **(E)**

66. **(D)** The patient account record, or ledger card, is used by the business assistant to record all financial transactions, including payments, charges, credits, and current balance information. Necessary information includes patient's home address and telephone number, work number and work address, and insurance information. The number of hours worked per week is not indicated as necessary information on a patient account record.

67. **(D)** A treatment plan is a systematic approach to accomplishing the dental needs of the patient. This plan is made after evaluating the diagnostic materials gathered from and about the patient (eg, medical and dental histories, radiographs, study models, clinical examination). Elements of a treatment plan include the procedure, the priority of the procedure, who will perform the task, and the amount of time the procedure requires.

68. **(A)** A running inventory is a system of altering the supply list to know what is present in the office. This list is updated continuously as the supplies are used. This type of system is especially important with disposable supplies.

69. **(B)** The advantage of purchasing a large quantity of a particular supply at one time is to save money. The drawbacks are the storage space needed and the shelf life of the material, which might expire before the material is used.

70. **(D)** When recalling patients by telephone, the business assistant should have the patient's recall record ready for reference.

71. **(A)** All account transactions should be entered promptly on the daily journal page and the patient ledger card. The patient ledger card keeps an ongoing record of all charges, payments, insurance reimbursements, and outstanding balance information that may be necessary for collections. Charge slips are a written form of interoffice communication relating information about the current account balance and the fees charged for the services performed at that visit.

72. **(C)** An office manual is most effective when it is organized by the dentist and the staff in keeping with the office's philosophy, goals, and objectives.

73. **(D)** Pegboard accounting materials do not include bank deposit slips. The bank deposit slip keeps an

itemized record of all the checks and cash payments. The deposit slip must contain the doctor's name, business address, and bank account number. After completion of the deposit slip, the money is ready to be deposited in the bank. A record of the deposit is recorded in the office account ledger.

74. **(D)** If the dental treatment has been completed and the account fully paid, the file is no longer considered active.

75. **(A)** The total fee for his dental treatment is $85.

76. **(B)** Money received in the dental practice must be placed in the bank. A deposit slip furnished by the bank is completed daily, detailing all of the checks and currency collected for that day. Checks and currency are listed separately on a deposit slip. Entries must be made in ink, legible, and in duplicate (carbon copy). The patient's account record must be adjusted to reflect the amount of the check written to the dental practice before depositing. Checks do not need to be listed in alphabetical order but must be endorsed properly in order to be deposited.

77. **(C)** A returned check (check that has bounced) must be charged back against the patient's account and subtracted from the office income bank balance. Allow the patient to clear the outstanding balance before proceeding with other dental treatment.

78. **(A)** A stop payment order on a check may be requested if there is reason to believe that a check has been lost. Payment can be stopped by filling out proper forms provided directly at the bank or by a telephone request to the bank. A stop payment order does not indicate insufficient funds.

79. **(A)** Daily proof-of-posting serves to double-check all entries and transactions made on the daily journal page. This system requires that each of the columns must be totaled and balanced to ensure accuracy. The cash drawer also must balance with the received on accounts entries. If daily record keeping procedures are handled by a computer system, the columns can be totaled automatically.

80. **(B)**

81. **(C)**

82. **(B)**

83. **(C)**

84. **(D)**

85. **(B)**

86. **(D)** The office manual does not include payroll records. Every office should have an office manual that is up-dated periodically to accommodate changes in office procedures and policies. The office manual may also serve as a procedural guide for training new staff members. Medical emergency procedures and the goals and objectives of the dental practice also are defined in the office manual.

87. **(D)** When a patient is injured by a dentist's employee, both the employee and the dentist are liable. Under the principle of respondeat superior, the dentist is automatically associated and brought into the legal suit with the employee.

88. **(C)** Using eye contact during an employment interview is important and a necessary part of effective communication. Immediately discussing salary and hours is not recommended at the start of an interview but are issues that do need to be addressed at some point during the interview. A professional appearance is required for employment success.

89. **(D)** Consent to an operation or to a course of treatment may be expressed or implied. A patient may approve of dental treatment by formally giving written consent by placing his or her signature on office consent forms or treatment plan forms. Implied consent is not as clearly defined but is interpreted by a patient's actions and behavior. When a patient offers to open his mouth for an examination, he is agreeing to treatment.

90. **(C)** Anything done to a person without his or her consent is termed a trespass. A trespass action may be interpreted by law as "an unconsented touching." The importance of obtaining patient consent either through an expressed contract (in writing) or an implied contract (mutual agreement by two persons) before rendering dental treatment is necessary to avoid possible charges of trespass.

91. **(C)** The most important piece of evidence used by the defense in most malpractice cases is the patient dental record. All patient dental records must be well documented and filled out in ink. Radiographs, laboratory reports, and study models also are part of the permanent dental record and must be correctly labeled. All entries should be dated and followed by a detailed description of each procedure performed. The initials or complete last name of the ancillary staff performing direct patient care should follow the dental entry. Medical health history questionnaires should be updated periodically and initialed by the reviewer.

92. **(C)** Professional liability claims are most likely to be based on the charge of faulty or erroneous diagnosis, based on the principle that the doctor's reasonable and prudent diagnosis determines the type and extent of dental treatment rendered to the patient. Every patient can expect the right to a reasonable standard of skill and care when they seek dental treatment. If this right is abused or neglected, a malpractice suit may be incurred.

93. **(D)** Negligence may be defined as the failure to exercise reasonable and ordinary care to avoid injury to another. In health care settings, the charge of negligence or lack of reasonable care in serving a patient by the health professional is termed malpractice.

94. **(D)** Receivables refer to money outstanding for treatment completed.

95. **(A)** Open accounts are the most difficult ones to collect, since statements on open accounts usually are sent to patients after treatment has been rendered. This gives patients the option of paying at their convenience, which can increase the office's accounts receivable status.

96. **(D)** Canceled checks are checks that have been paid and charged to the depositor's account. On receipt of the office bank statement, the canceled checks should be reviewed and verified against the office checkbook and bank statement. A record of all canceled checks should be kept on file for future reference, or the information should be stored in a computer system.

97. **(A)** Petty cash is a small amount of cash kept in the office to purchase miscellaneous inexpensive items for the office (eg, postage stamps,erasers). The business assistant may keep the petty cash vouchers, and a record of all transactions should be dated and recorded. The petty cash fund is determined and replenished according to the doctor and office needs.

98. **(B)** A cashiers check is drawn by a bank on its own funds in exchange for an individual's personal check or cash. Cashiers checks must be endorsed by the recipient.

99. **(D)** Bank service charges have been subtracted previously from the bank statement total by the banking organization and are NOT a step in reconciling a bank statement. Balancing (reconciling) the checkbook promptly against the bank statement is an important procedure and includes calculations involving outstanding checks, deposits in transit, and cross-checking canceled checks against the bank statement. All canceled checks and bank statements should be stored for future reference.

100. **(C)** The business assistant may often be involved in the initial or preliminary interview process and the supervision and training of new staff members in office policies and procedures.

101. **(E)**

102. **(D)**

103. **(B)**

104. **(C)**

105. **(A)**

106. **(E)** The interview is the process by which the potential employee (assistant) meets the employer (dentist or representative) and obtains information, such as job description, the office policy on working hours, vacation policy, salary, probation period, and benefits.

107. **(D)** On occasion, a disruptive patient or patients who present unusual behavior in the patient waiting room may require a firm direct approach. The auxiliary must always handle this type of situation in a professional manner. Patients suspected of substance abuse or disruptive patients who present irrational behavior should be rescheduled.

108. **(C)** Appointment control will prevent overcrowding, keep hours within desired limits, organize the dentist's production time, assign tasks to the proper individual, and provide patients with definite appointment information.

109. **(A)** Important reasons for record keeping are that it legally avoids possible malpractice involvement, provides an accurate history of treatment success and failure, provides production records, enables others to carry on treatment, and allows future treatment to be based on past performances, such as anesthesia and payment.

110. **(B)** During an office medical emergency situation the business assistant should assist the doctor and chairside assistant where needed and call for medical emergency support services if indicated. Each member of the office staff should be trained in medical emergency protocol.

111. **(E)** The dental auxiliary may seek employment opportunities through employment agencies, local and state dental assistant associations, dental assisting schools, and newspaper want ads.

112. **(A)** Postoperative calls usually are made at the end of the day to patients who have had difficult procedures performed during the day. The rationale for

these calls is to show the patients concern, to remind patients of their postoperative responsibilities (eg, taking medications, rinsing), and to remind them of their next appointment.

BIBLIOGRAPHY

Cooper TM, Di Biaggo JA. *Applied Practice Management.* St. Louis: CV Mosby Co, 1979.

Domer LR, Snyder TL, Heid DW, eds. *Dental Practice Management.* St. Louis: CV Mosby Co, 1980.

Howard WW. *Dental Practice Planning.* St. Louis: CV Mosby Co, 1975.

Ladley BA, Patt JC. *Office Procedures for the Dental Team.* St. Louis: CV Mosby Co, 1977.

Schwarzrock SP, Jensen JR. *Effective Dental Assisting,* 7th ed. Dubuque, Iowa: William C Brown Co, 1991.

Torres H, Ehrlich A. *Modern Dental Assisting,* 4th ed. Philadelphia: WB Saunders Co, 1990.

Woodall IR. *Legal, Ethical, and Management Aspects of the Dental Care System*, 3rd ed. St. Louis: CV Mosby Co, 1987.

NAME _____
Last   First   Middle

ADDRESS _____
Street

City   State   Zip

SOC SEC NUMBER

	0	1	2	3	4	5	6	7	8	9
	0	1	2	3	4	5	6	7	8	9
	0	1	2	3	4	5	6	7	8	9
	0	1	2	3	4	5	6	7	8	9
	0	1	2	3	4	5	6	7	8	9
	0	1	2	3	4	5	6	7	8	9
	0	1	2	3	4	5	6	7	8	9
	0	1	2	3	4	5	6	7	8	9
	0	1	2	3	4	5	6	7	8	9

DIRECTIONS Mark your social security number from top to bottom in the appropriate boxes on the right. Refer to the section "HOW TO TAKE THE PRACTICE TEST" in the introduction to the book for more information. PLEASE USE NO.2 PENCIL ONLY.

MAKE ERASURES COMPLETE

PAGE 1 2 3
TYPE 1 2 3

1 A B C D E   2 A B C D E   3 A B C D E   4 A B C D E   5 A B C D E   6 A B C D E   7 A B C D E   8 A B C D E

9 A B C D E   10 A B C D E   11 A B C D E   12 A B C D E   13 A B C D E   14 A B C D E   15 A B C D E   16 A B C D E

17 A B C D E   18 A B C D E   19 A B C D E   20 A B C D E   21 A B C D E   22 A B C D E   23 A B C D E   24 A B C D E

25 A B C D E   26 A B C D E   27 A B C D E   28 A B C D E   29 A B C D E   30 A B C D E   31 A B C D E   32 A B C D E

33 A B C D E   34 A B C D E   35 A B C D E   36 A B C D E   37 A B C D E   38 A B C D E   39 A B C D E   40 A B C D E

41 A B C D E   42 A B C D E   43 A B C D E   44 A B C D E   45 A B C D E   46 A B C D E   47 A B C D E   48 A B C D E

49 A B C D E   50 A B C D E   51 A B C D E   52 A B C D E   53 A B C D E   54 A B C D E   55 A B C D E   56 A B C D E

57 A B C D E   58 A B C D E   59 A B C D E   60 A B C D E   61 A B C D E   62 A B C D E   63 A B C D E   64 A B C D E

65 A B C D E   66 A B C D E   67 A B C D E   68 A B C D E   69 A B C D E   70 A B C D E   71 A B C D E   72 A B C D E

73 A B C D E   74 A B C D E   75 A B C D E   76 A B C D E   77 A B C D E   78 A B C D E   79 A B C D E   80 A B C D E

81 A B C D E   82 A B C D E   83 A B C D E   84 A B C D E   85 A B C D E   86 A B C D E   87 A B C D E   88 A B C D E

89 A B C D E   90 A B C D E   91 A B C D E   92 A B C D E   93 A B C D E   94 A B C D E   95 A B C D E   96 A B C D E

97 A B C D E   98 A B C D E   99 A B C D E   100 A B C D E   101 A B C D E   102 A B C D E   103 A B C D E   104 A B C D E

105 A B C D E   106 A B C D E   107 A B C D E   108 A B C D E   109 A B C D E   110 A B C D E   111 A B C D E   112 A B C D E

113 A B C D E   114 A B C D E   115 A B C D E   116 A B C D E   117 A B C D E   118 A B C D E   119 A B C D E   120 A B C D E

121 A B C D E   122 A B C D E   123 A B C D E   124 A B C D E   125 A B C D E   126 A B C D E   127 A B C D E   128 A B C D E

129 A B C D E   130 A B C D E   131 A B C D E   132 A B C D E   133 A B C D E   134 A B C D E   135 A B C D E   136 A B C D E

137 A B C D E   138 A B C D E   139 A B C D E   140 A B C D E   141 A B C D E   142 A B C D E   143 A B C D E   144 A B C D E

145 A B C D E   146 A B C D E   147 A B C D E   148 A B C D E   149 A B C D E   150 A B C D E   151 A B C D E   152 A B C D E

153 A B C D E   154 A B C D E   155 A B C D E   156 A B C D E   157 A B C D E   158 A B C D E   159 A B C D E   160 A B C D E

S O C / S E C — N U M B E R

| | 0 1 2 3 4 5 6 7 8 9 |
| 0 1 2 3 4 5 6 7 8 9 |
| 0 1 2 3 4 5 6 7 8 9 |
| 0 1 2 3 4 5 6 7 8 9 |
| 0 1 2 3 4 5 6 7 8 9 |
| 0 1 2 3 4 5 6 7 8 9 |
| 0 1 2 3 4 5 6 7 8 9 |
| 0 1 2 3 4 5 6 7 8 9 |
| 0 1 2 3 4 5 6 7 8 9 |

PAGE 1 2 3
TYPE 1 2 3

161 A B C D E 162 A B C D E 163 A B C D E 164 A B C D E 165 A B C D E 166 A B C D E 167 A B C D E 168 A B C D E
169 A B C D E 170 A B C D E 171 A B C D E 172 A B C D E 173 A B C D E 174 A B C D E 175 A B C D E 176 A B C D E
177 A B C D E 178 A B C D E 179 A B C D E 180 A B C D E 181 A B C D E 182 A B C D E 183 A B C D E 184 A B C D E
185 A B C D E 186 A B C D E 187 A B C D E 188 A B C D E 189 A B C D E 190 A B C D E 191 A B C D E 192 A B C D E
193 A B C D E 194 A B C D E 195 A B C D E 196 A B C D E 197 A B C D E 198 A B C D E 199 A B C D E 200 A B C D E
201 A B C D E 202 A B C D E 203 A B C D E 204 A B C D E 205 A B C D E 206 A B C D E 207 A B C D E 208 A B C D E

209 A B C D E 210 A B C D E 211 A B C D E 212 A B C D E 213 A B C D E 214 A B C D E 215 A B C D E 216 A B C D E
217 A B C D E 218 A B C D E 219 A B C D E 220 A B C D E 221 A B C D E 222 A B C D E 223 A B C D E 224 A B C D E
225 A B C D E 226 A B C D E 227 A B C D E 228 A B C D E 229 A B C D E 230 A B C D E 231 A B C D E 232 A B C D E
233 A B C D E 234 A B C D E 235 A B C D E 236 A B C D E 237 A B C D E 238 A B C D E 239 A B C D E 240 A B C D E
241 A B C D E 242 A B C D E 243 A B C D E 244 A B C D E 245 A B C D E 246 A B C D E 247 A B C D E 248 A B C D E
249 A B C D E 250 A B C D E 251 A B C D E 252 A B C D E 253 A B C D E 254 A B C D E 255 A B C D E 256 A B C D E
257 A B C D E 258 A B C D E 259 A B C D E 260 A B C D E 261 A B C D E 262 A B C D E 263 A B C D E 264 A B C D E
265 A B C D E 266 A B C D E 267 A B C D E 268 A B C D E 269 A B C D E 270 A B C D E 271 A B C D E 272 A B C D E
273 A B C D E 274 A B C D E 275 A B C D E 276 A B C D E 277 A B C D E 278 A B C D E 279 A B C D E 280 A B C D E
281 A B C D E 282 A B C D E 283 A B C D E 284 A B C D E 285 A B C D E 286 A B C D E 287 A B C D E 288 A B C D E
289 A B C D E 290 A B C D E 291 A B C D E 292 A B C D E 293 A B C D E 294 A B C D E 295 A B C D E 296 A B C D E
297 A B C D E 298 A B C D E 299 A B C D E 300 A B C D E 301 A B C D E 302 A B C D E 303 A B C D E 304 A B C D E
305 A B C D E 306 A B C D E 307 A B C D E 308 A B C D E 309 A B C D E 310 A B C D E 311 A B C D E 312 A B C D E
313 A B C D E 314 A B C D E 315 A B C D E 316 A B C D E 317 A B C D E 318 A B C D E 319 A B C D E 320 A B C D E